A Clinical Guide to Psychodynamic Psychotherapy

A Clinical Guide to Psychodynamic Psychotherapy serves as an accessible and applied introduction to psychodynamic psychotherapy.

The book is a resource for psychodynamic psychotherapy that gives helpful and practical guidelines around a range of patient presentations and clinical dilemmas. It focuses on contemporary issues facing psychodynamic psychotherapy practice, including issues around research, neuroscience, mentalising, working with diversity and difference, brief psychotherapy adaptations and the use of social media and technology. The book is underpinned by the psychodynamic competence framework that is implicit in best psychodynamic practice. The book includes a foreword by Prof. Peter Fonagy that outlines the unique features of psychodynamic psychotherapy that make it still so relevant to clinical practice today.

The book will be beneficial for students, trainees and qualified clinicians in psychotherapy, psychology, counselling, psychiatry and other allied professions.

Deborah Abrahams is a psychoanalytic psychotherapist and chartered clinical psychologist with over 25 years of clinical experience, including 15 years in the NHS. She is a dynamic interpersonal therapy (DIT) practitioner, supervisor and trainer as well as Programme Director of DIT at the Anna Freud Centre. Deborah is a senior member of the British Psychotherapy Foundation and has a private psychotherapy practice in North West London offering supervision, psychoanalytic and psychodynamic psychotherapy.

Poul Rohleder is a psychoanalytic psychotherapist and chartered clinical psychologist, as well as a dynamic interpersonal therapy practitioner. He has over 15 years' experience of working in public mental health care systems and in private practice. He is a trustee of the British Psychoanalytic Council and sits on several other professional committees and is currently a senior lecturer at the Department of Psychosocial and Psychoanalytic Studies, University of Essex, UK.

A Clinical Guide to Psychodynamic Psychotherapy

Deborah Abrahams and Poul Rohleder

Routledge
Taylor & Francis Group

LONDON AND NEW YORK

First published 2021
by Routledge
2 Park Square, Milton Park, Abingdon, Oxon OX14 4RN

and by Routledge
52 Vanderbilt Avenue, New York, NY 10017

Routledge is an imprint of the Taylor & Francis Group, an informa business

© 2021 Deborah Abrahams and Poul Rohleder

British Library Cataloguing-in-Publication Data
A catalogue record for this book is available from the British Library

Library of Congress Cataloging-in-Publication Data
A catalog record has been requested for this book

ISBN: 978-0-815-35265-5 (hbk)
ISBN: 978-0-815-35266-2 (pbk)
ISBN: 978-1-351-13858-1 (ebk)

Typeset in Baskerville
by Taylor & Francis Books

Contents

PART 3
Adaptations and practicalities   219

Illustrations

Figures

Tables

Acknowledgements

The authors would like to dedicate the book to our patients, from whom we have learned so much. We would like to thank our clinical supervisors for their wise guidance over the years. We are grateful to our colleagues with whom we have worked closely in the Camden & Islington NHS Foundation Trust, Anna Freud Centre, Tavistock Clinic and peer supervision groups at the British Psychotherapy Foundation. We are especially appreciative of the support and endorsements of Peter Fonagy, Alessandra Lemma, Bob Hinshelwood and Maxine Dennis.

Foreword

When I pick up this excellent introduction by Abrahams and Rohleder, I wonder what the secret ingredient might be that ensures the survival of the ideas and practices stated with brilliant clarity in this book. In principle, no scientific theory or clinical practice that is 125 years old has any right to be described as relevant to current practice. So, what has helped psychoanalysis and its offspring, psychodynamic psychotherapy, to survive all these years. In this Foreword, I would like to advance a few suggestions about the unique features of the approach which are all exceptionally well exemplified by Abrahams and Rohleder's book.

First, the idea that the mind is capable of generating mental disorder, the so-called principle of *psychological causation*, revolutionised psychiatry in the 19th century. The term 'dynamic' was used in the late nineteenth century by Leibniz, Herbart, Fechner, and Hughlings-Jackson to contrast with the word 'static' (Gabbard, 2000). As such, the word served to highlight the distinction between a psychological and a fixed organic neurological impairment model of mental disorder. Evidently, the approach continues to benefit from the flexibility this bridging of the mind-body divide generates. More recently, 'dynamic' has come to be contrasted with descriptive phenomenological psychiatry that has focused on categorising mental disorders in circumscribed ways, rather than emphasising the way mental processes (thinking, feeling, wishing, believing, desiring) interact to generate problems of subjective experience and behaviour. Psychodynamic Theory, as outlined in the first chapters of this book, is focused on understanding how we can meaningfully conceive of mental disorders as specific organisations of an individual's conscious or unconscious beliefs, thoughts and feelings. The rich case studies presented throughout illuminate the subtleties of this process and how the psychodynamic clinician, charged with the task of investigating the specific ideas and constructions, is able to elegantly explain a person's suffering.

Second, psychodynamic psychotherapy is unique in describing how psychological causation extends to the *non-conscious part of the mind*. Nagel, Wollheim, Hopkins and other philosophers of the mind (Hopkins, 1992; Nagel, 1959; Wollheim, 1995) have all pointed to the assumption of unconscious mentalisation as a key discovery within the psychoanalytic model. Implicitly or explicitly, psychodynamic models assume that non-conscious narrative-like experiences, analogous to conscious fantasies, profoundly influence an individual's behaviour, in particular their capacity to regulate affect and adequately handle their social environment. Whilst no modern cognitive scientists would restrict cognition to consciousness, psychodynamic approaches are alone in placing non-conscious functioning at the centre of its domain of interest. While such interactions go on consciously as well as outside of awareness, the psychodynamic model has been seen as a model of the mind that emphasises repudiated wishes and ideas which have been warded off and defensively excluded from conscious experience. The book illustrates how in the pursuit of understanding conscious experiences, we need to refer to mental states about which the individual is unlikely to be aware. What is more, the psychodynamic approach provides a roadmap for the likely location of those unconscious concerns and how these can be sensitively explored. It is in this last context that Abrahams and Rohleder's book is so valuable. The strategies that the clinician wishing to explore unconscious content should follow in order to achieve productive therapeutic change are neither simple nor obvious and demand careful committed study and opportunity, which the later chapters of the book helpfully present.

Third, as described in the initial chapters on the theoretical basis of psychodynamic work, the psychodynamic clinician generally believes that mental disorders are best understood bearing in mind that the mind is organised largely to avoid *unpleasure* which arises out of feelings and ideas that are incompatible and therefore are in conflict. Psychodynamic approaches consider that given the human condition, it is axiomatic that wishes, affects and ideas will be, at times, in conflict with one another. The psychodynamic therapeutic approach sees such incompatibilities as key causes of distress and the lack of a sense of safety. Clinical experience shows them to be frequently associated with adverse environmental conditions. For example, neglect or abuse is likely to aggravate an arguably natural but mild predisposition of the child to relate with mixed feelings to the caregiver who is perceived as vital to the child's continuing existence. While slight fragmentation of mental organisation was shown to be ubiquitous by existential philosophy (Gadamer, 1975; Heidegger, 1962), psychodynamic techniques often aim at identifying perceived inconsistencies, conscious or unconscious, in feelings, beliefs and wishes in relation to oneself and others with the aim of reducing the individual's distress. Not only are conflicts thought to cause distress, they are also considered potentially to undermine the normal development of key psychological capacities that in turn reduce an individual's competence to resolve incompatible ideas (Freud, 1965). Whilst it may seem obvious that we want to avoid unpleasure wherever we can, psychodynamic theories, and particularly the work of attachment theorists and also Joseph Sandler (2003), explain that it is not simply unpleasure that we want to avoid; rather, our minds are collectively and probably biologically organised to maximise a subjective sense of safety and belonging.

Fourth, psychodynamic theories are also used in describing the common set of mental operations that, whilst appearing to distort accurate depictions of reality and mental states, have the capacity to reduce anxiety, distress and displeasure. The term '*psychic defences*' may risk reification and anthropomorphism (precisely who is defending whom, and against what?). Notwithstanding this, the concept of self-serving distortions of mental states relative to an external or internal reality is generally accepted and frequently demonstrated experimentally (Lyons-Ruth, 2003; Shamir-Essakow, Ungerer, Rapee, and Safier, 2004). Further, individual differences in the predisposition to particular strategies may be helpfully examined and codified to groups of individuals and mental disorders in order to provide robust expectations about how a particular person is likely to behave, what they are likely to feel, and how they are likely to organise their thoughts (Bond, 2004; Lenzenweger, Clarkin, Kernberg, and Foelsch, 2001).

Descriptions of defences are invaluable when it comes to understanding the way individuals see the world they are in, sometimes minimising and sometimes exaggerating its dangers. This often leads those individuals to make suboptimal use of the opportunities they have available to them which can be altered when such self-serving distortions are surfaced in consciousness. The psychodynamic approach is a comprehensive view of human subjectivity, aimed at understanding all aspects of the individual's relationship with their environment, both external and internal. Freud's great discovery that is so often misinterpreted, namely "where id was, there ego shall be" (S. Freud, 1933, p. 80), points to the power of the conscious mind to alter radically its position with respect to aspects of its own functions, including the capacity to end its own existence. Psycho*dynamic*, as this book reveals, refers to this extraordinary potential for dynamic self-alteration and self-correction – seemingly totally outside the reach of nonhuman species.

Fifth, as outlined in the book, psychodynamic psychotherapies are conceived of in *developmental* terms. Of course, as the book also makes clear, varying assumptions are made by different psychodynamic approaches concerning normal and anomalous child and adolescent development. Nevertheless, the psychodynamic therapeutic approach is invariably oriented to the developmental aspects of the patient's presenting problems. In general, the belief that the past powerfully conditions an individual's present and future is a key assumption of all psychodynamic ideas. In essence, all psychodynamic psychotherapies are conceived of in developmental terms, with varying assumptions concerning normal and abnormal child and adolescent development (Fonagy, Target, and Gergely, 2006).

The sixth powerful general assumption underpinning the psychodynamic approach, one which runs right through this book like some kind of Brighton rock, is that *relationship representations* can be assumed to be linked with childhood experiences. Psychodynamic clinicians are by no means alone in considering interpersonal relationships, in particular the powerful bonds that are created within families, to be key in the organisation of personality. The specific focus of psychodynamic therapists, however, is the assumption that these intense relationship experiences are internalised and aggregated across time and come to form a schematic mental structure often metaphorically represented as a neural network. Childhood or adolescent experience, sometimes lazily referred to as early experience, is believed to influence interpersonal social expectations. This helps us understand why interpersonal strategies that are less than helpful for individuals may persist many years after their value has lapsed. As a strategy, it is not only obsolete: it is downright counter-productive. Interpersonal social expectations influence the relationship with the therapist (through the so called transference) in psychodynamic psychotherapy but perhaps also they emerge as parts of other approaches such as developmental social psychology (Mayes, Fonagy, and Target, 2007) or the currently popular examinative of ACEs (adverse childhood experiences) in adult relationships (Felitti and Anda, 2009) and health (Bellis et al., 2017).

The wish to understand this historical way of interacting with others in order to throw light on the conflicts an individual experiences in the here-and-now explains some of the peculiarities in the behaviour of psychodynamic psychotherapists. In order to allow expectations in relation to the therapist to emerge clearly, the psychodynamic psychotherapist is sometimes reticent to show too much of their own spontaneous way of acting and may appear so neutral in the face of distress as to attract accusations of being unkind. This is a criticism that perhaps can be accurately levelled at classical psychodynamic approaches. It cannot be levelled at this book. Here the therapist emerges as a rounded human being, with the capacity to act spontaneously at least to the point of making mistakes and saying things they regret. Perhaps the most important concept in the book focuses on relationship representations. Self–Other relationship representations are considered the organisers of emotion, as feeling states come to characterise particular patterns of Self–Other and interpersonal relating (e.g. sadness and disappointment at the anticipated loss of a person). The centrality of this idea, which emerges gradually within psychodynamic theory, helps us understand why the Self, a person's identity, cannot be understood except as a function of their relationships, how they are seen and their emotional experience of particular relationships. The combination of its developmental approach and the view that relationship experiences accumulate to create a sense of Self as well as a sense of generic Others is the appropriate clinical focus for this book. This so-called object relations theory has become the common language for psychodynamic psychotherapy, which has been fragmented historically by numerous individual approaches to theory and technique.

The seventh core feature of the psychodynamic approach that runs through this book, perhaps more clearly than most texts of the psychodynamic approach, is the *assumption of the complexity of meanings*. Whilst there exist key differences between psychodynamic approaches in terms of the specific meanings that are assigned by clinicians to particular pieces of behaviour, the general assumption psychodynamic approaches share is that behaviour may be understood in terms of mental states that are not explicit in action or within the awareness of the person concerned. Symptoms of mental disorders are classically considered as condensations of wishes in conflict with one another and that exist alongside defences against conscious awareness of those wishes. It is striking that different psychodynamic orientations find different types or categories of meanings 'concealed' behind the same symptomatic behaviours. Some clinicians focus on unexpressed aggression or sexual impulses, others on a fear of not being validated, yet others on anxieties about abandonment and isolation. Within the context of this book, it is the effort of seeking further personal meaning that would be considered more significant therapeutically, and that is shared by a range of psychodynamic therapeutic approaches (e.g. Holmes, 1998). Elaborating and clarifying implicit meaning structures, as opposed to giving the patient insight in the terms of any particular meaning structure, appears through these pages as the essence of psychodynamic psychotherapy.

And finally, the unique psychodynamic proposition that past relationship representations inevitably re-emerge in the course of psychodynamic treatments defines a further concern that preoccupies this book appropriately as it indeed preoccupies all psychodynamic psychotherapists. Within a psychodynamic framework, there is an extensive literature on both i) the *'transference'* relationship, in which non-conscious relationship expectations, repudiated wishes etc. are assumed to be played out and can be better understood through the shared experience of their enactment in a new context, and ii) the *'real'* relationship, which captures the generic factor referred to above, namely the therapeutic impact of having a relationship with an interested, understanding and respectful person, which may be a new experience for some.

However, this goes both ways. Psychodynamic therapists, like everyone else, have minds that are organised around avoiding unpleasure, are capable of generating defensive strategies to avoid challenges; they bring their own histories to the consulting room and their relationship representations dominate the way they form relationships with their clients. In other words, the non-conscious or indeed defended against dynamically unconscious part of the therapist's mind comes to psychodynamic treatment with the patient's capacity to use defences to protect themselves from unconscious conflict. Several things follow from this assumption. Most obvious is the recommendation for psychodynamic psychotherapists to have their own personal therapy in part to be able to share and empathise with the patient's experience that comes to see them but also to deal hopefully with the most problematic aspects of what they might otherwise bring to the consulting room. Second, is the absolute need for supervision at all levels of skill and expertise. Everyone, including the author of these lines, should be in supervision or at least have the opportunity to discuss their clinical work with fellow clinicians on a regular basis. Whilst this cannot prevent interference from parts of our mind outside of conscious awareness, it will avert an embedding of patterns of responding to a client that may not be in the client's or indeed the therapist's best interests.

Reflection on experience is a helpful corrective, as identified by most modern theories of consciousness (Fonagy and Allison, 2016). However, the most important parts of such unconscious reactions are in relation to the therapist's mind as a tool for discovery. An idea which now appropriately permeates psychodynamic practice is the common-sense notion that the way we react to fellow human beings tells us not just something about ourselves but also something about the other person. An emotional reaction of anxiety, boredom or hopelessness may be something that reflects not only our likely current state of being but also tells us something that has been triggered within our own minds which is of immense importance in trying to acquire an understanding of the person we are endeavouring to help. The systematic use of countertransference is explained well in this book alongside many other important psychodynamic techniques.

As an empirical researcher, I genuinely appreciate the unique efforts in this book to integrate scientific research with descriptions of clinical theory and technique. The epistemic framework of psychoanalysis, at least in the past, extruded empirical research. Experimental studies pertinent to psychoanalysis and psychodynamic psychotherapy are not simply randomised controlled trials, the strengths and weaknesses of which are well described in Chapter 3. The experimental method integrates anatomical, neurophysiological and genetic observations which are at the cutting-edge of our modern understanding of mental disorder (e.g. Holmes, 2020). The epistemic reach of psychodynamic theory goes significantly beyond the experimental and encompasses many aspects of psychology, particularly developmental psychology, cognitive science, computational psychiatry, feminist theory, sociology, queer theory, anthropology, pathology, evolutionary psychology, nonlinear dynamics and political science among others; in fact, very many domains of 21st-century thought intersect with it. Whilst its continued relevance is a puzzle to some, it also underscores the value of its study. In my view, psychoanalytic theory that underpins psychodynamic psychotherapy is the richest and most sophisticated set of ideas concerning the functioning of the human mind that we currently have available to us. It is a theory that is nested within psychotherapeutic practice. Without the experience of one mind getting to know another mind in real time interaction (both acting to make the best of the encounter yet both chained by their own history and the profound limitations that prior experience places upon spontaneous discovery) the theory would be arrested in its development and would not be able to nourish and inspire practitioners struggling to help those who have come to seek their assistance. Sure, now there are hundreds, probably over a thousand different kinds of psychotherapies. Why should anyone choose psychodynamic therapy? As a set of techniques, it is unlikely to be more effective than others. As an approach to understanding the human mind, it stands on its own. We have ample evidence that psychotherapy can effectively address human suffering and through it, we may learn about human nature in ways that are perhaps even more important in creating a better world, a world that is adequately understanding and kind to those people whose mental disorder exposes them to distress or whose actions generate distress in others. So, beyond the appropriate clinical call of helping individuals with mental disorders, I would commend to you the study of this book as you engage in a profession that will help you better understand others and thus fulfil a wider humanitarian call of creating a more generous and productive human environment for one another in this relatively new century where we need interpersonal understanding more than ever before.

Professor Peter Fonagy OBE
Professor of Contemporary Psychoanalysis and Developmental Science
at University College London (UCL), and
CEO of the Anna Freud National Centre for Children and Families
June 2020

References

Bellis, M. A., Hardcastle, K., Ford, K., Hughes, K., Ashton, K., Quigg, Z., & Butler, N. (2017). Does continuous trusted adult support in childhood impart life-course resilience against adverse childhood experiences - a retrospective study on adult health-harming behaviours and mental well-being. *BMC Psychiatry*, 17(1), 110. doi:10.1186/s12888-017-1260-z

Bond, M. (2004). Empirical studies of defense style: relationships with psychopathology and change. *Harvard Review of Psychiatry*, 12(5), 263–278.

Felitti, V. J., & Anda, R. F. (2009). The relationship of adverse childhood experiences to adult medical disease, psychiatric disorders, and sexual behavior: Implications for healthcare. In R. A. Lanius, E. Vemetten & C. Pain (eds), *The impact of early life trauma on health and disease: The hidden epidemic*. Cambridge, MA: Cambridge University Press.

Fonagy, P., & Allison, E. (2016). Psychic reality and the nature of consciousness. *International Journal of Psychoanalysis*, 97(1), 5–24. doi:10.1111/1745-8315.12403

Fonagy, P., Target, M., & Gergely, G. (2006). Psychoanalytic perspectives on developmental psychopathology. In D. Cicchetti & D. J. Cohen (eds), *Developmental psychopathology* (2nd edition, vol 1: Theory and methods, pp. 701–749). Hoboken, NJ: Wiley.

Freud, A. (1965). *Normality and pathology in childhood: Assessments of development*. Madison, CT: International Universities Press.

Freud, S. (1933). New introductory lectures on psychoanalysis. In J. Strachey (ed.), *The standard edition of the complete psychological works of Sigmund Freud* (vol 22, pp. 1–182). London, UK: Hogarth Press, 1964.

Gabbard, G. O. (2000). *Psychodynamic psychiatry in clinical practice* (3rd edition). Arlington, VA: American Psychiatric Publishing.

Gadamer, H.-G. (1975). *Truth and method*. New York: Crossroads.

Heidegger, M. (1962). *Being and time* (J. Macquarrie & E. Robinson, Trans.). New York: HarperCollins (Original work published 1927).

Holmes, J. (1998). The changing aims of psychoanalytic psychotherapy: An integrative perspective. *International Journal of Psycho-Analysis*, 79, 227–240.

Holmes, J. (2020). *The brain has a mind of its own: Attachment, neurobiology, and the new science of psychotherapy*. London: Confer.

Hopkins, J. (1992). Psychoanalysis, interpretation, and science. In J. Hopkins & A. Saville (eds), *Psychoanalysis, mind and art: Perspectives on Richard Wollheim* (pp. 3–34). Oxford: Blackwell.

Lenzenweger, M. F., Clarkin, J. F., Kernberg, O. F., & Foelsch, P. A. (2001). The Inventory of Personality Organization: Psychometric properties, factorial composition, and criterion relations with affect, aggressive dyscontrol, psychosis proneness, and self-domains in a nonclinical sample. *Psychological Assessment*, 13(4), 577–591.

Lyons-Ruth, K. (2003). Dissociation and the parent-infant dialogue: A longitudinal perspective from attachment research. *Journal of the American Psychoanalytic Association*, 51(3), 883–911. doi:10.1177/00030651030510031501

Mayes, L. C., Fonagy, P., & Target, M. (eds) (2007). *Developmental science and psychoanalysis*. London: Karnac.

Nagel, E. (1959). Methodological issues in psychoanalytic theory. In S. Hook (ed.), *Psychoanalysis, scientific method and philosophy* (pp. 38–56). New York: New York University Press.

Sandler, J. (2003). On attachment to internal objects. *Psychoanalytic Inquiry*, 23(1), 12–26. doi:10.1080/07351692309349024

Shamir-Essakow, G., Ungerer, J. A., Rapee, R. M., & Safier, R. (2004). Caregiving representations of mothers of behaviorally inhibited and uninhibited preschool children. *Developmental Psychology*, 40(6), 899–910. doi:10.1037/0012-1649.40.6.899

Wollheim, R. (1995). *The mind and its depths*. Cambridge, MA: Harvard University Press.

1   Introduction

When Sigmund Freud first began and developed psychoanalysis, it was referred to as 'the talking cure', a radical new approach to the treatment of mental health problems which were at that time treated through medicine and surgery. This new 'talking cure' formed the basis of much of the psychological therapies that we see today, which emphasise particular ways of talking, thinking, and listening as a means for understanding and working through traumatic or distressing experiences. Freud not only revolutionised ideas about the treatment of mental health problems, but he also developed a metapsychology of human development and behaviour. Thus, psychoanalysis is both a method of treatment as well as a theory of human development. We know a great deal about human development from biological disciplines about the body's growth over time while neuroscience focuses on the development and functioning of the brain. By contrast, psychoanalysis is a theory of human subjectivity, perhaps the most elaborate and developed theory of human subjectivity there is.

Freud's influence and legacy cannot be disputed. However, psychoanalysis has seen much criticism over the decades where short-term, evidence-based and solution-focused therapies have increasingly dominated public mental health service provision, most notably cognitive-behavioural therapy (CBT). In the United Kingdom, the National Health Service (NHS) predominantly provides CBT as the preferred treatment for many mental health problems. There are numerous reasons for this, including the greater availability of research evidence claiming CBT to be effective. This compares to psychoanalytic approaches which have thus far lagged considerably behind in accumulating research evidence into their efficacy. Thankfully there are recent changes in this regard, with important efficacy research published establishing psychoanalytic therapies to be as effective as CBT, and in some cases more enduring in effect. We will review this research evidence in the third chapter of this book.

Readers will note that the title of this book refers to 'psychodynamic psychotherapy', rather than psychoanalysis. Usually, 'psychoanalysis' refers to the theoretical corpus as well as the intensive form of treatment that involves being seen three to five times a week over a long-term period. The term 'psychodynamic' refers to therapy that draws on the theoretical framework of psychoanalysis and applies it to less intensive or short-term therapy. We use the term 'psychodynamic psychotherapy' to refer to a variety of ways of working psychoanalytically.

We may be witnessing a resurgence in recognising the important contribution of psychodynamic psychotherapy for mental health care. Fonagy and Lemma (Fonagy et al., 2012) in a debate about the relevance of psychoanalytic or psychodynamic therapies in the NHS, argue that psychodynamic therapies make three "valuable and unique contributions to a modern healthcare economy" (p. 19). They argue that psychoanalysis has a well-established model for understanding the developmental nature of mental health problems, stemming from childhood experiences, which few other models provide. Psychoanalysis also provides the theoretical foundation for a number of other applied interventions, including CBT. Furthermore, psychoanalysis, with its focus on interpersonal dynamics, helps healthcare staff better understand and manage their stressful, and at times distressing, reactions to the care work that they are involved in. They conclude that public mental health care cannot operate on a 'one size fits all' basis, dominated by CBT, and that other therapeutic modalities are needed. Recent critics have argued that CBT has not delivered the successful outcomes it has claimed to provide, and that mental health care requires a rethink to incorporate other approaches, including psychodynamic psychotherapy (e.g., Dalal, 2018; Jackson and Rizq, 2019). We the authors, Deborah Abrahams and Poul Rohleder, each trained firstly as clinical psychologists and then as psychoanalytic psychotherapists; we have both used a range of approaches in our clinical work. We are not here to advocate for psychodynamic psychotherapy over CBT or other approaches, recognising, as Fonagy and Lemma put it, that different therapies are needed for different difficulties and that people respond differently to different treatments. After all, as Fonagy put it in the 44th Maudsley debate (see Box 1.1), why would you throw out all your spanners and only keep the one you used most of the time in your proverbial therapy tool box?

What is psychodynamic psychotherapy?

All forms of counselling and psychotherapy involve the patient (please refer to our note below about our use of the term 'patient') talking with the therapist about their problems and life experiences and the therapist facilitating some form of understanding and insight into why things may feel so distressing for the patient at that moment; through this exchange of perspectives and understanding, the hope and possibility for change emerges. Individual therapies, such as CBT, tend to focus on psychological factors that contribute to distress in the present, such as problematic ways of thinking about issues (e.g. a tendency to perceive problems as bigger than they are or seeing problems in black-and-white terms) or problematic behaviours (e.g. avoidance behaviour, security seeking), or unreasonable perceptions about oneself and others (e.g. faulty cognitions or core beliefs). Psychodynamic psychotherapy is distinguished from other models in that it focuses primarily on unconscious aspects of our behaviour that lead to internal conflict, as well as how we experience, regulate and express our emotions in an interpersonal context, including in the therapeutic relationship (the transference, discussed in Chapter 9). The focus includes identifying repeated patterns of behaving or relating to others that we adopt from childhood and are then re-experienced in adulthood. We will elaborate on these and other distinctive features of psychodynamic psychotherapy in Chapter 3.

Many forms of treatment in mental health care attempt to rid patients of their symptoms. In psychiatry this is typically achieved through the use of medication. In CBT, this is achieved by recognising cognitive and behavioural factors that maintain symptoms, and focusing on ways of changing our thoughts and behaviours that help alleviate negative or fearful thoughts and experiences. In psychodynamic psychotherapy, we are not aiming for a cure or to rid patients of their symptoms, but rather to help patients understand how past experiences may have contributed to the distress they feel, and develop a more flexible and expansive way of relating to themselves and others. This is facilitated by attempting to bring together ambivalent and complex feelings of love and hate towards self and other. We help patients recognise dysfunctional or defensive patterns of relating that have developed over time, and to recognise their unconscious desires and impulses, in order to find a freedom, energy and playful creativity that would be otherwise diverted into defensive manoeuvres. Thus, we might say that the goal of psychodynamic psychotherapy is not so much symptom alleviation, but more personal growth, emotional maturity and increased affect regulation. Interestingly, research suggests that therapists, including CBT therapists, who seek personal therapy, usually select psychoanalytic or psychodynamic psychotherapy as the theoretical orientation of choice (Norcross, 2005). This may reflect the centrality of the 'personal growth' aspects of psychodynamic psychotherapy and our inherent preference to be treated as a whole person without being reduced to a constellation of symptoms.

Although all patients ostensibly enter therapy with the wish to improve their mental health, this is always easier said than done. If change were so easy, psychotherapists would be out of a job. Psychodynamic psychotherapy is not didactic or problem-solving. Indeed, most of our patients probably know what would be best for them to do – it is not about the advice per se but our inevitable resistance to following that advice. Alongside the conscious goals for help and the recognition of the need for change, there is also a strong, unconscious wish for homeostasis, to keep things as they are. It is this resistance that the therapist and patient will come up against repeatedly.

These aspects of psychodynamic psychotherapy make it difficult to develop a 'how-to-do-it' manual. In our experience of training clinical psychologists and counsellors, there is an expressed wish and anxiety about knowing precisely what to do and how to do it. This applies to all trainees, whatever the modality. However, while there are well-developed, circumscribed manuals for treating depression with CBT, for example, we do not have the same type of manuals for psychodynamic psychotherapy. There is no session-by-session psychodynamic psychotherapy protocol for treating a depressed patient. Furthermore, as we shall see in Chapter 2, there are many different theoretical schools of psychoanalysis, each with differing models for understanding psychic life, the ontogenesis of an individual, the development of mental health problems and therapeutic ways of working. While there are particular therapeutic techniques and skills that are shared across different modalities, practising psychodynamic psychotherapy cannot be reduced to defined techniques and exercises; rather, it entails holding a particular analytic attitude or relational stance that remains open to the patient's unfolding communications, both conscious and unconscious. A prescriptive approach will inevitably compromise the emergent quality of psychotherapy and inhibit unconscious communication. Yet there is a need to establish the common elements and skills across different schools of psychodynamic psychotherapy. In recent years, a team from University College London (Lemma et al., 2008) developed a set of core competences for psychodynamic psychotherapy, and we have drawn on these as a framework to underpin this book.

The core competences of psychodynamic psychotherapy

The core competences (see Figure 1.1) for psychodynamic psychotherapy were derived from existing manualised psychotherapy approaches that were then

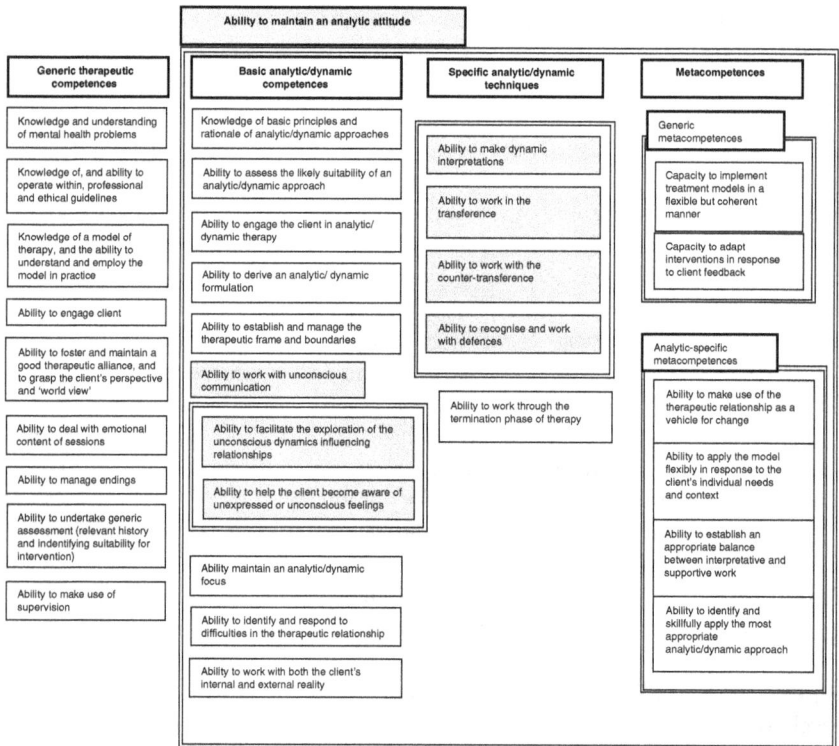

Ability to maintain an analytic attitude			
Generic therapeutic competences	**Basic analytic/dynamic competences**	**Specific analytic/dynamic techniques**	**Metacompetences**
Knowledge and understanding of mental health problems	Knowledge of basic principles and rationale of analytic/dynamic approaches		Generic metacompetences
Knowledge of, and ability to operate within, professional and ethical guidelines	Ability to assess the likely suitability of an analytic/dynamic approach	Ability to make dynamic interpretations	Capacity to implement treatment models in a flexible but coherent manner
Knowledge of a model of therapy, and the ability to understand and employ the model in practice	Ability to engage the client in analytic/dynamic therapy	Ability to work in the transference	
	Ability to derive an analytic/ dynamic formulation	Ability to work with the counter-transference	Capacity to adapt interventions in response to client feedback
Ability to engage client			
Ability to foster and maintain a good therapeutic alliance, and to grasp the client's perspective and 'world view'	Ability to establish and manage the therapeutic frame and boundaries	Ability to recognise and work with defences	Analytic-specific metacompetences
	Ability to work with unconscious communication		Ability to make use of the therapeutic relationship as a vehicle for change
Ability to deal with emotional content of sessions	Ability to facilitate the exploration of the unconscious dynamics influencing relationships	Ability to work through the termination phase of therapy	Ability to apply the model flexibly in response to the client's individual needs and context
Ability to manage endings	Ability to help the client become aware of unexpressed or unconscious feelings		
Ability to undertake generic assessment (relevant history and indentifying suitability for intervention)	Ability maintain an analytic/dynamic focus		Ability to establish an appropriate balance between interpretative and supportive work
Ability to make use of supervision	Ability to identify and respond to difficulties in the therapeutic relationship		Ability to identify and skillfully apply the most appropriate analytic/dynamic approach
	Ability to work with both the client's internal and external reality		

Figure 1.1 The core competences for psychodynamic psychotherapy
Source: Adapted from: www.ucl.ac.uk/clinical-psychology/competency-maps/psychodynamic-map.html. Reproduced here with permission.

checked and validated by a peer review process. A number of manuals for time-limited psychodynamic psychotherapy were identified that were associated with positive outcomes in research trials. A set of shared competences was extracted from those manuals and then validated by a peer review that included psychotherapists and psychoanalysts from a diverse range of theoretical orientations. The derived set of competences can be considered implicit to good practice of psychodynamic psychotherapy and despite divergence at the level of theory, there is great convergence when it comes to the application, i.e. the practice of psychotherapy. As such, these core competences offer a way of bridging differences across competing schools of thought in the area of psychotherapy in order to facilitate research, training and skills transfer. The competence set has been used consistently since it was developed.

When we focus on competences, we are trying to evaluate the level of the therapist's judgement and skill when delivering and implementing psychotherapy as it was intended; it forms part of an assessment of treatment fidelity that allows us to identify the key ingredients of a treatment approach and draw accurate conclusions about the efficacy of a treatment. Interestingly, it has been shown that an intermediate level of adherence, representing a balance between manual adherence and clinically flexible deviation, predicted better outcomes than did overly rigid adherence on the one hand, or loose treatment adherence on the other (Henry et al., 1993; Frank et al., 1991; Barber et al., 1996). This relates to the generic meta-competences in Lemma et al.'s (2008) framework for flexibility and adaptation. The therapist requires the ability to judge when to intervene and when to abstain by weighing up the appropriateness and timing of interventions in a dynamic way based on transference and countertransference moment to moment in the session. The concept of adaptive flexibility is a fundamental component of competence as it entails the ability of the therapist to intuitively adjust, improvise and reshape the understandings and therapeutic strategies in agreement with the continuous changes of the therapy (Binder, 1999; Schön, 1983, 1987) Assessing competence should also take into account knowledge of the patient and the therapeutic context. As you can see, it is a complicated process to identify these elements, which probably explains why psychoanalytic psychotherapy did not readily engage in this type of research. More recently, there have been attempts to pinpoint the critical ingredients for a psychoanalytic/dynamic approach such as David Tuckett's European Psychoanalytic Federation (EPF) Working Party on Comparative Clinical Methods in order to identify the essential ingredients of psychoanalysis and Tamara Ventura's (2019) doctoral work that develops a competence framework underpinning Dynamic Interpersonal Therapy.

Competences are a useful way of articulating the required standards for profession accreditation. Focusing on a competence-based approach represents a way of demystifying the acquiring of psychotherapy skills and allows training courses to be more transparent about the expectations and evaluation of their students. Notwithstanding the challenges, it is important that we are able to identify the key ingredients associated with therapeutic impact in psychotherapy. This will aid in evaluation and delivery of psychotherapy trainings as well as therapeutic outcomes and future research. The competence in the green box in Figure 1.1 is the overarching psychodynamic competence, namely maintaining an analytic attitude. Permeating the psychodynamic stance is an emphasis on unconscious processes and being able to listen on different levels to the latent as well as the manifest content of what our patients bring.

Aim and outline of the book

This book aims to provide an accessible, hands-on introduction to psychodynamic psychotherapy for students and trainees from psychology, counselling, psychotherapy, psychiatry and other allied professional backgrounds. From our experience in teaching and supervising clinical and counselling psychology trainees among others, we were often asked for accessible resources on psychodynamic psychotherapy that give helpful and practical guidelines for responding to the plethora of situations, clinical choices and dilemmas that arise in this line of work. Existing textbooks tend to focus on the intensive end of treatment, namely psychoanalytic psychotherapy and psychoanalysis, and tend to require an in-depth knowledge of psychoanalytic theory in order to grasp the concepts. At the other extreme, there are textbooks directed at entry level skills in psychodynamic counselling. Our hope in writing this book is to bridge this gap for an applied text on psychodynamic psychotherapy and to bring attention to contemporary issues facing psychodynamic psychotherapy practice in the 21st century, such as the role of the technology in our practice and an analytic view of diversity. By taking a practical approach to this topic with minimal use of jargon, we aim to introduce these psychodynamic concepts to a wider audience, including undergraduate students. Each topic discussed in this book could be the subject of a book in its own right, and so the various chapters serve as an introduction to thinking about how these aspects may become salient in the therapist's work. We have ended each chapter with recommended readings as well as useful resources (including YouTube clips) if you wish to further your understanding of each topic.

The book is organised into three sections:

Part 1 focuses on theory and research. There is an overview of the different theoretical schools in psychoanalysis, identifying differences and points of similarity between then. The second chapter focuses on efficacy and outcome research for psychodynamic psychotherapy.

Part 2 explores key concepts and competences that underpin psychodynamic work, namely: exploring the analytic setting and analytic frame; carrying out an assessment for psychotherapy and arriving at a psychodynamic formulation; understanding defences against anxiety; introducing the idea of mentalising in the clinical setting; interpreting different forms of unconscious communication; looking at the therapeutic relationship through the concepts of transference and countertransference; and working with endings.

Part 3 examines adaptations and practicalities facing the practice of psychodynamic psychotherapy. There is a chapter that outlines the specific adaptations required for brief psychodynamic therapy. This is followed by a chapter that explores different challenges and dilemmas a therapist may encounter in their work with patients. We also look at matters of diversity: thinking about and working with differences. Finally, we have included a chapter on technology and social media and its implications for psychotherapy.

Notes on terminology and use of clinical material

In the main text of the book, we have chosen to use the word 'therapist' to refer to the clinician, psychologist, counsellor, psychiatrist or whatever your core profession is. In doing so, we do not wish to imply that you, the reader, are required to have a psychotherapy training to use this book. When referring to the patient, we have chosen to use gender neutral, third person pronouns ('they' or 'them'), aside from the clinical material where we used pseudonyms and suggested a gender.

There are times in the book when we may refer to terms such as 'psychopathology' or use diagnostic terms such as 'neurosis' or psychiatric diagnoses that are relevant to the topic at hand. However, as will be evident in the chapter on assessment and formulation (Chapter 5) and elsewhere, we have not adopted a diagnostic or psychiatric focus in this book, rather taking a more holistic view of understanding distress and mental health problems.

We have chosen to use the term 'patient', the term that is most frequently used in the psychoanalytic literature. There are many debates about what terminology should be adopted, with some preferring the term 'client' while others favour 'service user'. These debates tend to centre around issues of power and passivity, dignity and autonomy (Neuberger and Tallis, 1999). We have selected this term mindfully, to reflect the psychoanalytic tradition, and, like Nina Coltart (1993), feel that the alternative descriptors of 'client' or 'service user' represent attempts to rewrite and deny the reality that someone is coming for help, and that there is an inevitable power differential in the therapeutic setting. We feel that the term 'patient' also reminds us of our ethical obligations in working with people who are often vulnerable, distressed, or experiencing shame. As Coltart (1993) eloquently states:

> To me, 'patient' is an honourable old word, stemming from the Latin root, *patio*, 'I suffer'. People who come to us *are* suffering. It feels to me far more careful of their dignity if we allow for that, rather than trying to cloak their pain under some false notion that we are the vendors of something without emotional colouring, or that people are not really in sometimes desperate need, which we are trying to meet. (p. 26)

In order to ensure confidentiality and anonymity, we have written clinical material in the form of composites of patients we have seen in our working life. We have drawn on aspects of different patients where there are some similarities in their presenting difficulties, experiences and circumstances and we have disguised any identifiable data. One of the benefits of co-authoring a book, is that it provides us with opportunities to draw on each other's work and experiences in a combined way, so as to protect the confidentiality of our clinical work. Nevertheless, there may be patients of ours who recognise themselves in the material as well as those who may feel disappointed not to find themselves here. We have had to weigh up the benefits of including clinical vignettes to illuminate the work with providing absolute privacy and excluding any details. In the clinical material, we have used the pronoun 'I' to refer to ourselves as the therapist, in order to provide a further level of anonymity. What is not possible to convey is the non-verbal communication and the tone of voice of both patient and therapist. Something can be said in a cold and harsh way that sounds certain and judgemental, or it can be offered in an attuned, warm way that conveys concern. Inevitably a textbook about psychodynamic psychotherapy will struggle to convey these sub-textual aspects of the work, the nuanced way that an interpersonal relationship comes to be formed and where the therapeutic alliance is established as the bedrock of future work.

When embarking on the journey of becoming a psychodynamic psychotherapist, we want to keep in mind the words of eminent psychoanalyst and paediatrician Donald Winnicott (1971):

> One could compare my position with that of a cellist who first slogs away at technique and then actually becomes able to play music, taking the technique for granted. I am aware of doing this work more easily and with more success than I was able to do it thirty years ago and my wish is to communicate with those who are still slogging away at technique, at the same time giving them the hope that will one day come from playing music. There is but little satisfaction to be gained from giving a virtuoso performance from a written score. (p. 6)

Psychodynamic psychotherapy is improvised, dynamic and unpredictable. As such, it can never be manualised in the same way that music can be scored. We can develop a set of competences but that does not mean they are all present in every session to the same degree or that this obviates the clinician from the responsibility of deciding what to take up with the patient at any point in the process. Just as in the metaphor of the cellist, to become a 'virtuoso' psychodynamic therapist requires practice, practice and more practice, alongside the ability to learn from our mistakes. We hope that this book helps guide you in that journey.

Box 1.1 Useful resources

Readings

The following two popular books provide a good, accessible look into psychodynamic psychotherapy:

The Examined Life by Stephen Grosz, is a bestseller and features a range of beautifully written short case studies that provide thoughtful glimpses into the consulting room.
Couch Fiction by Philippa Perry and Junko Graat, is a graphic novel following the journey of a psychotherapist and her patient.

Online resources

The UCL competences framework for psychodynamic psychotherapy can be found on the UCL website: www.ucl.ac.uk/drupal/site_pals/sites/pals/files/migrated-files/PPC_Clinicians_Background_Paper.pdf

The 44th Maudsley Debate, entitled "Wake up to the unconscious" is available to listen to on the Kings College London website, dated March 2012: "This house believes that psychoanalysis has a valuable place in modern mental health service". Chaired by Prof Sir Robin Murray. For the motion were Prof Peter Fonagy and Prof Alessandra Lemma. Against the motion were Prof Lewis Wolpert and Prof Paul Salkovskis. www.kcl.ac.uk/ioppn/news/special-events/maudsley-debates/debate-archive-31-50

Part 1

Theory and research

2 An overview of psychoanalytic theory

For many unfamiliar with psychoanalysis and its theoretical canon, psychoanalytic theory starts – and ends – with Sigmund Freud. Introductory psychology text-books often refer to a handful of Freud's key theories, only to critique him, thereby joining a chorus that declares Freud – and thus psychoanalysis – dead. Any book dealing with psychoanalysis and psychodynamic psychotherapy needs to start with Freud, the father of psychoanalysis. However, more than a hundred years have passed since Freud first espoused his theories, and psychoanalytic theory as a whole has developed considerably since then. It is beyond the scope of this chapter to consider all those developments in the United Kingdom, Europe, North and South America and elsewhere. We will provide an overview of some of the psychoanalytic schools of thought that have had a particular influence on psychodynamic psychotherapy practice in the UK. Having an understanding of the theoretical framework and model of psychodynamic psychotherapy is a basic competence of an analytic approach. Indeed, having a theoretical framework is a generic competence for any therapy. Most of the chapters in this book outline clinical aspects of psychodynamic psychotherapy, with reference to theoretical works. This chapter serves as a theoretical foundation for the psychodynamic model, and contains discussions of theorists and concepts that we will return to in future chapters.

A history of splits

One of the ironies of the psychoanalytic profession is that it is characterised by significant rifts and splits into differing, at times warring, schools of thought. One would think that a profession with a focused interest in understanding human emotional life would be able to manage conflict and disagreement, however, the history of psychoanalysis shows this not to be the case! Notwithstanding substantial conflict, shared themes and trends are evident. The body of theory has shifted from a biological and intrapsychic understanding of the human mind and human beha-viour, to a developmental focus, and more recently, to an interpersonal/relational and intersubjective focus.

Freud began his career in 1880s Vienna, Austria, as a neurologist and neu-roanatomist. He took an interest in a particular group of patients who were presenting with what was referred to as 'hysterical symptoms'. He began working closely with general practitioner, Josef Breuer, who was using hypnosis to treat a patient presenting with hysterical symptoms of unexplained paralysis and mental confusion. This was the famous case of 'Anna O' (Breuer and Freud, 1895). Freud collaborated with Breuer on this and other cases, using hypnosis and talking as a cure for treating hysterical symptoms. However, Freud became uncertain about the effectiveness of hypnosis, troubled by its suggestive possibilities, and started to break away from Breuer to pursue a talking treatment for hysteria. This was the genesis of psychoanalysis as both a technique and a theory of psychic development.

As Freud began to publicise his ideas and clinical observations, other physicians took an interest in his ideas, and a first group of psychoanalytic practitioners developed: Freud, Jung, Adler, Stekel, Abraham, Ferenczi, Jones and Rank (Bateman and Holmes, 1995). Freud's theories of development focused on sexual instinct as central to understanding the psyche and its development. His insistence on the centrality of infantile sexuality made his followers uncomfortable, and some began to diverge from Freud. Most notable was the rift between Freud and Jung. Jung was Freud's protégé, and he had been named as the first head of the newly formed International Psychoanalytic Association. Jung and Freud began to disagree on the fundamentals of Freud's theory. Jung de-emphasised the importance of sexual instinct for development, instead privileging the influence of religion and spirituality. They also diverged on their understanding of the nature of the unconscious, with Jung introducing the idea of a collective unconscious. A schism developed between Freud and Jung, with their relationship eventually breaking down in 1912. The theories of Jung and his followers have become known as Analytic Psychology, whereas Freud and post-Freudian theory forms the basis of psychoanalytic and psychodynamic psychotherapy, which we outline in this book. It is beyond our remit to expand on the theories of Jung; instead we have recommended some introductory texts in Box 2.1 should you wish to read more of his work.

Freud and his family, together with many of the early psychoanalytic practitioners in Europe, had to flee Nazi persecution in the 1930s because they were Jewish. Freud settled in London in 1938 and, sadly, died a year later. The arrival of the Freud family in London meant that Britain became an important centre for psychoanalysis. His daughter and trained psychoanalyst, Anna Freud, both continued and extended her father's work by pioneering the psychoanalytic treatment of children.

One of the earlier tensions within the profession was around eligibility to train as a psychoanalyst. At first the profession was only open to medical practitioners, but in Britain, Ernest Jones, then president of the British Psychoanalytic Society, was in favour of allowing non-medical practitioners, or 'lay' persons to train as psychoanalysts. One such 'lay' analyst was Melanie Klein, who quickly became a key figure in British psychoanalysis. She also pioneered a method for analysing children, namely play therapy. Klein began to focus on the mother–infant relationship, and placed a greater emphasis on the early origins of psychic life, claiming that Oedipal conflicts existed in the first year of life, much earlier than Freud had stipulated (see below). She also placed greater attention on the role of aggression in infant development.

Klein's theories conflicted with key aspects of Freud's theories and Anna Freud's work, leading to increasing tension and disagreement between Anna Freud and her followers on the one hand, and Klein and her followers, on the other. This led to a major split in the psychoanalytic movement in Britain. A series of talks were held at the British Psychoanalytic Society, which became known as the 'controversial discussions', where attempts were made to thrash out these disagreements in order to find common ground. This was not achieved, and the society split into followers of Freud and followers of Klein. The theories of Klein and her followers formed the beginnings of what became known as the British Object Relations School. Later, a third group emerged from this split, declining to align themselves with either camp; they became known as the Independents, or 'middle group'. This group led by Donald Winnicott, Harry Guntrip, Ronald Fairbairn and others, emphasised the role of the maternal environment in psychic development. These three groupings remain a key feature of British psychoanalysis to this day, however, the differences are now less stark with more collaboration and integration having been achieved.

In the USA, psychoanalysis became a major force within psychiatry. Unlike in the British Society, only medical professionals could train then as psychoanalysts. Psychoanalysis in the USA was first influenced by Freud's visit to the States in 1909. By 1952, 64% of members of the International Psychoanalytic Association (then located in the USA) were from North America. The predominance of psychoanalytic practitioners in the USA led to further developments in psychoanalytic theory, with influences from varying perspectives. There was an early emphasis in the USA on ego development, influenced by the ego psychology of Heinz Hartmann. This emphasis remained a Freudian one, until later theorists progressed psychoanalytic theories in different directions particular to the USA. These neo-Freudians differed from Freudian orthodoxy in emphasizing the importance of social and cultural factors in psychic development. One such development came from Harry Stack Sullivan and his interpersonal school of psychoanalysis in the 1920s and 1930s in which he repudiated drive theory and emphasised the role of external factors such as culture and society together with interconnectedness. His work and writings synthesised contemporary ideas of psychiatry and social science and formed the basis of social psychiatry and the community mental health movement. Another development came in the 1970s with Heinz Kohut's Self Psychology theories. Subsequent feminist thinkers such as Horney, Chodorow and Benjamin were influential in the growing emphasis on the interpersonal and intersubjective nature of psychodynamic development and psychoanalytic technique.

Owing to the world wars in the first half of the 20th century, many psychoanalysts of Germany, Austria and nearby countries immigrated to Britain or to the Americas, escaping Nazi persecution. In Germany and Austria, psychoanalytic thinking was depicted as a 'Jewish Science', something Freud repeatedly denied. In Europe, France went on to become a centre for psychoanalytic thought, and remains so to this day. Influenced by French philosophers, French psychoanalysts critiqued the determinism of Freud's theories. Lacan became a dominant figure in French psychoanalysis, calling for a return to the pre-structural model of Freud, and viewing the unconscious as a form of language. Lacanian psychoanalysis has its own distinct flavour and training methodology. Other, more 'mainstream' French psychoanalysts include André Green who extended the work of Winnicott to develop the concept of the analytic 'space' – the creative space between the analyst and patient where growth can occur, but also where despair can be held. Laplanche and Pontalis were influential post-Freudian French psychoanalytic thinkers, best known for their comprehensive dictionary of psychoanalysis. In Italy, psychoanalysis also has some prominence, tending to follow a Kleinian tradition. A strong psychoanalytic tradition can also be found in the Scandinavian countries as well as The Netherlands and Belgium. Germany has several schools of psychoanalysis and intensive analytic treatment can be obtained there on the public health service.

In the remainder of this chapter, we will focus on the psychoanalytic theories of Freud and post-Freudians, the Kleinian School, The British Independent School, and finally the influential schools from North America. We focus on these particular groups because they provide the theoretical framework on which this book is based. We acknowledge that in doing so, we are leaving out many important psychoanalytic theorists by necessity. What is immediately evident in the very brief outline above is how psychoanalysis is dominated by the Global North, although there are thriving psychoanalytic centres in the Global South, particularly South America (a place where many analysts settled after leaving Europe).

Freud's structural and developmental theories

Freud not only founded the practice of psychoanalysis as a 'talking cure', but also presented a metapsychology of human development and behaviour. Freud was not the one to 'discover' the unconscious, but he was the first to explore and understand the central role that the unconscious plays in human development and mental life. The unconscious was central to Freud's model of the mind, which went through two significant theoretical phases: the topographical model of the mind, and later the structural model of the mind.

The topographical model of the mind

Freud initially understood the mind as having different functions, that are located in different places or topographies. The topographical model depicts the mind as divided into three different systems: the systems unconscious, pre-conscious and conscious (Freud, 1900). This is commonly represented by the analogy of the iceberg: the visible part of the iceberg above the surface of the water represents the *System Conscious*; the larger part of the iceberg that is submerged under water and invisible to the eye represents the *System Unconscious*; and the parts of the iceberg that bob up and down the water line representing the *System Pre-conscious*. The conscious is that part of the mind containing aspects of our experience of which we are fully aware. The unconscious, by contrast, contains aspects of our experience which are repressed, and which remain outside our awareness. The pre-conscious is that part of the mind which contains things of which we are at any one time unaware, but can become aware of when necessary (e.g. our familiarity with driving a car that is done seemingly automatically, without conscious awareness but which we can articulate if we focus on what it is we are doing; by contrast, a learner driver is very much conscious of every step and decision they are making).

Freud articulated two principles of mental functioning within the topographical model of the mind (Freud, 1911), which he referred to as primary and secondary process thinking and that belong to the systems unconscious and conscious respectively. *Primary process thinking* is irrational and follows no logic; whereas *secondary process thinking* is rational, logical and organised. Primary process thinking is typically reflected in the irrational and illogical nature of dreams. In primary process thinking, there is no linear sense of time, with events of the past and present occurring simultaneously or in reverse, as often happens in dreams. The unconscious operates with primary process thinking, which means that we are unaware of what is contained within it. Notwithstanding this, Freud observed that the unconscious frequently reveals itself through communications such as dreams, slips of the tongue or parapraxes, non-verbal gestures and other means.

The structural model of the mind

Later, Freud (1923a) proposed a structural model of the mind comprising three separate structures or components of personality: the id, the superego and the ego. While he never updated his earlier, topographical model of the mind, it leaves us to consider these two theoretical models side by side, and how they inform each other.

The *id* is the basic, primitive part of the mind, mostly in the unconscious, which contains the instinctual drives. Freud's theories were rooted in a biological understanding of human behaviour, and he first conceptualised psychological processes as dominated by instinctual drives. The drives are innate instincts that push us into particular behaviours in an attempt to satisfy these urges. Freud understood that, like most animal species, we have a sexual and an aggressive instinct or drive. Later he broadened his understanding of the instincts to refer to the life instinct (or *Eros*) and the death instinct (or *Thanatos*). The life instinct includes self-preservative drives that encompass sexual and procreative drives. The death instinct includes aggressive and destructive urges. Freud understood these instincts as having a chemical energy or impulse which builds up and leads to a physical (behavioural) discharge that needs to find connection with an object in the world in order to achieve its aim. Freud laid emphasis on the sexual instinct as the primary force behind human development (we will elaborate this below when looking at Freud's psychosexual stages of development). Freud understood that the instinctual urges demand gratification, and thus operate according to what he termed the *pleasure principle* (Freud, 1911; 1920). The id is completely governed by the pleasure principle, whereby the mind avoids pain or 'unpleasure' and seeks 'pleasure'. In this context, 'unpleasure' is understood to result from accumulation of instinctual tension and conversely, pleasure from the discharge of this tension.

The *superego* refers to our conscience and ideals. These include social and cultural moral values, norms and ideals that we internalise, primarily derived from the role models served by our parents and other significant adults. They are internalisations of our relationship to our parents and other authority figures. Since they are internal representations of these figures and relationships, they are based both in reality as well as distorted and modified by fantasy. Freud similarly conceptualised the superego as involving energies that exert an internal pressure on the individual. Distorted internalised representations may, for example, result in a very harsh superego, with the individual struggling with intense feelings of guilt and moral conflict. Aspects of the superego can be in our conscious mind, while other superego parts can be unconscious.

The *ego* is that rational, executive part of our personality. The ego is mostly conscious but also has unconscious parts. The ego operates according to what Freud termed the *reality principle* (Freud 1911), and mediates between the demands of the id, the superego and external reality. This capacity develops with time as ego functions strengthen. The ego seeks gratification in external reality and not merely by hallucinatory wish-fulfilment and thus has to take into account the availability of gratifying objects, safety of discharge and potential benefits of postponement of instinctual gratification. In many ways, the marshmallow test illustrates this reality vs pleasure principle emerging in young children: can the ego delay gratification or will the id win out if the child cannot resist eating the marshmallow? These intrapsychic and external demands can be in conflict with one another, resulting in considerable anxiety or 'unpleasure' for the individual, which they then need to manage or adapt to by means of the defence mechanisms. Anna Freud took particularly interest in understanding more about the ego and extended Freud's understanding of anxiety and defence mechanisms in her important book, *Ego and the Mechanisms of Defence* (Freud, 1954; first published in 1936) (see Chapter 6).

The structural model of the mind does not supersede the topographical model, nor does it map directly onto the later model. As outlined above, the id operates at the unconscious level, but the ego and the superego have both conscious and unconscious (or indeed pre-conscious) aspects. This is represented by Freud as shown in Figure 2.1.

Stages of psychosexual development

As mentioned earlier, Freud (1905a) placed the sexual instinct at the centre of his understanding of human development, which he conceptualised as progressing through five sequential stages: the oral, anal, phallic, latency and genital stages of psychosexual development. This covered the ages from birth through childhood, puberty and into adulthood. As discussed earlier, Freud understood instincts, and the sexual instinct in particular, as a form of biological urge or impulse which exerts a pressure on the organism, demanding release. Freud observed that this

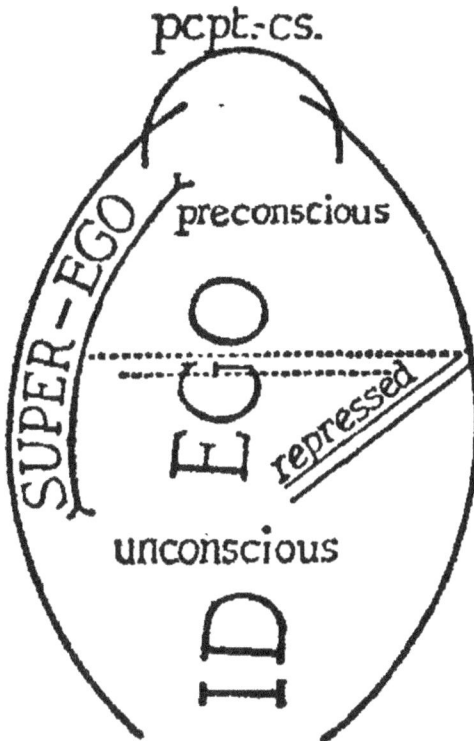

Figure 2.1 Freud's model of the mind
Source: Freud, 1933, p. 78

sexual instinct is primarily located in different areas of the body as the individual develops, thus the psychosexual stages of development are differentiated by the physical location of the instinctual urges. According to Freud, the baby is born with only an id, dominated by primitive sexual and aggressive instincts. The ego, and subsequently the superego, develop during the first years of life as the child engages more and more with the objects (people) in their environment. Freud put this succinctly, as follows: "Where id was, there ego shall be" (1933, p.80) and "the ego is first and foremost a bodily ego" (1923a, p. 26), thereby locating the development of the self in the body and its functions.

The *oral stage* of development occurs in the first year of life when the infant's libidinal (sexual instinct) energy is focused on the mouth. The infant explores their environment and derives pleasure primarily through sucking, whether this is the nipple of mother's breast or a teat, their hand, thumb and other objects they put in their mouth. During this first year, the baby moves from a purely subjective state (or what Freud referred to as primary narcissism) to a gradual recognition of the primary caregiver as an object separate to themselves. The *anal stage* occurs during the second and third years of life when the anal zone becomes the focus of libidinal energy. Toddlers experience pleasure through the sensations of their bowel movements and mastery of this during toilet training by releasing or holding in their faeces. Around the ages of three to four, during the *phallic stage* of psychosexual development, children make a salient discovery of their genitals. The sex organs become the zones of libidinal energy as the child plays with their genitals and becomes aware of sameness and difference, recognising gender differences and developing a secure sense of their own sexual identity.

Freud's (1905a) theory of the child's sexuality during the *genital or Oedipal stage* between the ages of four to six, introduced the importance of resolving the Oedipus Complex for the male child and the Electra Complex for the female child. According to Freud, during this stage the child's libidinal desires are directed towards the opposite-sex parent. Boys are typically unconsciously attracted to their mothers, perceiving father as a rival for mother's affection with resultant feelings of hostility towards him. The boy, fearing that his father will punish him by means of castration, renounces his desire for his mother, and begins to identify with father, wishing to become just like him so as to attract an object just like his mother. Freud's theory of female sexuality was less developed than his theory of male sexuality. His theory of female sexuality centred on her 'lack' of a penis. The girl becomes aware that she does not have a penis. Envying her father's penis, the girl renounces her primary desires for the mother, whom she blames for her own lack of a penis, and turns her affection towards the father. We have provided here a very brief outline of the Oedipus and Electra complex – the Electra complex is not taught or adhered to in psychoanalysis and the focus on the Oedipal complex has broadened to think about triangulation, with Ron Britton (1989) having developed this further, namely, that the Oedipal complex is a model of triangulated relationships, where the child is excluded from the parental relationship, and each individual parent has a relationship to their child that differs from the relationship that the other parent has. Much has been written to critique and contest Freud's theories of these complexes, which is beyond our discussion here. One thing to note though is its heteronormative focus, and we will examine this in Chapter 13 when considering diversity and difference. We want to underline that according to Freud, the superego develops out of the resolution of the Oedipus complex, as the child internalises their parents' rules and through them, society's moral laws about sexuality and sex roles. Resolution of the Oedipal stage leads to greater ability to accept intergenerational differences, tolerate disappointment and identify with the perspective of a third person.

Between the ages of six and eleven years, Freud said that children go through the *latency stage*. With the development of the superego during the phallic stage, the child's sexual and aggressive energies are now sublimated. The child gains greater control of their instincts and directs their energies towards social pursuits, such as friendship, games, learning and adapting to reality. However, those working with pre-teenagers today have recognised that this latency age is less and less present in our world of sexualised clothing, images, internet and tv, leading Alessandra Lemma to rename it the 'blatancy' stage (Lemma, 2017, p. 44). The sexual libidinal energies re-emerge in full force during *puberty*, the final stage of psychosexual development. This flourish of sexual energy threatens the established ego defences. It is typically a time of emotional upheaval. Oedipal struggles around desire, inclusion and exclusion are recapitulated as the child enters into competition with same-sex peers for the affections of opposite sex peers (in heterosexual adolescents). The child begins to explore romantic relationships, which gradually allows them to free themselves from their parents. This is a period of increasing maturity and independence.

Anxiety and psychopathology

Freud rooted his theories in a biological model of psychology, understanding the human body and psychic life in terms of energies and forces. The biological organism constantly attempts to achieve a state of homeostasis. Freud understood anxiety to be a state of 'unpleasure' within the organism as homeostasis is disrupted. Anxiety is caused by the libidinal forces exerting pressure on the organism, resulting in intrapsychic conflict between the id, ego and superego; such conflict threatens to break into consciousness and endanger the ego's resources. The individual manages these anxieties by deploying various defence mechanisms, such as repression or denial. However, in the case of repression, what is repressed is not necessarily deleted, and 'threatens' to return thereby creating anxiety, what Freud (1896) referred to as the "return of the repressed" (p. 169); what is repressed often 'returns' as an inexplicable symptom or an unconscious communication (we will expand on this in Chapter 8). Psychopathology arises when defence mechanisms are used in unhelpful and dysfunctional ways as well as when those defence mechanisms break down. We shall discuss anxiety and defence mechanisms in more detail in Chapter 6. Freud (1914a) argued that we are prone to repeat our early traumatic experiences that we have tried to repress within current relationships. Freud states that

> the patient does not *remember* anything of what he has forgotten and repressed, but *acts* it out. He reproduces it not as a memory but as an action; he *repeats* it, without, of course, knowing that he is repeating it. (p. 150)

He goes on to give the example of a patient's past, unremembered difficulty with the authority of their parents being repeated in their current behaviour towards authority figures, or early experiences of being shamed, being repeated in feelings of shame in current relationships. This forms the basis of the transference, which we will discuss at length in Chapter 9.

Psychopathology may also be caused by a fixation at – or regression to – any of the five stages of psychosexual development. At each psychosexual stage, new conflicts arise. Fixation at a particular stage may occur as a result of excessive gratification or frustration. A child or adult may also regress to a fixation at an earlier psychosexual stage during times of stress. When fixated to a particular stage, the child or adult maintains a preoccupation with the libidinal pleasures of that particular stage. For example, a fixation at the anal stage may be expressed in preoccupations with issues of control, cleanliness and order, which can manifest pathologically in obsessive-compulsive difficulties. Fixations at the oral stage are expressed in preoccupations with oral pleasure, such as smoking, thumb-sucking, drinking and eating, and in their more problematic forms, may manifest as eating disorders and substance abuse.

Freud stressed the importance of successfully passing through the various stages of psychosexual development for healthy psychic life in adulthood. The significance of childhood experiences for adult functioning is also implicit in Freud's concept of transference; that is, we transfer past, unresolved and unconscious experiences with our primary objects onto others in the present, including the therapist. We shall discuss transference in more detail in Chapter 9, along with countertransference, the feelings and responses engendered in the therapist by the experience of being with the patient.

Anna Freud's concept of developmental lines

Anna Freud furthered the developmental aspects of Freud's work, in particular the development of psychopathology. While Sigmund Freud worked mainly with adults and attempted to trace their psychopathologies by looking towards the past, Anna Freud worked mostly with children and was concerned with childhood development and healthy development looking forwards towards adulthood. She argued that the journey to healthy adulthood follows a coherent "developmental line" (Freud, 1963, p. 130). In her model, conflicts were not just intrapsychic, but also arose at different stages of development where there are maturational steps involving the interaction between drive (id) maturation, ego functioning, superego demands and the influences of the environment. As the child matures into adulthood, they would typically move forward along certain developmental lines, but they may also regress backwards along these lines in times of stress or challenge. This backwards and forwards movement implies a certain optimism in the capacity of children to overcome difficulties and reach maturation. Anna Freud delineated several different developmental lines, for example, the development of the adult's ability and capacity for work develops from the child's capacity for play: first with their mother's body and by themselves, through to playing with toys, then playing with peers in the form of role plays and games, then developing hobbies. and finally, the ability to work.

One important developmental line is the move from infant dependency to adult emotional self-reliance and mature relationships, which Anna Freud (1965) argued involved eight stages. First, there is unity between the infant and their mother, where the infant does not yet have the capacity to perceive the mother as separate to themselves. Through a process of gradual initial separation, the child moves into the second stage where they have a relationship to the mother that is primarily based on the fulfilment of their biological needs. In this stage, the need for the object increases with the arousal of the bodily drives (e.g. hunger) but recedes when the needs are satisfied. In the third stage, the child is able to perceive the mother as entirely separate to them and forms a representation of their mother in their mind. This stage forms the basis for reciprocal relationships. In the fourth stage, the child exercises more ambivalent feelings towards the mother, is able to be frustrated and disappointed with her, and so starts to exercise some basic independence from the mother. Stage 5 corresponds with the phallic-Oedipal stage where the child understands that there is a triangular relationship between themselves and their mother and father, developing possessive feelings towards the opposite sex parent and rivalrous feelings towards the same-sex parent. In Stage 6, the child transfers their libidinal drive from their parents to their peers, including teachers and other significant adults. In the pre-adolescent Stage 7, Anna Freud described a regression from the relatively reasonable behaviour of latency period, to the self-centred, demanding behaviour of adolescence. Finally, in Stage 8, representing maturity, the individual is able to master their sexual and aggressive drives, withdraw libidinal investment in their parents, and form libidinal attachments with others. Anna Freud suggested that these stages entail resolving conflicts related to the shifting aggressive and libidinal drives felt towards the object, and the tolerance of increasing separation and independence from the primary objects.

The beginnings of Object Relations theory: Melanie Klein and Wilfred Bion

Melanie Klein developed her psychoanalytic work and theories on the foundations of Freud's theories. Like Anna Freud, she too was a pioneer in the development of a psychoanalytic technique for working with children. Klein has been an influential thinker in psychoanalysis and her work was furthered by others such as Paula Heimann, Hanna Segal, Betty Joseph, Donald Meltzer, contemporary Kleinians like John Steiner and Ron Britton and notably, Wilfred Bion's writings in relation to working with adults and groups. The theories of Klein and Bion were the beginnings of what has become known as the British Object Relations School.

Although Klein founded her thinking on Freud, and seemingly agreed with Freud's theories of instinct, she placed less emphasis on instinctual and libidinal theories, instead focusing on the infant's development of the self in relation to their primary objects (caregivers). This was a departure point from drive theory towards object relations theory, notwithstanding that Klein was mostly concerned with internal objects coloured by phantasy, as opposed to later object relations theorists who paid more attention to the external environment and interpersonal objects. Klein also differed with Freud in her view of the infant as born with a rudimentary, developing ego structure, including the existence of Oedipal object relations from the very first year of life. These fundamental differences with the Freudian model led to a split in the British Psychoanalytic Society, as mentioned earlier.

Klein's writing tends to be filled with jargon, which readers can find unpalatable, and as a result, her ideas are not easy to grasp. One of the more influential ideas developed by Klein involves her developmental understanding of the self and its objects, focused primarily in the first year of life. She is most known for her formulation of two developmental positions that occur during the first years of an individual's life, and which recur reflexively in later life, namely the *paranoid-schizoid position* and the *depressive position*. Readers unfamiliar with the theories of Klein may interpret such terminology (phrases such as 'paranoid' or 'depressive') as referring to psychiatric disorders. However, Klein used these terms to capture the infant's unconscious emotional response to their environment. Before discussing these two positions, it is important to first consider Klein's understanding of the subjective mind.

Unconscious phantasy and internalised objects

Klein (1932) distinguished between an outer world (environment) and inner world (psychic reality) that affect our subjective experiences. She theorised that the individual makes unconscious mental representations of their subjective experiences in their mind, which she terms unconscious phantasies. She spelled it with a *ph* – phantasy – to distinguish it from *fantasy*, a term that refers to a narrative genre. Klein argued that from birth, unconscious mental representations of our bodily sensations and emotional experiences exist as phantasies through which we experience the outer world, as well as our inner world. Klein understood our capacity for phantasy to be innate, in that we are born with some innate proto-typical knowledge. Klein argued that the infant is born with innate knowledge – albeit poorly formed – about sexuality and the existence of the mother's breast (food), for example. Phantasies are experienced as *internal objects* with which we then relate to our inner world, hence the term object relations. For example, a baby who experiences hunger, will experience bodily sensations of pain in their stomach and this is felt to be an object inside them that is causing this pain rather than it originating from themselves. As the baby matures and develops a more coherent sense of self, so a clearer and integrated sense of what is 'me' and 'not me' can take shape.

The inner world is created and built up through repeated processes of introjection and projection. Introjection involves things from the outside being taken in and incorporated into the inner world in the form of mental representations. Projection refers to what is eliminated through expulsion into the outside world. The inner world is made up of object representations that are built up through repeated processes of introjection (incorporation). These introjections are distorted by the feelings and mental states with which they were projected. Thus, what exists in our inner world – our internalised objects – is not an accurate representation of the objects that exist in the outer world, but rather a distorted version of them. We relate not only to the object in the external world, but more to our internalised object representations in the inner world. For example, we may have an internalised object of a critical parent, which affects our experience of relating to our actual parent. At first, we introject aspects of an object, which are internalised as *part-object* representations. Over time as we introject more aspects of an object, with all their complexity and nuances, we then have a whole, albeit distorted, internalised object.

Another important concept that Klein (1946; 1957) discussed in relation to the creation of object representations in the inner world is *projective identification*. Projection, as already mentioned, involves the expulsion and externalisation of emotions and mental states which are then attributed to the outside. Identification refers to the process when aspects of the object are introjected and become self-representations. Projective identification, as the term suggests, combines projection and introjection is a complex single mechanism or process. In projective identification, a phantasy of something that the infant experiences as a 'bad' part of the self (e.g. their aggression) is split off and projected *into* the object (the mother, in the case of the infant) so that the object then becomes a split off bad part of themselves. The difference is whereas feelings or experiences can be projected *onto* an object so that they are experienced through the distortion of that projection, in projective identification, a part of the self (not just a feeling) is projected *into* the object in a more powerful way such that this part is disowned and the object is seen 'in reality' as if it were that part-object. The primary purpose in projective identification is communication and it represents a primitive form of communication that infants use to convey states of great distress. Yet, it is a form of communication that becomes problematic in later life since it depletes the self and often leaves the individual extremely paranoid that some form of retaliation will follow.

We will discuss projection and projective identification in more detail in Chapter 6 when looking at different defence mechanisms. It is important to touch on them here, because for Klein, these mechanisms and processes form the foundations of psychic development in the first year of life, during the paranoid-schizoid and depressive positions.

The Paranoid-Schizoid Position

Klein (1932; 1959) argued that the early experience of the infant involves anxiety arising out of their dependence on the mother as primary caregiver. The infant is governed by their internal sensory experiences together with interchanges with their primary caregiver. Klein focuses on the subjective state of self in the infant's relationship with the mother, in particular the infant's relationship with the breast during feeding. Because the infant has not yet acquired an understanding of space and time, they cannot tolerate the sensory experience of hunger and cannot yet hold on to the expectation or knowledge that they will soon be fed. The infant is not yet able to experience the mother as a separate, whole person, only experiencing her as disparate parts. When hungry, the infant's subjective experience includes pain, distress, fear of perishing and angry frustration among other feelings. When the mother feeds the infant, the feelings of hunger are gradually satisfied. The infant takes in (or incorporates) the feelings of goodness and nurturance of the mother as if it were their own; the infant has a good experience of self, with the mother experienced in turn as 'good'. For example, when the infant is hungry and frustrated, the sensation of hunger is externally attributed to the withholding breast of the mother. The 'bad' internal feelings (in this case hunger pains and frustration) are projected onto the withholding breast/mother and so the mother is perceived as 'bad' (withholding and hurtful). Similarly, with other sensations, when the baby is in need of comfort, the 'bad' feelings of discomfort are projected onto the mother who withholds this comfort. This creates a polarised experience of the mother (breast), experiencing her as a frustrating, hated object (the 'bad breast') and a separate nurturing, loved object (the 'good breast') depending on the infant's experience. This split experience of the mother serves a defensive function – the 'bad' experience of the mother is split off and kept separate from the 'good' mother in order to preserve the good. The term 'schizoid' is used to refer to the fragmented mental state of experiencing the environment as part objects, while the term 'paranoid' is used to describe the persecutory feelings associated with the frustrating 'bad' object (Hinshelwood, 1989).

The depressive position

As the infant matures, they begin to experience their mother as a whole object, and the infant comes to realise that the mother is both the 'good', nurturing mother, as well as the 'bad', withholding mother. The infant is now better able to tolerate these ambivalent feelings, and so does not have a split experience of the mother (and in turn, of the self). When the infant is hungry, for example, they can tolerate their frustration more, in the knowledge that mother will soon appear to feed them. Klein (1935; 1937) referred to this as the depressive position, because she theorised that the infant, aware now that the mother is both 'good' and 'bad', feels unconsciously guilty (and remorseful) for the hatred felt towards the mother when previously frustrated. What may result is an unconscious wish to make reparation for the 'damage' caused by the aggression felt towards the 'bad' mother of the paranoid-schizoid position.

Although these positions are understood as following a developmental sequence, they are not considered to be developmental stages, since an individual continues to vacillate between these positions throughout their lives, particularly during times of stress (Segal, 1992). In moments of tension, we often move into a paranoid-schizoid position, defending our experience of a 'good' self from perceived 'bad' experiences or objects. There is then a splitting of the ego, where the 'bad' parts of the self are split off and projected onto an object (or person) through projective identification where they are then attributed as belonging to another. At other times, we operate from the depressive position and are able to acknowledge both good and bad aspects in ourselves and in others.

As mentioned earlier, Kleinian theories marked a shift from Freudian drive theory and the focus on intrapsychic conflict towards considering the impact of the external world. However, her emphasis was primarily an intrapsychic one, in that Klein emphasises the way the impact of the external world is affected by our internal phantasies. Thus, it is our internalised object representations with which we have a relationship and which influence our behaviour, rather than the actual objects of the external environment. The influence of real external experience was developed further by members of the British Independent group such as

Winnicott and Fairbairn. Contemporary Kleinian theorists and psychotherapists have shifted away from considering object relations only in terms of the inner world of phantasies, most particularly as this manifest in the patient's transference to the therapist, and towards acknowledging the role of environmental trauma and failure in the psychic development of the individual. Thus, the focus for post-Kleinian analysis is on the interplay between environmental trauma and inner phantasy.

Wilfred Bion: on containment and thinking

Bion (1962a) was a significant proponent of Klein who expanded on her understanding of projective identification in particular by emphasising the importance of the mother-infant relationship and the impact of the environment on the individual. He introduced the notion of the mother acting as a *container* for the infant/child's projections, and how she provides emotional *containment*, when these projections are metabolised by the mother and the experience is returned to the infant in a nurturing way, helping them feel *contained*. So, for example, an infant feels anxiety and fear and in the paranoid-schizoid position, projects this into the mother who is experienced as 'bad'. The infant's experience is often beyond words and requires the mother to receive these projections of the infant's experience of anxiety and fear and make sense of them. She contains these feelings, metabolises them and can then respond to the infant's anxiety and fear in a soothing, nurturing way. The infant is thus able to introject the 'good' feelings of being held, understood and cared for. This concept of 'container-contained' in the earliest relationship of mother and baby has applications in the therapist-patient dyad, where the therapist serves as the container for the patient's projected anxieties, fears, and destructive feelings of hatred. Being able to receive these projections and respond to them in an empathic way, rather than with retaliation or denial, allows the patient to feel understood and helped. Psychopathology results when containment breaks down, for example if the mother is depressed and unavailable, or responds to the infant with anger or frustration. The infant's emotional experiences are returned to the baby without being modified or metabolised and in fact, may now be augmented by the mother's distress or frustration. For the mother to be a container, she adopts a state of maternal *reverie*, a mental state of free-floating attention where she can absorb her infant's projections, feel them and make sense of them, and process them in her response to the baby.

Bion's concept of containment emphasises a much more interactional model of object relations than Klein's formulation. It is more than the infant projecting and introjecting object representations, but rather the objects playing an intrinsic role in influencing and having an impact on the quality of what the baby introjects. The object is an active component in the infant's metabolising of mental states.

Bion (1962b) also wrote about the process of thinking, and made an important theoretical contribution towards understanding how raw bodily/instinctual sensations are transformed into mental representations (an important aspect underpinning Klein's notion of unconscious phantasy). Bion referred to this conversion process as '*alpha function*'. In alpha function, raw bodily sense data (sounds, smell, touch and so on) are generated into mental contents of meaning, or *alpha elements*, which Hinshelwood (1989) refers to as "the furniture for dreams and for thinking" (p. 229). Bion understood this conversion process as occurring through stages involving an initial pre-existing anticipation, or pre-conception of something, which is then followed by its realisation when an occurrence in actual reality matches that preconception. This in turn creates a conception or mental representation, which can then be thought about (Hinshelwood, 1989). So, for example, when an infant is hungry, they experience hunger pains (bodily sensations) and we can hypothesis that they have some instinctual pre-conception of 'food' (the existence of the mother's breast). The infant's pre-conception of 'food/breast' is then realised when the mother gives them a feed. This matching of internal phantasised experience with outer reality, then allows the infant to develop the conception of 'food/breast' as a mental representation which can then be thought about. When this process of alpha functioning does not occur – that is, when bodily sense data are not converted into mental content – the sense data remains unassimilated. Bion referred to this as *beta elements*, that are usually evacuated through projective identification. In other words, beta elements consist of sense data that cannot be thought about. This is the basis of projection and projective identification.

Object Relations Theory: the British independents

As mentioned earlier, there is an independent group of British psychoanalysts within the British Psychoanalytic Society, that chose to identify with neither the Freudian nor the Kleinian traditions, instead taking the middle ground where they could be influenced and inspired by a wide range of theoretical approaches. On the whole, the independent group placed much more emphasis on the influence of the environment, and so can broadly be considered object relational theorists (rather than drive theorists). Two of the most notable early figures in this group are Fairbairn and Winnicott, whom we will discuss here.

Fairbairn and object-seeking motivation

William Fairbairn, a Scottish psychoanalyst, initially focused on libidinal drive theory. However, rather than agreeing with Freud that the libido was essentially pleasure-seeking, Fairbairn (1952) proposed that the libidinal drive was object-seeking, and that this object-seeking was the key motivation in life. This emphasis on object-seeking laid the foundations for the object relations school of thought. In his model, pleasure is not the result of the satisfaction and release of libidinal energy, but rather is felt as the outcome of good quality self-object relationships, that are both represented internally and exist externally. Fairbairn understood repetition compulsion in terms of object-seeking: because the libido is motivated to attach to objects, the child forms an attachment bond to the parent, in whatever form that bond takes, whether nurturing, lacking or at its worst, iatrogenic.

Fairbairn differed from Klein in his conceptualisation of internal objects. Whereas Klein understood internal objects as unconscious phantasies that are always a feature of mental life, Fairbairn (1952) held that internal objects develop as a result of external frustrations. For Fairbairn, the child who receives good parenting will be outwardly directed onto the real relationships of their external environment. Where the child is disappointed, neglected or frustrated by the parental object, they will turn away from the external environment and form internal objects with whom they maintain fantasised relationships.

Fairbairn (1952) focused in his writings on schizoid personality functioning and the associated splitting of the ego. When a child has an experience of neglectful parenting as a result of a depressed, bullying or narcissistic parent, they will internalise these aspects of the parent as internal objects, with whom the self identifies and maintains a relationship with (as internal objects). However, part of the ego remains outwardly orientated, maintaining a relationship with the actual external parent, seeking real responses from them. This creates a further split in the object between an exciting object (with whom hoped-for responses are still sought) on the one hand, and a rejecting object that has been internalised, on the other.

Winnicott: the holding environment and the 'good enough mother'

Donald Winnicott expanded on the early object relational theories of Klein, Bion and others, and became an important and influential theorist in developing a more relational, social model of psychic development. Winnicott moved away from instinct theory, emphasising the primacy of early environmental (maternal) experience for psychological development. Winnicott was a paediatrician prior to training as a psychoanalyst, and this specialist medical background greatly influenced his understanding that the quality of the mother-infant relationships holds the key for healthy development. He is most known for his notion of the *good enough mother* and the *holding environment*, that are related to the development of a *true, authentic* or *false self*.

Winnicott (1960) stated that "there is no such thing as an infant" (p. 586), emphasising that we cannot think of an infant as separate from the mother. He viewed the mother and infant as being in a merged state of oneness, where the infant only exists within an environment of maternal care. The mother is attuned to the infant's needs, thereby providing the necessary environment for the infant to thrive. This is what Winnicott (1965) referred to as the *holding environment* – the physical and emotional environment in which the infant is held. The mother is able to do this by falling into a state of 'primary maternal preoccupation', in which her subjective state is partly merged with the mental state of the infant. Winnicott helpfully recognised that a mother cannot be perfect, because she is inevitably her own, flawed person with her own needs. Mothers inevitably grow tired, frustrated and need to be (pre)occupied with other matters: she can never be perfectly available to the infant. Winnicott stressed that what was important was for the mother to provide 'good enough' mothering. Frustrations also facilitate healthy development for the infant, who learns that there are limits to their needs and what the environment can provide. As the infant experiences such limits and frustrations, so they become aware of mother as a separate person with her own subjectivity. The level of frustration introduced to the infant should be at an optimal level and not overwhelm the infant with despair. At the other end of the continuum of parenting is the mother who is *not* good enough; who is unable to, or does not care to, respond adequately to the infant's needs. This may include a mother who impinges on the infant's subjective experience by being an intrusive, frightening, or even threatening and hostile object, or a mother whose needs overshadow the needs of the infant.

Although Winnicott's notion of the good enough mother provides some degree of sympathy for the challenges facing mothers, his writing places great emphasis on the importance of maternal qualities to understand healthy development, and conversely, to explain the development of psychopathology. However, Winnicott recognised that the mother is not alone with this responsibility. He wrote about the importance of the father – and more broadly the social environment – in providing a supportive environment for the mother. Society has its responsibilities too. Contemporary theorists point out that Winnicott's emphasis on maternal care and the 'good enough mother' should not preclude the father from playing a significant role; indeed, fathers can also provide the sort of 'maternal' function and good enough parenting that Winnicott describes.

In this state of merged oneness with the mother, the infant is totally dependent. For a separate subjectivity to develop, the infant must move from this state of infantile dependence on the object to a state of mature dependence, where they have a relationship to the object, yet can survive in its absence. Winnicott (1953) emphasised the importance of what he called 'transitional objects' to help the infant move from infantile dependence to mature dependence. A transitional object allows for the fantasised presence of the mother in her absence by standing in for her, thereby allowing the infant to gradually tolerate the disillusionment of mother's periodic absences. For example, a young child may have a favourite teddy bear or blanket that they cannot do without and feel comforted by when mother is not around. Transitional objects are not just a phenomenon of infant life, they can also be a feature of adulthood. For example, a person feels the presence of a deceased loved one by wearing that person's favourite jumper or perfume. Transitional objects allow for the painful, gradual separation with the object and represent the start of symbolic thinking and creative processes.

Winnicott: the development of the true self or false self

Winnicott (1965) was primarily concerned with the quality of subjective experience and the development of personal meaning and sense of self. Winnicott was interested with understanding patients who did not *feel* themselves to be their own person despite being able to function reasonably well enough. He understood there to be an inherent uniqueness and potential with which we are born, that if allowed to develop and flourish, facilitates the development of a sense of a 'true self'. He was concerned with the early years of infancy, where the infant gradually learns to make sense of their own subjectivity, prior to the resolution of the Oedipal complex and triangulated relationships. Winnicott linked the development of the true self to good enough mothering.

Winnicott described the development of the false self when there is an inadequate holding environment that is intrusive or neglectful. Impingement was Winnicott's (1965) term for environmental acts and events that disrupt the infant's and later the child's authentic 'going on being'. Not all impingement is bad. A small amount can be assimilated and lead to ego growth; however, premature and intense impingement causes the infant to become reactive and leads to the formation of the false self. The infant, on learning that the maternal environment does not respond in a way that feels congruent with their internal experience, adapts their behaviour and feelings in response to that environment. For example, a baby whose cries when hurt are met with an angry, hostile response, may eventually stop crying and dull their sense and expression of hurt, in order not to elicit the angry, hostile response from the object. The false self refers to that part of psychosocial functioning that results from accommodating and responding to environmental demands and not one that comes from inner spontaneity. The false self serves a defensive function, a form of protective shield and we can see this in adult patients who adopt a clowning, joker persona for example, or others who are hard-working, pleasing others or overly self-sufficient. Some degree of false self is inevitable and may even be necessary. Too much, however, leads to a life lived only for others. The purpose of the false self is to "search for the conditions in which the true self can come into its own" (Winnicott, 1960, p. 138)

North American developments: a greater focus on the Self

The early years of psychoanalysis in America was dominated by the work of Anna Freud and her focus on the ego and defence. This extended to the work of other post-Freudians, notably Heinz Hartmann (1939), who became interested in the development and functioning of the ego, and understanding the process of healthy development. This led to an increased focus on issues of identity.

Psychoanalysis thrived in North America, particularly since it had a much closer relationship to psychiatry than in the UK. Over the years, this prominence has waned, but there have been many significant practitioners and theorists that have developed psychoanalytic theory in directions that emphasise a more social and relational understanding. Fonagy and Target (2003) usefully distinguish between object-relational and interpersonal-relational psychoanalytic models from North America. While we cannot do justice to all these developments here, we will provide a brief outline of these approaches drawing on Heinz Kohut, Otto Kernberg, Harry Stack Sullivan and Stephen Mitchell as key theorists.

Object-relational models: Kohut and Kernberg

Heinz Kohut (1971; 1977) departed significantly from Freud's drive theory and Freud's approach to psychopathology as arising from intrapsychic conflict between the id, ego and superego. Kohut placed greater emphasis on ego and identity development and understood psychopathology as resulting from the self's experiences of isolation and alienation. Kohut's work forms the foundation of a school of psychotherapy known as Self Psychology.

Kohut was interested in the development and experience of the self; in particular, he was interested in issues of narcissism and disorders of the self. For Kohut, narcissism was not in itself pathological. Classical Freudian theory understood (secondary) narcissism as related to the immature fantasies of omnipotence and grandiosity of early childhood, fantasies which have not been overcome nor challenged as unrealistic. Instead, Kohut viewed these grandiose fantasies as elements of aliveness and creativity, which if supported and encouraged, provide the basis of healthy narcissism. Kohut referred to others (or the objects) in an individual's life as 'self-objects', deriving from the experience of others in infancy as part of the self, rather than as differentiated objects. Self-objects are people, or abstract concepts such as society or culture, that provide the basis from which the individual develops a sense of self. Healthy development of the Self results from experiences with self-objects that provide recognition and affirmation, through experiences of mirroring and idealisation. However, the child will gradually learn for themselves, through everyday disappointment, that their grandiose fantasies are unrealistic, but in the process, they will have developed a sense of self-confidence and enjoyment in themselves that is more realistic. Where parents as self-objects have failed in their empathic mirroring, recognition and affirmation of the child, the child will not develop a sufficiently cohesive sense of self. In psychotherapy, the therapist is understood as acting as a new self-object, and may be sought in the transference to provide the patient with the sort of mirroring or idealisation that they failed to adequately receive. Through this process, the earlier failures are worked through, and gradually a more cohesive self can develop.

Otto Kernberg is one of the more prolific and important contemporary psychoanalytic theorists in North America. His work (1976) has attempted to synthesise the structural model of Freud with the object-relational model of Klein, as well as integrating ideas from developmental or ego psychology. Kernberg (1982) regarded two primary affective states as key features of early life: namely, affective states that are pleasurably and involve gratification; and affective states that are unpleasurable and involve frustration. At first, the infant has a merged experience with their maternal environment, and through a process of development, they begin to differentiate self from object and form internalised representations of both; that is, self-representations and object-representations. These representations are linked by an affective state (pleasurable or unpleasurable; 'good' or 'bad'), forming an object relational unit (self + object + affect), which is internalised. These relational units are then organised as libidinal or aggressive motivational drives. The structures of the id, ego and superego are internalisations of these self- and object-representations and linked affective states. At first the linked affective self- and object-representations are kept separate by the process of splitting. Thus, positive self- and object-representations with linked affective states of pleasure, love, and gratification are experienced as distinct from negative self- and object-representations with linked affective states of frustration and aggression. As the infant develops and begins to experience their objects as whole objects, including both 'good' and 'bad' qualities, so their self-representations also become integrated, with both 'good' and 'bad' aspects. The older infant is able to model the self after objects through their identifications, thus self-representations are flexible and complex. An ego identity develops from these combined internalisations and identifications. These ideas of Kernberg have been applied to the model of Dynamic Interpersonal Therapy and are explained in greater detail in Chapter 11 in relation to the interpersonal and affective focus in DIT.

Interpersonal-relational models: Sullivan and Mitchell

In the past two decades, there has been a growing influence of the relational approach in psychoanalysis, which emphasises the interpersonal and inter-subjective dynamic between self and other (including patient and therapist). Relational psychoanalysis has developed from an integration of British object relational theories and their focus on the internalisation of relationship dynamics, with the interpersonal school of Harry Stack Sullivan (1953) and his stress on the important role played by actual interpersonal interactions.

In the interpersonal model of psychoanalysis, the mother-infant relationship is seen as central to the development of the self and personality. However, unlike the British object relational theories, the internal world of the infant is not regarded as a driving force; rather the interpersonal environment is seen as the determining influence. In this model, the internal world is shaped and determined by the interpersonal context. Affective states such as anxiety are stimulated by the external interpersonal environment, rather than seen as arising from frustrated internal drives or wishes. In this model, psychological needs are not determined biologically (as in Freud's model), but rather by the responses of others to our developing behaviour. This starts in infancy where the biological needs of the infant (such as to eat when hungry) is responded to by the mother with 'maternal empathy' (Sullivan, 1953): she recognises and understands the biological needs of the child as if they were her own. This maternal empathy is experienced as love and tenderness by the baby, which in turn creates a psychological need for love and tenderness. This need is seen as an interpersonal need, not a biological one. The child tends to group interpersonal experiences with the mother as either 'good mother' (tender, loving) or 'bad mother' (anxious, disapproving). Rather than seeing the self as existing in a merged state with the object from which the self has to separate, in the interpersonal model the self develops out of these 'good mother' and 'bad mother' experiences, to form 'good me' and 'bad me' self-representations, based on the responses of the mother/other.

Jay Greenberg and Stephen Mitchell (1983) wrote a synthesis of the various object relational psychoanalytic theories together with the interpersonal theory of Sullivan, to demonstrate a relational/structural model of psychoanalysis, which they differentiated from the drive/structural model of Freud. Their work formed the basis of the contemporary interpersonal-relational psychoanalysis that has a growing influence today. Mitchell criticised psychoanalytic models that emphasised intrapsychic aspects of the individual (Freudian, Object Relations and Self Psychology). For Mitchell (1988), relational experiences are central to psychoanalysis, and include both individual subjectivity and intersubjectivity. In the relational model, the mind or psychic reality of the individual is a relational matrix. For example, according to Mitchell and later relational theorists, sexuality and aggression are not understood as innate biological drives, but rather are seen within a relational context as "powerful vehicles for establishing and maintaining relationship dynamics" (Fonagy and Target, 2003, p. 212).

In a relational approach, the subject matter of psychoanalysis and psychodynamic psychotherapy are the relational bonds and dynamics of the patient. The subjectivity of both self/patient and other/parent/therapist is taken into account as having a mutual influence on each other. In this approach, the therapeutic encounter is co-constructed by the subjectivities of the patient and therapist in relation to each other, creating what Ogden (1994) refers to as 'an analytic third' space. There is not one unconscious mind (the patient's) being observed, but rather two unconscious minds (the patient's and the therapist's) co-constructing a dialogue and relationship. Popular contemporary theorists in the USA include Thomas Ogden and Jessica Benjamin, amongst others. In the UK, Christopher Bollas can be considered to adopt a more relational approach to psychoanalysis.

Related theoretical developments

In addition to the classical and contemporary psychoanalytic theories, there have been offshoots of theoretical developments that apply and extend psychoanalytic concepts and ideas. For example, Cognitive Analytic Therapy is a therapeutic modality developed by Anthony Ryle (1990) in the UK, which attempts to integrate cognitive-behavioural theories with psychodynamic theories. Schema Therapy is another development by Jeffrey Young (1990) that blends elements from cognitive-behavioural, attachment, Gestalt, object relations, constructivist, and psychoanalytic schools into a treatment model designed mostly for patients with diagnoses of personality disorders and characterological difficulties.

We focus here on three avenues of theoretical development which have drawn on or incorporated psychoanalytic ideas: namely attachment theory, mentalisation and neuropsychoanalysis. The first two provide a useful introduction to the brief model of psychodynamic work, Dynamic Interpersonal Therapy (see Chapter 11) and we have expanded on mentalising theory and techniques in Chapter 7. We also provide a brief introduction to neuropsychoanalysis, an exciting new field that is bridging advances in neuroscience and the psychoanalytic model of mind.

Attachment theory

John Bowlby (1969; 1973; 1980) was a British psychiatrist and psychoanalyst who became interested in the emotional bonds between mother and baby, as well as other close interpersonal relationships. Rather than placing importance on the sexual and aggressive drives that underpin the work of Freud and Klein, Bowlby emphasised the view of the infant as inherently object-seeking, in keeping with Winnicott and Fairbairn. Bowlby saw the need to form attachments (i.e. emotional bonds) to others as instinctual and innate. He considered the relationship between mother and baby to be the most powerful relationship in all the animal kingdom. This was the basis of attachment theory, which became a dominant body of work in developmental psychology.

Bowlby's theories were based on his observation of children's reactions to being separated and deprived of parental attachment during the Second World War as a result of evacuations during the Blitz as well as those children who were orphaned following the war. He was also working with children who were hospitalised and institutionalised. Bowlby employed James Robertson to assist with this work and it resulted in his moving 1953 film, *A Two-Year-Old Goes to Hospital* (available on YouTube – the link appears at the end of this chapter). This had a revolutionary impact on the practise of enforced parental separations during periods of childhood hospitalisation and resulted in parents being allowed to stay with their children. Bowlby viewed attachment as involving a series of behaviours that orientate the baby to others and motivate the formation of their emotional bonds. The mother's attuned responsiveness to the infant plays an important part in attaching infants to their mothers. The quality of that attachment can be observed by a system of behaviours, such as being clingy, protesting or distant.

Mary Ainsworth and colleagues (1978) developed an experiment to observe these different types of attachment behaviour patterns, that led to the categorising of attachment behaviour. The 'strange situation' experiment consists of a laboratory-based observation of how a one-year old infant behaves when they are separated and then reunited with the primary caregiver. We have included a link to this in Box 2.1. What is observed in this experiment is the pattern of proximity seeking behaviour that the infant displays when reunited with their caregiver. The caregiver becomes a secure base from which the child can then explore the world safely. Four different displays of behaviour patterns can be observed that map on to the following four attachment styles:

1   *Secure Attachment*: this is demonstrated by the infant being upset by the separation, and when reunited seeking proximity with the caregiver, showing signs of missing them, but then returning to exploration of the environment (e.g. returns to play with toys). In the adult relationship questionnaire developed by Bartholomew and Horowitz (1991), this is described as follows: "It is relatively easy for me to become emotionally close to others. I am comfortable depending on them and having others depend on me. I don't worry about being alone or having others not accept me" (p. 244).

2   *Insecure-Avoidant Attachment*: this is demonstrated by the infant showing little or no distress at the separation, and when reunited they ignore or avoid the caregiver, seemingly unemotional. This has been developed by Bartholomew and Horowitz's (1991) adult attachment styles into Fearful Avoidant and

Dismissive Avoidant attachment styles. The fearful avoidant style in adults is represented by the following statement: "I am somewhat uncomfortable getting close to others. I want emotionally close relationships, but I find it difficult to trust others completely, or to depend on them. I sometimes worry that I will be hurt if I allow myself to become too close to others" (p. 244), while the dismissive avoidant style is characterised by the following statement: "I am comfortable without close emotional relationships. It is very important for me to feel independent and self-sufficient, and I prefer not to depend on others or have others depend on me" (p. 244).

3   *Insecure-Ambivalent or Preoccupied Attachment*: this is demonstrated by the infant being upset by the separation, but when reunited, they both seek some proximity to the caregiver and also resist emotional contact and comfort. They appear to fail to settle upon being reunited, continuing to cry and be upset with the parent. In the adult attachment questionnaire referenced above, this corresponds with the preoccupied style, characterised by the following statement: "I want to be completely emotionally intimate with others, but I often find that others are reluctant to get as close as I would like. I am uncomfortable being without close relationships, but I sometimes worry that others don't value me as much as I value them" (p. 244).

4   *Disorganised Attachment*: this is demonstrated by a disorganised behaviour in the presence of the parent. For example, the infant may freeze when the parent returns to the room, they may rise, as if to approach the parent but then turn away or collapse to the floor. The infant shows signs of fear in approaching the parent, or being in their company, which usually relates to abuse. This is an unusual attachment pattern and usually arises when the parent is both the source of comfort and of danger.

These attachment patterns develop in the first years of life and different patterns will develop in respect of each significant attachment figure. Thus, the attachment style reflects the parents' different sensitivities. The best predictor of secure attachment in a baby is the parent's own secure attachment style. The attachment patterns form what Bowlby referred to as 'internal working models' of relationships that become templates by which we relate to people in adult life and that are in keeping with these attachment patterns. Studies have shown that around two thirds of children in the general population are securely attached to their primary caregiver (Van Ijzendoorn et al., 1999).

Bowlby's work on attachment incorporated ethology, cybernetics, information processing and developmental psychology alongside psychoanalysis. This widening influence, together with his emphasis on observations and real experience rather than the internal world, led to his eschewing psychoanalysis and developing his ideas outside the British Psychoanalytic Society. He fell out of favour as a psychoanalytic theorist, however, in recent years, there has been a resurgence of interest in attachment theory. There is a robust body of research that supports Bowlby and Ainsworth's theories including the attachment styles, adult attachment interviewing technique and internal working models. Later research (e.g. Steele et al., 1996) has called into question the original conceptualisation of attachment patterns as relatively fixed and stable once formed, conceived as being determined primarily by the infant-mother bond. We now know that attachment patterns can shift and change over time, and that individuals have different attachment patterns with different figures.

Mentalisation theory

Fonagy, Target and colleagues (2002) have developed a theory of mentalisation that is centred on the development of affect regulation and reflective capacity. We will discuss mentalisation in more detail in Chapter 7, but it is helpful to provide a brief outline of this theory here. Fonagy et al.'s (2002) theory is informed by an integration of object relations psychoanalytic theory (particularly Winnicott), attachment theory and theory of mind research. Theory of mind refers to the ability of an individual to recognise and reflect on their own mental states and the mental states of others. They suggest that it is not the physical environment that affects development (although it does play a role); rather it is the psychological environment that is most important, namely the way we experience the world through the filter of our mental representations and interpretations.

A key feature of healthy, human development is the capacity to mentalise, which they refer to as "the process by which we realize that having a mind mediates our experience of the world" (p. 3). The ability to mentalise is not inherent; it is learned socially by the individual in early attachment relationships, through the way their mental states are mirrored back to them by significant others. This draws on Winnicott's notion of the holding environment and good enough mothering, as well as attachment theory. The ability to mentalise permits the capacity to reflect on oneself and others, to be able to identify the mental states of self and others, and to appreciate that they are representations of reality that are subject to change. Mentalising refers to the capacity for introspection and self-awareness as well as understanding and empathy for the mental states of others. Mentalising is key for healthy relationships. Poor mentalising is associated with emotional dysregulation, where an individual has difficulty in recognizing their own mental states and that of others, becoming overly certain or vague. It is implicated in various 'personality disorders', violent and self-destructive behaviours and Mentalisation Based Therapy (MBT) was developed particularly to work with patients who have received a diagnosis of Borderline Personality Disorder or Emotionally Unstable Personality Disorder.

How does mentalisation develop? As Winnicott indicated, a child learns to be aware of their own mental state and subjectivity through parental mirroring. According to Winnicott, the baby finds themselves not by looking within but rather by turning outwards towards other people who reflect back a version of the self. Attuned 'affect mirroring' from a parent will reflect the baby's emotional states accurately while also ensuring those states are recognised in a marked, theatrical way, so that the baby recognises that this is their own emotion and not the parent's emotional state. For example, the baby starts to cry and the mother presents 'sadness' in a marked way by her downturned mouth and pouting lip while making sounds that represent sadness, rather than by responding with her own crying and sadness. This allows the baby to link the parent's marked affective display to their own affective state, thereby validating the baby's emotions and sense of self.

Where affective mirroring has not taken place, as a result of childhood trauma or abuse, the ability for mentalisation will not develop, and the child does not have the experience of learning to reflect on both their own and others' mental states and how to make sense of them. In adulthood, such individuals are likely to have problems with mentalisation, especially when stressed, or in the context of significant attachment relationships where interpersonal anxiety throws mentalising off-line. Mentalisation is a useful framework and technique in psychodynamic psychotherapy, whereby the therapist facilitates the patient's ability to develop mentalisation.

Neuropsychoanalysis

Neuropsychoanalysis, although not a separate school of psychoanalysis is worthy of mention here since it is a significant development in psychoanalytic research, attempting to map psychoanalytic theories and concepts with new neuroscientific research methods. It has been spearheaded by Jaak Panksepp, Allan Schore, Antonio Damasio, Joseph LeDoux, Mark Solms, Oliver Turnbull and others. Schore's book *Affect Regulation and the Origin of the Self* (1994), Panksepp's (1998) *Affective Neuroscience*, LeDoux's (1998) *The Emotional Brain: The Mysterious Underpinnings of Emotional Life*, Damasio's (1999) *The Feeling Of What Happens: Body, Emotion and the Making of Consciousness* and Solms and Turnbull's (2002) *The Brain and the Inner World* are important seminal texts in this growing field.

As Solms and Turnbull (2011) point out, while some may view with scepticism the merging of psychoanalysis with neuroscience, this is not a new endeavour. Freud himself began as a neuroscientist, wanting to map his theories of the functioning and structure of the mind with that of the brain, yet he recognised that he did not have the scientific research tools to do so at the time. In psychoanalytic theory, the mind itself is unknowable; that is it can only be inferred or represented by our phenomenological experience of consciousness. In this way, we develop theoretical models about how the mind works based on subjectivity, the defining feature of psychoanalysis. With the emergence of techniques for studying the activity of the brain such as MRI, PET and CAT scans, interest grew in research of psychology and neuroscience (the discipline of neuropsychology and cognitive neuroscience). However, this work has mostly focused on behaviour, cognitive processes, learning and memory. Only recently has there been an emerging interest in using neuroscience to look at affect, another key preoccupation of psychoanalysis.

Psychoanalysis is the most elaborate theory of subjectivity there is. However, Solms and Turnbull (2002; 2011) argue that to rely on subjectivity alone renders psychoanalysis a 'weak' science. Indeed, many critics of psychoanalysis state that it cannot be considered a science at all. Solms and Turnbull contend that psychoanalysis can only be strengthened by using neuroscience to correlate psychoanalytic concepts with brain anatomy. This allows us to study mental apparatus in two different ways: if we look at our mental apparatus with our eyes, we see a brain, and if we look at our mental apparatus through our subjective experience (i.e. introspectively), we observe the mind (Solms and Turnbull, 2011, p. 137).

By way of introduction, Solms (2018, p. 2) outlines three core claims made by psychoanalysis about the emotional mind, for which there is compelling neuroscientific evidence, as follows:

1   We are all born with innate biological needs that are felt as emotional and bodily affects. Solms suggest that these innate needs are what Freud referred to as the drives of the id. However, while Freud theorised that the drives exist at the unconscious level, Solms argues that the felt affects associated with these needs are conscious. Solms outlines that neuroscientific observations suggest the existence of various *emotional* needs (based on Panksepp's research): the need to engage with the world through seeking (felt as curiosity); the need to find sexual partners (felt as lust); the need to escape danger (felt as fear); the need to attack against frustration (felt as anger); the need for attachment; the need to nurture others; and the need to play. We will return to consider these further in Chapter 7 (see Table 7.1). As discussed above, Freud conceptualised two drives: the sexual and aggressive drives. These expanded needs could be mapped on to the drives, and also include the need for attachment, emphasised by attachment theory.

2   The main aim of mental development is to foster methods for meeting these affective needs. These methods are learnt when we establish predictions as to when the needs are met and satiated, and when they are not. When needs are unsatiated, they continue to be affectively felt. This learning involves various types of memory systems, including short-term and long-term memory. Short-term memory is a small resource, only able to hold a small range of five to seven items of information at any one time. Memory that is not required for a specific action is then repressed (thereby becoming unconscious). An unmet need would activate memory traces of unsuccessful attempts to satisfy the need. These are the sorts of functions that Freud considered to be part of the ego.

3   Most of the methods we use to meet our needs occur unconsciously, and so, in order to change them, they have to be brought into consciousness. Because short-term memory is a small, limited resource, the mind is under pressure to consolidate what has been learnt and to make implicit and automatic the various types of methods learned to meet these needs. Thus, these methods start to operate at an unconscious level. There is significant neuroscientific evidence to support the claim that much of our mental life occurs via unconscious processes.

It is beyond the scope of this introductory chapter to outline the many developments and findings in the exciting and emerging field of neuropsychoanalysis. Readers are encouraged to approach Solms and Turnbull's (2002) book as an accessible introductory text to this area, including neuroscientific findings about topics including mental conscious and unconscious processing, dreams, memory and representation.

Thinking about theory and practice

In this chapter, we have outlined a range of key psychoanalytic theories and approaches. There are many others we have not discussed, notably Jung and post-Jungian theorists, French psychoanalysis and many of the American psychoanalytic theorists. For readers who want to expand on their knowledge, we recommend further reading and resources at the end of this chapter. We conclude this chapter by thinking about theory and its links to practice.

Theory in psychodynamic psychotherapy can be regarded as an important, and necessary, 'third' presence (Tuckett, 2011), alongside the patient and therapist. This 'third' presence, includes theories about the mind and development (as outlined above and revisited in other chapters), theories about affective coping and functioning (discussed in Chapter 6 on anxieties and defence as well as Chapter 7 on mentalising), theories about listening and communication (discussed further in Chapter 8 on unconscious communication), and theories about the therapeutic relationship and therapist-patient dynamic (discussed in Chapter 9 with regard to transference and countertransference). Many practitioners align themselves with specific theoretical schools (e.g. Contemporary Freudian or Kleinian) and work strictly within this theoretical framework. Others may take a more pluralistic and integrative approach, drawing on various theoretical schools. There is a diversity of theories, and as we have seen, there has been a shift from a biological, drive model of the human mind, to a more relational, interpersonal model. There are many differences, but what unites these theories as psychoanalytic?

In an attempt to define the foundations of contemporary psychodynamic theory, Fonagy and Target (2003) have suggested the following six propositions and central core ideas that unite all psychodynamic theories:

1   that there exists an unconscious level of our experiences that motivates and drives us towards feeling and acting a certain way;
2   that our early childhood experiences, attachment processes and internal models of relationships impact upon adult functioning;
3   that internal and external processes influence our minds and our perceptions of ourselves in relation to others;
4   that there exists both unconscious projective and introjective processes underpinning our experiences of relationships;
5   that we all experience conflicts that create psychic unpleasure and therefore need to utilise different defence mechanisms in order to protect ourselves from such conflicts and states of unpleasure; and

6   that transference influences the way in which we respond to others, including a psychotherapist and therefore is an important source of clinical information, requiring exploring, challenging and revising.

These propositions and ideas are fundamental to many of the core competences for working as a psychodynamic therapist, particularly having a knowledge and understanding of the basic theoretical principles of a psychodynamic approach and applying the most appropriate psychodynamic approach to the needs of the patient; having an ability to recognise and work with unconscious communication; having an ability to work with a patients internal world as well as external reality; having an ability to recognise and work with different defence mechanisms; and to recognise and work with the transference, and make use of the therapeutic relationship to effect change (Lemma et al., 2008, p. 14).

Box 2.1 Useful resources

Readings

The following books provide an informative overview of the different schools of psychoanalytic theory:

Mitchell, S. A. and Black, M. J. (1995). *Freud and beyond: A history of modern psychoanalytic thought*. New York: Basic Books – this is now dated, but nevertheless provides a very useful and accessible outline of the various important earlier psychoanalytic theoretical schools.

Fonagy, P. and Target, M. (2003). *Psychoanalytic theories: Perspectives from developmental psychopathology*. London: Whurr Publishers – this book provides a comprehensive analysis of the various psychoanalytic theories, and looks specifically at what is said about development and psychopathology.

For readers interested in learning more, we recommend the following introductory text on Jung and Jungian analysis:

Goss, P. (2015). *Jung: A complete introduction*. London: John Murray Learning.

Online resources

British Psychoanalysis Yesterday and Today – this video by the British Institute of Psychoanalysis provides a useful illustration of some of the particularly British developments in psychoanalytic theory: https://vimeo.com/156705216.

The School of Life has a series of helpful introductory film clips that illustrate key psychoanalytic theorists and concepts, including clips on Anna Freud https://youtu.be/v80Nd8w1uts; Melanie Klein https://youtu.be/HU3iSW6WTo8; Donald Winnicott https://youtu.be/ZaZkvvB367I; John Bowlby https://youtu.be/3LM0nE81mIE among other topics.

Robertson's 1958 short film clip of A Two-Year-Old Goes to Hospital can be found at https://youtu.be/s14Q-_Bxc_U

The Strange Situation experiment is illustrated in this YouTube clip: https://youtu.be/QTsewNrHUHU

The Melanie Klein Trust has a helpful theoretical section on their website: www.melanie-klein-trust.org.uk/theory/

Introductory videos on neuropsychoanalysis by Mark Solms are available here: www.therapyroute.com/article/what-is-neuropsychoanalysis-by-m-solms

Introductory video attachment theory and brain development by Dr Alan Schore available on YouTube: https://youtu.be/c0sKY86Qmzo

3 Efficacy and outcome research

In the next chapters of this book, we will outline the various competences of psychodynamic psychotherapy. But before we explore these, an important question to answer for our patients, as well as other mental health professionals, is whether psychodynamic psychotherapy works. We live in a time where there are many different therapeutic approaches that claim to help, even cure, mental health difficulties. In many countries (including the UK), anyone can call themselves a 'psychotherapist' or 'counsellor' and offer consultations to help people experiencing depression or anxiety. Increasingly, emphasis is (mis)placed on 'evidence-based' therapy (Shedler, 2018), namely only offering interventions that have been shown by robust research studies to have an evidence base for reducing symptoms of emotional distress. For psychodynamic therapists working in the public sector as well as in private practice, we need to be able to discuss with confidence whether what we do works, and the mechanisms for that change. In this chapter, we will examine the research evidence for psychodynamic psychotherapy, and how it compares with other therapeutic modalities. In doing so, we will identify the hallmarks of a psychodynamic approach that differentiates it from other therapies, and what types of therapy may work best for particular patients and presenting difficulties. However, it is not enough for psychodynamic therapists to familiarise ourselves with the research findings; it is incumbent on us to practice in ways that reflect and evaluate whether our interventions are working or not, and to base our clinical decisions on those evaluations.

The rise of evidence-based practice

In the UK, USA and many other countries, public mental health services increasingly aim to ensure that the therapeutic interventions offered are *evidence-based*. What is meant by *evidence-based practice*? In short, this means that interventions have been shown to be effective in robust, published research studies. It is not enough for an intervention to be demonstrated as effective in one single research study, but rather that a number of studies have repeatedly shown that the intervention is effective. So, if you offer psychodynamic psychotherapy to people with depression, for example, evidence-based practice means that research has consistently shown that the therapy you offer will help with reducing symptoms of depression.

How does research measure efficacy? Let's continue to use depression as an example. If we wanted to conduct a research study to show that psychodynamic psychotherapy is effective in reducing symptoms of depression, then we need to find a way of measuring the improvement in the severity of depression after therapy. In order to do this, we first need a way to measure depression symptomatology. In research, this is done through the use of standardised questionnaires that ask patients to rate the severity of their symptoms as per the official medical diagnosis of depression published in the American Psychiatric Association's (2013) *Diagnostic and Statistical Manual of Mental Disorders* (the DSM), currently in its 5th edition or alternatively, the World Health Organisation's (1992) *International Classification of Diseases* (ICD), with the 11th edition published in 2019. There are many different questionnaires that can be used to measure depression in this way. In the UK, an outcome measure of low mood that is typically used within the National Health Service (NHS) is the Patient Health Questionnaire (the PHQ-9), which includes nine questions related to depression symptoms (e.g. feeling down, tiredness and low energy, having sleep and appetite disturbances) where patients are asked to rate the severity of each, in terms of frequency of experience, on a scale from 0 to 3. The completed questionnaire is scored, and the overall score indicates whether the patient has no depression, mild, moderate or severe depression. There are obvious critiques to be made of this 'measurement' of depression, including what Dalal (2018) calls the "objectification of subjectivity" (p. 151). This is beyond the scope of our discussion here.

With these measures, we could then conduct a study where patients struggling with depression are given the PHQ-9 to complete before receiving any form of therapy, and then again after finishing a course of therapy. We are interested to see whether their scores on the PHQ-9 improved after the intervention. However, while we might attribute the improvement in scores to the therapy, clearly any number of other things may have happened during the intervening period that may have influenced the scores, such as a change in job resulting in less financial anxiety and improved mood. Research studies have to be conducted in such a way that demonstrates that it is the intervention associated with an improvement in depression, rather than other extraneous or unknown factors.

In medical and psychotherapy research, such research evidence is typically collected through studies known as randomised control trials (or RCTs). In an RCT, a group of patients, all with a similar diagnosis, are indiscriminately allocated into two groups that are matched in terms of demographic characteristics (e.g. age, gender, socio-economic status). One group is provided with an intervention (the treatment group), whilst the other group does not have any treatment (the control group). There needs to be a large enough number of patients in each group for it to have statistical significance (i.e. statistical *power*). Each patient is given a measure at the start and end of the trial period. Scores are compared between each group, and if the treatment group showed an improvement that was not apparent in the control group, then we can conclude that the improvement is owing to the intervention. So, an RCT to measure the efficacy of psychodynamic psychotherapy for depression might resemble what is depicted in Figure 3.1. In this diagram, while Group B (the control group) showed some minor improvement in average PHQ scores

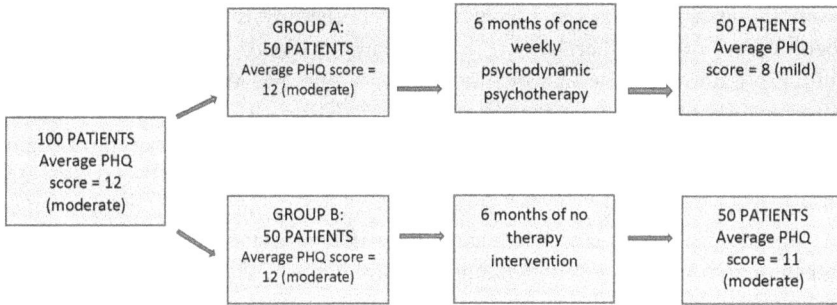

Figure 3.1 A diagrammatic representation of a randomised control trial

over the 6-month trial period, the scores for Group A (the treatment group) showed greater improvement, suggesting that psychodynamic psychotherapy was effective with this group.

We said earlier that it is not enough to show that an intervention worked in one RCT. Evidence-based practice is indicated when an intervention is shown to be effective across a number of RCTs. This is studied through a method known as meta-analysis, which involves collating the results of a number of RCTs and measuring the overall effectiveness for the intervention across the group. This analysis is conducted by measuring the average effect size of the composite studies. The *effect size* refers to the statistical difference between the mean scores of the treatment and control groups, as expressed in standard deviation units, where an effect size of 1.0 refers to the mean for a treatment group being one standard deviation healthier than the mean of the control group. A large effect size would be a score of 0.8, while a medium effect size would be a score of 0.5 and a small effect size a score of 0.2 (Shedler, 2010).

However, such an RCT as depicted in Figure 3.1, does not prove that it is *psychodynamic* psychotherapy in particular that was effective. In this trial, the control group received no intervention, so the improvements shown in the treatment group may have been attributed to the interaction with a psychotherapist. We cannot tell if it is *psychodynamic* psychotherapy in particular that resulted in this improvement. Thus, what we need to know is how treatment in psychodynamic psychotherapy compares to another type of intervention. We are interested to know if (a) psychological therapies work in comparison to psychiatric medication, and (b) whether psychodynamic psychotherapy works in comparison to other approaches such as cognitive-behavioural therapy.

The efficacy of psychodynamic psychotherapy

In 2010, Jonathan Shedler published an important review on the efficacy of psychodynamic psychotherapy in the *American Psychologist* journal. Shedler cites a number of published meta-analyses on different treatments for various mental health problems. He concludes that there is empirical support for psychodynamic psychotherapy, and that psychodynamic psychotherapy is at least as effective as cognitive-behavioural therapy, which has a large evidence base. Shedler quotes a number of studies, some of which appear in Table 3.1. We have included citations of studies that look at the efficacy of psychotherapy in general, the efficacy of anti-depressants and the efficacy of psychodynamic psychotherapy and cognitive behavioural therapy, with each of the respective effect sizes. If you compare the effect sizes measured in the various meta-analysis, you can see that the effect size for psychotherapy is much greater than that of anti-depressant medication, and the effect size for psychodynamic psychotherapy is slightly greater than that for cognitive-behavioural therapy.

There are several caveats that need to be considered, which Shedler flags in his article. First, although the effect size for anti-depressants is small, it does not mean that it is not effective in treating mental health problems such as depression. While the overall effect size is small, medication can be prescribed to a much larger number of people than psychotherapy can reach, and thus it is likely to benefit a larger number of people, on average. Shedler also discusses a number of methodological issues which make it difficult to derive generalisations from these meta-analyses. Often, there is no real 'like for like' comparison of the delivery of therapy and the mental health problem measured. He also observes that many studies rely on highly selective samples. It should be noted that there are many more studies on the efficacy of CBT, with far fewer on psychodynamic psychotherapy. Dalal (2018) details substantive criticisms about the science behind such efficacy studies. He discusses this in relation to CBT efficacy research, but they apply equally to all efficacy research. Leaving aside these criticisms, if we consider the research evidence (perhaps with a pinch of salt), Shedler argues that at the very least we can conclude that psychodynamic psychotherapy is as effective as cognitive-behavioural therapy.

Table 3.1 Comparisons of meta-analysis studies on treatment effectiveness

Research	Studies looked at	Overall effect size
Efficacy of psychotherapy generally		
Smith et al., 1980	475 individual studies	0.85
Lipsey and Wilson, 1993	18 meta-analyses	0.75
Robinson et al., 1990	37 studies for depression	0.73
Efficacy of anti-depressant medication		
Turner et al., 2008	Studies of anti-depressants	0.31
Moncrieff et al., 2004	Meta-analyses of studies on anti-depressants	0.17
Efficacy of psychodynamic psychotherapy vs cognitive-behavioural therapy		
Abbass et al., 2006	23 RCTs of psychodynamic psychotherapy vs 'treatment as usual'	0.97
Haby et al., 2006	33 studies of CBT vs 'treatment as usual'	0.68

Where things become more promising and significant for the efficacy of psychodynamic psychotherapy, is the emergence of research that demonstrates the superior lasting effects of psychodynamic psychotherapy, particularly longer-term psychodynamic psychotherapy, as compared to other forms of treatment. A meta-analysis (Abbass et al., 2006) of 23 RCTs of 1431 patients showed that the effect of short-term psychodynamic psychotherapy compared to 'treatment as usual' was 0.97, and at long-term follow up, this effect size increased. Similar increases in effect sizes for psychodynamic psychotherapy at long-term follow up were found by other studies (cited in Shedler, 2010). These findings suggest that psychodynamic psychotherapy "sets in motion psychological processes that lead to on-going change, even after therapy has ended" (Shedler, 2010, p. 101). This is sometimes referred to as the 'sleeper effect', when the improvements following long-term psychodynamic psychotherapy only emerge several years after the conclusion of treatment, as compared to CBT, as we will see below.

Since Shedler's review paper, two further reviews summarised the growing evidence of psychodynamic therapies for various DSM-classified mental health 'disorders' (Fonagy, 2015; Leichsenring and Klein, 2014), and both concluded that psychodynamic therapies have been found to be effective for the treatment of depression, social anxiety, generalised anxiety and panic disorders, anorexia, somatic disorders, and personality disorders, but are not effective for post-traumatic stress disorder, obsessive compulsive disorder, bulimia, and drug dependence and in the longer term for psychosis.

In 2015, the first UK randomised-control trial study for long-term psycho-analytic psychotherapy for treatment-resistant depression carried out at the Tavistock Clinic was published (Fonagy et al., 2015). The study compared 67 patients who received long-term psychoanalytic psychotherapy (60 once-weekly sessions delivered over 18 months by experienced psychoanalytically trained practitioners) with 62 patients receiving 'treatment as usual' over the same period. Treatment as usual consisted of various interventions provided to the patient by the referring practitioner, and included counselling, CBT or medication. It is worth noting that this patient group was made up of chronically depressed patients who had all had failed previous courses of treatment for depression such as CBT and medication. The patients were assessed for symptoms of depression at the start of treatment, then at six-months intervals at 6, 12 and 18 months as well as at 24, 30 and 42 months follow up. Results indicate that psychoanalytic psychotherapy was as effective as treatment as usual by the end of the 18-month treatment phase, but the impact of psychoanalytic therapy was significantly more enduring, with 30% remission rate at 42 months for psychoanalytic therapy, compared to only 4.4% for the control group. Those patients who received psychoanalytic psychotherapy also showed greater improvements in measures of social adjustment at 42 months' follow up as compared to the control group (i.e. evidence of the sleeper effect).

Most recently in 2019, findings from the first randomised control trial for Dynamic Interpersonal Therapy (DIT), a brief-term psychodynamic psychotherapy were published (Fonagy et al., 2019). The study compared outcomes for patients who had received DIT for moderate to severe depression (n = 147) with patients who had received low-intensity treatment (which comprised guided self-help based on CBT principles). The analysis of outcomes data indicated that 51% of DIT patients showed clinically significant reduction in their symptoms of depression. This outcome was superior to those patients who had received low-intensity treatment (9% of patients) and equivalent to CBT patient outcomes in IAPT. An audit of clinical outcomes of DIT provision at a specialist NHS psychotherapy service at tertiary level, for patients with more severe levels of depression and complex mental health needs, suggests that DIT may be effective (Douglas et al., 2016).

As mentioned earlier, there is a paucity of published research on the efficacy of psychodynamic psychotherapy – particularly long-term psychodynamic psychotherapy – as compared to other forms of treatment like psychotropic medication or CBT. However, this recent research provides a strong and growing evidence base that psychodynamic psychotherapy does work, particularly for depression, anxiety and personality disorders. However, Shedler (2010) alerts us to an important caveat in that the label of 'psychodynamic psychotherapy' or 'cognitive-behavioural therapy' is used in this research as if representing something comparable across different therapists. There are variances in how therapists practise. So, how do we know if it is the theoretical underpinnings of different therapies that work in these studies, or not? Or is it the experience of being with a therapist, regardless of their theoretical modality, that benefits patients?

The 'active ingredients' of therapy

To examine what therapists actually do in therapy sessions, Jones (2000) and Ablon and Jones (1998) developed a method of analysing therapy sessions called the Psychotherapy Process Q-Sort (PQS). The Q-Sort consists of 100 statements, representing specific variables that assess the therapist's technique and the therapy process. It includes variables related to different behaviours, actions and verbal comments that a therapist can make. Ablon and Jones (1998) conducted a study using the PQS on hundreds of hours of recorded psychodynamic and CBT therapy sessions. They asked an expert panel of CBT and psychodynamic therapists to construct a prototype of a typical, ideal CBT and psychodynamic psychotherapy session. These are presented in Box 3.1.

Box 3.1 The 'active ingredients' of psychodynamic psychotherapy vs CBT (Shedler, 2010, pp. 103–104)

Prototype for psychodynamic psychotherapy described as:

- an unstructured approach using open-ended dialogue
- identifying recurring patterns in the patient's experience
- drawing attention to patient's emotions that the patient may find unacceptable (e.g. anger or envy)
- observing defensive behaviours

- linking the patient's emotions and current perceptions to experiences of the past
- interpreting avoided or unconscious thoughts, wishes, or feelings
- focusing on the therapy relationship, and drawing connections between the therapy relationship and other relationships

Prototype for CBT described as:

- a more structured approached with a more focused dialogue
- discussing and setting treatment goals with the patient
- the therapist being more didactic and teacherly in their manner
- explicitly explaining the treatment rationale and techniques
- the therapist offering advice or guidance
- maintaining a focus on current difficulties
- focusing on cognitions (thoughts and beliefs)
- use of 'homework' tasks and activities for patients to do between sessions

In Albon and Jones' (1998) study, 'blind' raters (i.e. raters who were not familiar with the type of therapy offered in sessions) then rated recorded therapy sessions using the Q-Sort and each session was evaluated in terms of containing psychodynamic and/or CBT prototypical techniques. In this approach, a CBT session could be found to contain psychodynamic prototypical techniques and vice versa. The analysis of the results indicated that therapists' adherence to psychodynamic prototypical techniques predicted successful therapy outcomes in *both* psychodynamic and CBT treatments, whereas therapists' adherence to CBT prototypical techniques predicted little or no relation to outcome in both psychodynamic or CBT sessions.

In another study, Castonguay and colleagues (1996) measured three variables against outcome success in randomly selected therapy transcripts of 64 patients. The three variables were: the quality of the working/therapeutic alliance; implementation of the cognitive model (e.g. challenging dysfunctional cognitions); and a focus on the patient's 'experiencing', including emotions and thoughts about the self as well as "*previously implicit feelings and meanings*" (Castonguay et al., 1996, p. 499). The last variable has an obvious link to a psychodynamic approach, while the first variable – therapeutic alliance – has its roots in a psychoanalytic approach although now is recognised as a common 'ingredient' of all types of therapy. Their findings show that adherence to the cognitive model variable predicted poorer outcomes, compared to the therapeutic alliance and focus on experiencing, which both predicted good outcomes.

As Shedler (2010) notes, these findings do not suggest that CBT techniques are harmful. There are plenty of RCTs that indicate that CBT is effective. Rather, what they show is that the more effective therapists (including CBT therapists) practise techniques that can be considered prototypically psychodynamic (e.g. focus on feelings, the patient's subjective and interpersonal experience, and the therapeutic relationship).

Research on patient experience of therapy

While randomised control trials and the abovementioned studies tell us something about the effectiveness of psychodynamic psychotherapy and how that compares favourably to other interventions, they tell us little about what patients themselves find beneficial about psychodynamic psychotherapy. Qualitative research provides additional, useful forms of evidence for the effectiveness of psychodynamic psychotherapy.

Binder et al. (2010) conducted a qualitative interview study involving ten former psychotherapy patients in Norway who were asked what they considered to be good outcomes of psychotherapy. The participants did not explicitly name the types of therapy received, although three described their therapy as clearly psychoanalytic. The interview transcripts were analysed and four themes were identified that depict the patients' view of a good therapeutic outcome, namely: developing new, improved ways of relating to others; a change in patterns of behaviour that resulted in less symptoms of distress; greater insight and improved self-understanding; and being able to accept and value oneself. This study concluded that although reduction in distress was reported as a significant positive outcome, personal growth in the form of greater insight and improved interpersonal experiences was regarded as a key constructive outcome.

Binder et al.'s study is interesting because it explores what patients themselves consider to be good outcomes, rather than the typical RCT studies that predetermine good outcomes to equate with symptom reduction. It gives an indication of what could be important for patients, rather than what is determined to be important by therapists or public health services. The study did not look at patients' experiences of psychodynamic psychotherapy specifically, however, all of the perceived good outcomes reported in the study are relevant for psychodynamic psychotherapy with its distinctive focus on emotions, patterns of relating, insight and self-understanding.

An interesting study by Nilsson and colleagues (2007) from Sweden compared the reported experiences of satisfaction and dissatisfaction of a more or less equal sample of patients who had undergone CBT and patients who had received psychodynamic psychotherapy. While the quantitative levels of reported satisfaction and dissatisfaction for both groups were similar, they observed notable differences in the quality of satisfaction and dissatisfaction. Both groups of patients described feeling satisfied that their perceived levels of anxiety were lessened as well as feeling more emotionally stable. However, patients who had completed CBT related feeling satisfied that they had gained skills and techniques to help them better cope with specific problems, whereas patients who had received psychodynamic psychotherapy reported feeling satisfied as a result of becoming more self-reflective and observing wider changes to their personality. Where dissatisfaction was reported, it was related to unhappiness with the therapist: dissatisfied CBT patients experienced their therapists as rigid and intrusive and feeling overly restricted; while dissatisfied psychodynamic psychotherapy patients experienced their therapists as too aloof, withdrawn and disengaged, leaving them feeling on their own.

In the UK, Leonidaki, Lemma and Hobbis (2016; 2018) published a qualitative interview study with a small sample (five patients) who had completed a course of Dynamic Interpersonal Therapy. They analysed patients' experience of DIT and found that this brief psychodynamic therapy helped them feel more empowered to attend and respond to their own needs, increasingly able to reach out for help and support as well as unblock interpersonal obstacles, thereby enriching their relationships and lifestyle. The patients also reported an increase in insight and understanding of their interpersonal difficulties, and aspects of their self-experience previously shut off to them, which enabled them to formulate a more coherent narrative about themselves and their life story. Of course, we do need to note that this was based on a very small sample, but it does provide some useful pointers to what patients themselves might find useful about DIT.

Distinctive features of psychodynamic psychotherapy

Many therapists are not comfortable with the language of research. Many do not enter the profession because of a stated scientific interest in their practice, rather they have an empathic curiosity about human behaviour and a wish to help patients with their distress. Therapists tend to be more interested in what happens *in* the room, between the patient and themselves. Some of you may be less interested in the statistical and research-based discussions included in this chapter. However, it is important to know what research has to say about our practice. Psychoanalytic teaching methods seldom include the evidence base for the theories presented. In turn, psychodynamic practitioners tend to be unaware of the research base for our profession, and this leaves them unqualified to defend their therapeutic practice, not only to other professionals but also to potential patients who are grappling with which type of therapist and approach will help them.

It is useful to know that psychodynamic psychotherapy has an evidence base. Now that we have identified the 'active ingredients' of therapy, it is important to distinguish the distinctive features of psychodynamic psychotherapy as compared to other forms of therapy. Blagys and Hilsenroth (2000) identified seven core characteristics of psychodynamic psychotherapy that differentiate it from other forms of therapy (usefully summarised by Shedler, 2010). They compiled these characteristics after careful analysis of hundreds of hours of transcripts of recorded therapy sessions. The following seven factors are distinct to psychodynamic psychotherapy:

1 Psychodynamic psychotherapy focuses on affect and the expression of emotion. Now at first reading, this may seem like an odd distinctive characteristic, because aren't all therapies concerned with how people feel? On one level yes, but psychodynamic psychotherapy focuses on affect and feelings at a deeper, more sustained level than other therapies do. Cognitive-behavioural therapy, as the name suggest, focuses much more on thoughts and behaviours and how these in turn influence our mood. In CBT, feelings are described in generalised terms, like feeling 'down', 'upset', 'sad', 'anxious',

and so on. A psychodynamic therapist typically wants to know more about what 'upset' or 'anxious' means to the patient; we work at a deeper level of affective experience. We will explore some of this in greater detail in Chapter 7 when considering mentalising and affect regulation as well as in Chapter 8 when looking at forms of unconscious communication. What is important in a psychodynamic approach is to help the patient develop *emotional* rather than intellectual insight.

2   Psychodynamic psychotherapy explores attempts to avoid distressing feelings or thoughts. As we will elaborate in Chapter 6, we make use of defence mechanisms to protect ('defend') ourselves against consciously experiencing distressing memories, thoughts and feelings. In psychodynamic psychotherapy we aim to understand these defences and the purpose they serve so that what is being avoided can be worked through, rather than continually repressed or enacted.

3   Psychodynamic psychotherapy aims to identify recurring themes and patterns of behaviour and experience. As Freud (1914a) observed, we have a compulsion to repeat our traumas and difficulties in an effort to master them. However, typically we are not consciously aware of these repeated patterns of relating, behaving or thinking that we fall into. Psychodynamic psychotherapy aims to identify these unhelpful patterns and to understand them. Typically, this happens in the transference (as discussed in Chapter 9).

4   Psychodynamic psychotherapy has a developmental focus, with discussion of past experiences. As we learned in Chapter 2, much of our adult interpersonal experience and individual functioning has its roots in childhood experiences. In psychodynamic psychotherapy, we actively explore the past, particularly early attachment relationships, in order to better understand and gain insight into a patient's current experiences, including through understanding the transference. We cannot undo the past, however, by helping patients free themselves from the shadow of the past, they can be released to live more unencumbered lives in the present.

5   Psychodynamic psychotherapy focuses on interpersonal relationships. Most of psychoanalytic theory (particularly object relations theory) concentrates on the patient's experience of relationships and their interpersonal context. Difficulties are understood as primarily linked to interpersonal dynamics, i.e. how the patient relates to others and the role the patient plays in interpersonal dynamics. Identifying and exploring recurring interpersonal patterns of relating is a core focus in Dynamic Interpersonal Therapy (see Chapter 11).

6   Psychodynamic psychotherapy focuses on the therapeutic relationship. A crucial feature of psychodynamic psychotherapy is the exploration of the interpersonal dynamic between patient and therapist. This involves more than just developing a working alliance. Rather, it includes particular ways in which the patient relates to the therapist that echo repeated patterns of relating found in other, earlier relationships, namely the transference. The therapeutic relationship provides a live example of the patient's embedded past relationship experiences. This is discovered through working with transference and countertransference (to be discussed in Chapter 9).

7   Psychodynamic psychotherapy involves the exploration of fantasy life. Psychodynamic psychotherapy uses an unstructured, open-dialogue approach in order to encourage the patient to speak freely about whatever is on their mind, including thoughts, feelings, wishes, dreams, desires and fantasies. It encourages the exploration of unconscious communications (to be discussed in Chapter 8). This gives fresh insight into the patient's experiences and meanings.

Reflecting on these distinctive features of psychodynamic psychotherapy, we can see that the overall aim in psychodynamic psychotherapy is not relieving of symptoms per se (which one might say is the goal of CBT). Rather, psychodynamic psychotherapy endeavours to free the patient from the constraints, fears, defences and inhibitions that prevent them from living a more creative and meaningful life. It provides them with the insight and psychological strength to make better use of their resources and have more satisfying relationships. Using Freud's model of the mind, we can say that psychodynamic psychotherapy aims to help the patient develop a less constricted id (by freeing up desires and urges), to experience a more humane super-ego (with the lessening of more punitive standards), and to develop a stronger, expanded ego capacity. We will return to these considerations when thinking about assessment for suitability for psychotherapy in Chapter 5.

Neuroscientific evidence for the benefits of psychotherapy

In the previous chapter, we provided a brief introduction to neuropsychoanalysis and the increased dialogue between neuroscience and psychoanalytic theory. Neuroscientific research has provided support for key psychoanalytic principles, such as the prevalence of unconscious processes and the existence of innate biological needs. Neuroscience has also been utilised to examine the biological effects of therapies. Most notably, this has been in the area of psychiatry and psychiatric medication. However, recent neuroscientific research has been conducted to investigate the possible biological benefits of talking therapies, including CBT and psychodynamic psychotherapy (see Karlsson, 2011).

Neuroscientific research has demonstrated that the brain has a degree of plasticity; that is the chemistry of the brain is able to change in response to environmental influences, whether these are stressors or nurturing experiences (Gabbard, 2000). Some studies have begun to show that psychotherapy (CBT or psychodynamic psychotherapy) alone (i.e. without the combined use of psychiatric medication) can have beneficial effects on the chemistry of the brain. For example, Gabbard cites studies that suggest that psychodynamic psychotherapy and CBT result in chemical changes to the neurotransmitters of the brain leading to reduced symptoms of depression and improvements in mood. Neuroscientific studies have also demonstrated how learning affects neural plasticity. Thus, the learning that occurs in a psychotherapy session – through increased insight, memory and associations – leads to changes in neural functioning in the brain (Beutel et al., 2003). More studies have been conducted on the neurological benefits of CBT, while studies comparing patients undergoing psychodynamic psychotherapy compared to a control group have shown similar improvements in neurological functioning for treating anxiety (Beutel et al., 2010).

As mentioned in Chapter 2, neuropsychoanalysis is a new, emerging field of study. The research is still in its infancy, but there are some exciting suggestions and implications for psychodynamic theory and therapy. Some readers may be uncomfortable by the links to biological models of distress, instead considering this to belong to the terrain of psychiatry. While Freud attempted to ground his theories in biological explanations, psychoanalytic theory has moved further away from the biological model towards an interpersonal-social model, linking the causes of distress to experiences such as early trauma, loss and interpersonal conflicts. However, as the studies on the neuroscientific research on the impact of trauma and the benefits of psychotherapy demonstrate, the interpersonal and social factors have an impact on biology.

Working with outcome measures

If you are working in a public mental health care setting, such as the NHS, you are probably expected to use sessional outcome measures as part of your psychotherapy practice. Some health insurers also require some kind of outcome measure to indicate the severity of the patient's difficulties. Typically, outcome measures have not been a part of private practice and have been seen as interfering with the analytic setting. However, some practitioners are starting to use them, particularly when offering brief psychodynamic therapy. As mentioned previously, in primary health care in the UK, the Patient Health Questionnaire (or PHQ-9) is commonly used to measure depression, and the Generalised Anxiety Disorder scale (or GAD-7) for anxiety. Usually, patients are invited to complete the measures at the start of every session. Over the course of therapy, the clinician will track changes in the scores, with a reduction in the scores usually seen as evidence of the effectiveness of therapy. Increasingly in secondary health care in the UK, psychotherapy departments and personality disorder services employ a range of outcome measures to establish the evidence base for their work and justify the continued existence of these services, for example by measuring the number of hospital admissions or medical doctor (referred to as the GP or general practitioner in the UK) visits with patients diagnosed with Borderline Personality Disorder; or by administering the 34 question CORE-OM (Clinical Outcomes in Routine Evaluation – Outcome Measure) at the start and end of psychotherapy, as well as occasionally mid-treatment.

A psychodynamic therapist may well ask why these measures would be used if the aim of psychodynamic psychotherapy is not symptom reduction per se, but rather understanding and working through experience and patterns of relating? Some claim that the use of outcome measures in psychodynamic work muddies the analytic setting. However, one of the distinctive features of psychodynamic psychotherapy (as discussed above) is a focus on emotions and linking emotions to past and present experience as well as patterns of relating and behaving. The therapist can usefully work with these measures to help the patient see links between their interpersonal experiences and their emotions; in this way, as interpersonal dynamics improve over time, so mood will also improve. It can convey the impact of the 'work' of psychotherapy on the patient's life. Sometimes, it is possible to use measures that are better suited to the hoped-for outcomes of psychodynamic psychotherapy, like the Schwartz Outcome Scale which is a measure of well-being rather than ill-health, as well as the Inventory of Interpersonal Problems that measures the extent of interpersonal difficulties. There are also specialised scales to evaluate group therapy interventions as well as the Reflective Functioning scale that was developed by Fonagy et al. (2016) in order to capture the dimensions of mentalising.

Rather than see the measures as intrusions, it is important to reflect psychodynamically on the measures as sources of information and springboards for discussion in therapy. It would be unhelpful to invite the patient to complete the measures, and then not make any comments on it. In a psychodynamic approach, the measures represent an important communication to the therapist and often include information about risk that may not otherwise come to light in the course of the work. It is useful to make links between the reported scores and the intervening events from the previous session. In brief psychodynamic therapy, this is particularly useful as a way of maintaining a here-and-now interpersonal focus. The therapist may observe: "I see your scores have gone down this past week. What do you think has contributed to this?" Or the therapist may make a connection between an interpersonal dynamic that the patients goes on to discuss and a change in the sessional measures, such as: "You have been talking about how your boyfriend's response left you feeling insecure and uncertain. I wonder if this might explain your increased anxiety over the past week, as indicated by your scores?"

How the patient completes the outcome measures can also be considered a form of communication to the therapist. Does the patient score at the high end of the measures, suggesting a possible negative transference? Or is the patient's sudden improvement in their scores a manic flight to health that defends against approaching anything painful by appearing to be much better. The patient may also have an unconscious investment in maintaining certain scores, believing this to be the only way they can stay in the mind of their objects. These all become avenues to explore what the patient may be expressing interpersonally and intrapsychically when we approach the outcomes measures from a psychodynamic perspective. The therapist should also consider issues of timing when interpreting the outcome measures. It is often the case that scores worsen slightly when the patient and therapist are approaching a break as well as the ending of therapy, since anxieties about dependency and separation are often activated. You may want to give the final outcome measures as you approach the ending rather than in the final session for this reason.

The use of outcomes measures in your work will depend on your work context and the organisational requirements. If you are working in private practice, you will need to consider your reasons for choosing to use outcome measures, for example, does the medical aid require an objective evaluation of the extent of the patient's difficulties? It is important to have a clear rationale as well as a vested interest in its usefulness. Doing something as a token gesture or as a 'tick box' exercise is never useful. You may want to adopt different practices with different patients. In our private practices, we have used outcome measures mostly when working in the DIT model of brief therapy but we don't used questionnaires when working in longer-term and open-ended psychotherapy.

Box 3.2 Useful resources

Readings

Jonathan Shedler has written an accessible article about the effectiveness of psychodynamic psychotherapy, intended for a non-academic audience in the November/December 2010 edition of Scientific American Mind. The article is available from his personal website here: https://jonathanshedler.com/PDFs/Shedler%20Scientific%20American.pdf

Shedler has also written an accessible introduction to contemporary psychodynamic psychotherapy practice, available from his personal website here: https://jonathanshedler.com/PDFs/Shedler%20(2006)%20That%20was%20then,%20this%20is%20now%20R9.pdf

These are useful readings for those new to psychodynamic psychotherapy, or as information for patients:

Karlsson, H. (2011). How psychotherapy changes the brain. *Psychiatric Times*, *28*(8), 1–5.

Online resources

There is a recorded lecture on evidence-based psychotherapy by Jonathan Shedler on YouTube: www.youtube.com/watch?v=3UpHl9kuccc

There is an interview with Nancy McWilliams about the evidence base for psychotherapy and the challenges in research on YouTube: https://youtu.be/ptvbUjjdJ8E

Part 2

Competences

4 The setting and the analytic frame

The therapeutic encounter is an unusual type of relationship. Some patients may find it strange that we refer to it as a 'relationship' – yet there is an emotional connection between patient and therapist. It is a strange relationship because as many patients observe, it is a one-way relationship where the patient is invited – even encouraged – to share their most private thoughts and feelings as well as their unexpressed fears and desires. The therapist's role is to listen and abstain from sharing in turn. It is a relationship like no other, and it invites the patient to be vulnerable in the presence of a so-called stranger (for over time, the therapist becomes a very significant person yet one who remains a rather shadowy figure). As we discussed in the opening chapter with reference to our use of the term 'patient', this inevitably results in a power dynamic that needs to be understood and respected. Like any other relationship between parent and child or between close friends, the dynamics and form of relating are framed by a set of rules and customs. This framework for the therapeutic relationship is referred to as the *analytic frame*.

The ability to establish and maintain a therapeutic or analytic frame is one of the basic competences for working as a psychodynamic therapist. However, at a more fundamental level, the ability to maintain an analytic attitude is the backdrop against which all the various activities of psychodynamic psychotherapy outlined in this book are carried out. The defined competences state:

> Activities in all domains of psychoanalytic/psychodynamic therapy competence need to be carried out in the context of an overarching metacompetence: the ability to approach all aspects of the interaction with the client, and of the management of the therapeutic setting, with an 'analytic attitude'. (Lemma et al., 2008, p. 16)

Why is this so important that we have dedicated an entire chapter to this topic? The analytic frame within which the therapeutic relationship takes place is not only essential in terms of professional standards and conduct in creating a safe container for both patient and therapist, but it is also fundamental to facilitating psychic change. The aims of psychodynamic psychotherapy are to explore the unconscious aspects of our interpersonal life and to bring unconscious conflicts into awareness so that we may be less restricted by our anxieties and fears, unexpressed wishes and desires. A useful and simple way of conceptualising this is by applying Freud's structural model of the mind, whereby we can conceptualise the aim of psychodynamic psychotherapy as facilitating the development of a less constricted Id alongside a more humane and less punitive Superego, which in turn allows for the development of a stronger, freer Ego. This can be a long-term aim, or it can serve as a guiding goal for short-term work that is focused on a particular central issue.

One avenue in which we are able to explore and work through these dynamics of the patients' interpersonal life is within the therapeutic relationship, where these dynamics are likely to be re-experienced in the transference and counter-transference (see Chapter 9). In order to facilitate this happening, we have to create a particular therapeutic environment of safety and trust (the therapeutic alliance) whereby the patient can become vulnerable, and express their authentic feelings and thoughts without punitive consequences or external judgment. A useful theoretical framework for this is Winnicott's (1960) concept of the *holding environment* provided by the parent for the infant and child. A 'good enough' mother is one that is able to provide an environment where the infant and child feels emotionally held and responded to in a way that allows for their sense of self to emerge with minimal impingements, so that they can develop a secure and confident sense of self and realise their true potential within the parameters of society. This is a useful framework for thinking about the analytic frame as a holding environment where the therapist responds to the patient in a facilitative manner. Of course, this is not to say that the therapeutic relationship is identical to that of a parent and child one, but the analogy is useful. In psychoanalysis or psychoanalytic psychotherapy where the patient is coming for three to five sessions a week over an extended period of time, this is a more pertinent analogy, because such intensive treatment involves a degree of regression to early childhood experiences and is more likely to introduce the dynamics of the parent–child relationship into the consulting room. Psychodynamic psychotherapy is at a lower intensity and should involve fewer regressive aspects. Notwithstanding this, we continue to focus on the way childhood experiences impact or inform current interpersonal experiences, so some form of emotional regression is unavoidable.

So how do we establish and maintain an analytic frame? In this chapter, we discuss the various aspects of the analytic frame, focusing on characteristics of the external setting, and thereafter the core qualities of the analytic attitude (i.e. the therapist's internal setting). It is important to note that these are guiding principles, not absolute rules. Ultimately, there must be a degree of flexibility depending on the realities of the patient and therapist as well as the place of work. In this chapter we consider some differences between working privately versus in public health systems and larger organisational settings. Some psychoanalysts and psychotherapists have been known to stick so rigidly to the 'rules of engagement', that their manner can feel quite alarming or alienating for patients unfamiliar with these expectations. We will return to considering the analytic frame in relation to Winnicott and the 'good enough' therapist who responds to the unique needs of each patient. In this chapter, we have outlined a range of issues to consider, many of which will be elaborated in subsequent chapters including Chapter 12 on challenging situations that confront the analytic frame. This chapter will also consider the professional responsibility of maintaining competences through continuing professional development (CPD) activities and supervision, as well as the need for the therapist to reflect on their own self-care. These are important professional components of maintaining an effective analytic frame.

The setting

The setting refers to the practical arrangements and physical environment in which the therapeutic encounter takes place. This is the physical holding environment, and within it there are various aspects to consider.

Contracting

The therapeutic relationship is a professional relationship that increasingly needs to be defined by the boundaries of a contract in today's world of boundary violations and data protection. Contracting will be discussed further in Chapter 5 in the context of assessment and agreement about a way forward. Here, we want to consider the contract as a core component of the analytic frame.

A clear contract should be discussed for all forms of consultation, including initial consultations and assessments as well as psychotherapy sessions. With an initial consultation, it is important to be clear about what this will involve, how long it will take and to address the goals and expectations around assessment, including issues of confidentiality. It may also be useful for the therapist to convey to the patient a sense of the different forms of therapy available and to articulate how and why psychodynamic psychotherapy would benefit them (as discussed in the previous chapter). If, following this consultation process, you decide to offer the patient a vacancy with you, it is important to have a clear contract in place going forward. The therapist needs to explain what this form of therapy typically involves, how long it is likely to last, what can and cannot be addressed in therapy, and the rules around the contact such as fees, payment, holiday breaks and managing cancellations (see below). In the era of social media, smart phones and increased digital presence, it is important to clarify rules around forms of communication, data protection and privacy (see Chapter 14). Some therapists find it useful to give patients a 'terms and conditions' document when contracting for therapy, outlining some of the basic arrangements for working together. We have included an example of this in Appendix 1 of this book.

The contract also extends to the role and responsibilities of the patient in therapy. The therapist should encourage the patient to bring whatever is on their mind, including their dreams and to associate freely to dreams, memories and feelings. It should be made clear that the therapists' input is less structured and directive than would otherwise be expected in CBT, for example. Many patients may expect some sort of question-answer format in which they are prompted by the therapist, and while the initial consultation should aim to give the patient some sense of the analytic frame, during the assessment invariably the therapist may be more active in asking questions than normal. Thus, we should help orient the patient from the outset as to what is expected of them once therapy sessions begin. Bollas (2009) goes further by suggesting that the therapist helps the patient develop this capacity to speak freely of the daily 'quotidian', by which he means the moment-by-moment minutiae of our life, thereby allowing the unconscious processes of the mind to reveal themselves. After all, the injunction to 'free associate' will invariably be met by resistance and some clinicians do not instruct the patient to do so, as a result.

Physical space

Therapy cannot take place anywhere. A particular kind of physical space is needed. The primary consideration is that the space is quiet and confidential. The space should be one where there are minimal disruptions from outside noise and inter- ruptions from other people. This may seem obvious but in reality, this can be quite difficult to ensure, particularly when you are working in public health systems or bustling cities. The therapist cannot always be in control of the environment, and the multiple noises of a busy public health service will always be present. Working in private, whether in a consulting room at home or elsewhere, does not ensure the space will be quiet either. There will always be noises coming in from outside: traffic, people shouting unexpectedly, nearby construction work, children playing, dogs barking, to name just a few. One of us had a consulting room in a practice where different types of therapists worked. In the adjoining consulting room, a Body Psychotherapist at times made use of techniques that resulted in loud bang- ing. It did not happen often, but when it did, it was very disruptive.

The therapist would want to ensure there are no interruptions from other people. You don't want someone bursting into the room in the middle of a session. A system of having an 'occupied/vacant' sign on the door helps avoid this but is no guarantee. We have both worked in busy public health services with real pressure on rooms and multiple part-time honorary therapists, where occasionally someone has mistakenly interrupted a session when looking for a room. In our experience, it is often the therapist who is left more disturbed by the intrusion than the patient. One of us was based in a busy, poorly resourced community medical clinic, which included a mental health service. During one session, a nurse walked into the room, looking for a file. Alarmed, the therapist pointed out that there was a confidential session going on. The nurse replied that she would be quick and persisted in retrieving the file from a filing cabinet. Meanwhile, the patient continued to talk to the therapist while the nurse was in the room, seemingly unperturbed by the interruption.

It is useful to bear in mind Winnicott's enumeration of Freud's setting:

> This work was to be done in a room, not a passage, a room that was quiet and not liable to sudden unpredictable sounds, yet not dead quiet and not free from ordinary house noises. This room would be lit properly, but not by

a light staring in the face, and not by a variable light. The room would certainly not be dark and it would be comfortably warm. The patient would be lying on a couch, that is to say comfortable if able to be comfortable, and probably a rug and some water would be available. (1955, p. 21)

While we would endeavour to choose a consulting room that it is as quiet and confidential as possible, we have seen that noises and interruptions cannot be avoided. It is important to check with the patient how they experience particular aspects of the setting and to enquire about the personal meaning it has for them. Sometimes, this can lead to fruitful sharing of past experiences, conjuring up infantile memories of the primal scene and evoking prurient interest in what is going on behind the wall. Ideally you should try to use the same room each time and for the contents of the room to remain consistent. In setting and maintaining the analytic frame, consistency is key, as we will repeatedly come to see. A sense of security and trust is best achieved when there is a stable environment, including the physical space. This may be challenging in a busy public health service, so it is important for the therapist to plan ahead and block off the room bookings if the service culture does not support analytic work.

Other practical aspects of the physical space such as a waiting area and access to a toilet, are important to bear in mind and communicate to the patient. It is not always possible to have a waiting area in busy locations or if working from home. This should be made clear to the patient, so that they can make appropriate arrangements about arriving on time. Patients need to know where the available toilets are. If working from home, there should ideally be a separate toilet for patient use and the bathroom cabinet we would suggest either be locked or emptied of personal effects.

Therapists working in the public health service usually have little influence on room decor, although some therapists may choose to bring a few decorative objects for their rooms in order to create a more inviting environment. However, this can cause difficulties for other therapists who use the room. One of us shared a room in the NHS with another therapist who placed a gold leafed Buddha in a prominent position. This felt very personal and so the Buddha ended up in the cupboard while we were using the room, to be returned to its position at the end of the day. For those therapists working in private practice, décor needs to be given careful thought since this inevitably reveals something of the therapist's personality that they should feel comfortable with disclosing. Ideally, we are striving for a therapy room that is relatively neutral in style. It is important to think about the possible impact on the patient of items that may reflect the therapist's personal life, such as photographs, paintings, books and so forth. If you are able to visit the Freud Museum in London, you will see Freud's consulting room transposed from Vienna to Hampstead, and it is jam-packed with archaeological finds, classical busts, antiquities, oriental rugs and cigar fumes among other personal relics from Freud's life and travels. Today, we adopt a somewhat different approach. Personal family photographs should be avoided in the effort to remain open to the patient's projections. In psychodynamic psychotherapy, the therapist works with the patient's transference and if the therapist has too much of themselves on display, this can impact negatively on the fantasies the patient may form about the therapist that make for fruitful exploration and provide insight into the patient's internal world. It is important also to consider the appropriateness of artwork on display. For example, what would an erotic or violent artwork suggest to the patient? While we need to consider the décor for therapeutic reasons, it is also important that the room is comfortable. After all, it represents our working environment, a place where we may spend a lot of time and we do want to have a supportive chair, enough lighting to read or make notes. However, do bear in mind that this is a professional space, not a personal one.

One piece of furniture of particular relevance to psychoanalytic ways of working is the analytic couch, as indicated in the above quotation of Winnicott's. Sometimes, people will respond as if the couch is out of vogue and belongs to the 'good old days'. However, the analytic couch is very much in use today and is typically used in longer-term, intensive psychoanalytic work. Occasionally a once-weekly patient will elect (or it is suggested) to use the couch too, perhaps because it facilitates their ability to talk about shameful topics like sex, aggression or past abuse. The couch is situated against a wall with the therapist's chair behind, out of sight of the patient but in close physical proximity to them. Winnicott (1947) writes that:

> For the neurotic, the couch and warmth and comfort can be symbolical of the mother's love; for the psychotic it would be more true to say that these things are the analyst's physical expression of love. The couch is the analyst's lap or womb, and the warmth is the live warmth of the analyst's body. And so on. (p. 72)

The couch facilitates a particular holding environment: it encourages regression and free association. It affords the patient (and therapist) more privacy and facilitates space for both patient and therapist to think freely without the distraction of the other's gaze or facial expression, or having to follow the usual conversational cues that take place when sitting face-to-face. Freud was said to have encouraged patients to lie down because "I cannot put up with being stared at by other people for eight hours a day" (Freud, 1913, p. 134), however, he goes on to elaborate that he didn't want his facial expressions to unduly influence the patient and that using the couch allowed the transference to be isolated so that it could come forward more clearly. One would certainly not use a couch in brief-term applications, as the interaction is very much in the present and the therapist is more active and supportive. Jeremy Holmes (2012) has written about the use of the couch in light of attachment needs to be seen and mirrored by the therapist and argues the benefits and drawbacks of being both seated upright and recumbent. In sitting face-to-face, the face of the therapist may provide an important visual mirror to the patient, but, he argues, the therapist can equally provide a mirror through tone of voice, utterances and responses to the patient on the couch. The important point is to explore with the patient what the experience of sitting up or lying down (on the couch) means to them.

Lone working

Lone working refers to any situation where someone works by themselves without a nearby colleague or when working out of sight or earshot of another colleague. This is a constituent part of working as a psychotherapist. Most psychotherapists in private practice are lone workers without much thought to the safety aspects of the setting, particularly when working after hours or on weekends. Those psychotherapists working in public health or organisational settings would usually have nearby colleagues and a staffed reception area, panic buttons installed in offices and attend regular training in managing risky situations. Given that lone working is an essential part of our work, we all need to carry out a dynamic risk assessment. Most of the time, you may feel with a patient that there would be minimal risk to your own safety, and you would feel comfortable about seeing them in your consulting room, where you are lone working. However, you may assess a patient where you are left uneasy or unsure about an issue of safety, based on aspects of their presentation or history. You would need to give careful consideration as to what help would be available to you, if you were to take on such work.

In such instances, it is best to have other people working nearby for your own safety. When meeting a new patient for the first time, you can't be sure whom you may be faced with, so you may want to decide to see new potential patients at a time when you are not on your own in the building. Part of the risk assessment will include ascertaining whether the patient has posed any risk to others (including the therapist, going forward). It is important to establish if the patient has any forensic history.

Does anyone have access to your diary and know which patients you are seeing? This may fall to the colleagues who hold your *living will* (discussed in the section on holidays and cancellations). You may want to let someone know that you are meeting a new patient and check back with them at the end of the consultation, for example. Can you establish communication systems around sharing any risk concerns with your colleagues? Make sure you have an appropriate means of communication in your office. This includes your mobile phone or you may want to set up a mobile panic button if you are very isolated in your working environment. Bear in mind that your mobile phone is not a protection device. Alarms and panic systems do need to be tested regularly to make sure they are in working order and need to be easy to access, rather than tucked away in a drawer or bag. Phones should also be charged. Pay attention to how you can get out your office should you urgently need to do so – it is advisable to avoid walking in front of the patient or positioning yourself in the consulting room in such a way that it is difficult to escape. It is equally important not to impede the patient from leaving should they choose to do so. You may want to look around the room to be aware of items that could potential be used as a weapon.

> When working in the NHS, I saw a patient that generated some concern in me, and I used to ensure that my scissors were safely put away in my drawer during those sessions. At another time, I was aware of my countertransference during an initial assessment of a man

who described his violent and intrusive nightmares. I felt a sense of alarm and noticed his large hands and how vulnerable I felt. In that instance, I was able to consider whether it would be better for him to be seen by a male therapist.

There are additional considerations in the event you carry out any home visits, not something that typically would happen in psychodynamic psychotherapy. If you feel at risk at any time, you should feel able to call an end to the consultation. You should have the number of your emergency and ambulance services to hand if you have to make an urgent referral and it is important to add an 'In Case of Emergency' number on your mobile phone.

Time, frequency and regularity

The therapy encounter is framed by the structure of time and frequency. There is a limit to the availability of the therapist which the frame makes explicitly clear. Some patients have a wish for more and will try to contact the therapist between sessions and extend their session time, wanting a therapist on tap, so to speak. The therapist's limited availability is a reality or 'fact of life'; the therapist after all has their own life outside the consulting room. This limited availability may very well evoke feelings of frustration and neglect that as part of the work, will need to be understood and interpreted. This is not a bad thing; part of any healthy relationship is being able to be with someone and tolerate their independence as an individual. Winnicott (1969) observed that a crucial aspect of development is the ability for the child to have a relationship with their parents and others, knowing that they have a separate mind and life to their own.

The psychodynamic psychotherapy hour is 50 minutes long; what Greenson (1974) refers to as 'the 50-minute hour'. Initially, for Freud, there was no symbolic significance to this number, it was more a matter of practicality than anything else, allowing Freud to see patients on the hour with a short break in between to write quick notes or take a comfort break (Will, 2018). Later, the 50-minute hour became an important component of the therapeutic frame as it allows for regulation of the patient's emotional experience, but is also stretching enough to create a degree of pain (Will, 2018). In psychodynamic psychotherapy, with its focus on unconscious fantasies, adhering to the 50-minutes, and thus providing consistency, is what is most important. If the therapist sometimes extends the session beyond the 50 minutes, what might this communicate to the patient: is the therapist feeling guilty, or are they being nice to their 'favourite' patient, giving rise to fantasies of feeling special? If on the other hand, the therapist occasionally ends a bit short of 50 minutes, what might this be communicating: is the therapist feeling irritated with the patient, wanting to cut short the session? If the session is consistently 50 minutes in duration and then there is a sudden change, the patient may wonder about this. Of course, applying this aspect of the analytic frame does not mean that the patient must be stopped mid-sentence at the stroke of 50 minutes. However, if there is a change in consistency, it is important for the therapist to consider what is going on in terms of their counter-transference, and whether they are acting out something unconsciously in their transference towards the patient, whether this is favouritism or antipathy, or whether something is being communicated by the patient.

The ending of the session may have different meanings for patients, and this can change over time. Some may experience the end of the session with relief, while for others it is a painful reminder of the therapist's limited availability. Sometimes this feeling is accentuated when patients start talking about something painful and emotionally charged in the last few minutes of the session, thereby repeating an experience of being prematurely cut off. Let's look at a clinical example:

> *Carl came to therapy because he was depressed and lonely. He struggled with maintaining relationships, feeling unwanted and unable to trust in his partner's fidelity. Carl was the oldest of three brothers. He described growing up with a sense that his father was disappointed in him for being something of a 'softy' and a bit effeminate. He felt his father preferred his younger brothers, who were more masculine and enjoyed the same sports as their father. Carl was closer to his mother, although once his brothers were born, he felt he had less attention from her. After three months of therapy, Carl took the step to end his intimate relationship, tired of the frequent arguments and suspecting that his partner was seeing someone else. During a session, Carl spoke about his loneliness and ensuing despair that he will always be alone. He became very tearful and flooded with emotion. When I gently announced the end of the session, he seemed surprised, saying he wanted to continue speaking and reminding me of how very distressed he felt. He asked whether I had another patient after his session, or not. I did not answer his question but stated that the time was up, acknowledging his difficulty accepting the end of the session and his wish for more time. Carl arrived slightly late to his subsequent session and seemed quieter. I interpreted that he may feel angry with me, perhaps feeling rejected at being cast out at the last session in favour of another patient (like his favoured siblings, and the suspected infidelity of his partner). Carl was able to admit he had felt angry and had considered not returning to his sessions. This allowed us to address his feelings of being side-lined, and cast aside in the transference and for the therapy to offer him a different space in which his challenging feelings could be understood and addressed.*

In addition to consistency in the location and duration of sessions, equally important is the frequency and regularity. Ideally, sessions should be at the same time and day each week. When contracting for psychotherapy, this is an important consideration: can the patient commit to attending at the same time each week during term time? This is not always possible in cases where someone's work arrangement change week on week, for example, those who work shifts or travel frequently or have sporadic employment and need to take jobs as they arise. With these prospective patients, it is important to consider the practicalities of making a commitment to attending psychotherapy. Sometimes, this may lead the therapist to offer brief therapy if that is the most viable way forward for the person. The consistency of regular sessions allows for a sense of security and trust to develop in the knowledge that the therapist can be found at the same time and place each week. The patient becomes able to tolerate the inevitable frustration of the therapist's limited availability in the knowledge that the therapist will be there as expected next time. Of course, therapists are human too, and sometimes may run late because of transport delays or they may need to cancel at short notice owing to an unexpected emergency or illness. It is useful in such cases for the therapist to have the patient's phone number to hand (or another agreed method of communication) so that they can let them know about the delay or cancellation. Part of holding the analytic frame requires the therapist to privilege their clinical work over other commitments and to keep their work diary protected and free from interference in other areas of their life as far as possible.

As Lemma (2016) states, the frame itself – including how it is set up, managed and used – is a form of therapeutic intervention. Thus, any change to the consistency of the frame has an impact on therapy, and needs to be understood and addressed. The work of therapy should also be contained within the framework of the session. Some patients may try to establish contact outside the setting, via phone calls, email or even social media. Others may try to strike up small talk as you accompany them to and from the waiting area. It is important to establish clear boundaries from the start. You can explain that this is a different form of conversation and that the session begins when you enter the consulting room; this also protects their confidentiality.

Every now and then, the therapist may encounter their patients in a public setting, such as a restaurant, lecture or other event. This is more likely if your paths cross at work or in a training organisation, for instance. These sorts of overlaps need to be considered at the initial consultation as part of a consideration about the viability of working together if there are obvious shared connections at first meeting, most notably connections with existing patients of yours. If you work in a small town, then bumping into each other is usually unavoidable and it is advisable to discuss with the patient what you will do in these circumstances, as part of the contracting process. It is best not to greet the patient first, rather you can discreetly acknowledge having seen them once they have acknowledged you. The reason for this is that you cannot be sure who the patient may be with and your greeting may put them in a difficult position as to how to explain to others who you are. Inevitably, it makes for useful material to reflect on at the next session – something you would want to bring back if your patient does not raise it themselves.

Confidentiality

Confidentiality is one of the essential requirements of therapy. In order to invite patients to be honest and open about their private internal worlds, we need to provide a confidential space. Yet, confidentiality is also not something we can assure in the absolute because there are necessary limitations. An obvious limit to patient-therapy confidentiality is where the patient reveals a potential threat of harm to themselves (such as self-harm or suicide) or someone else (such as acts of violence, sexual abuse or safe-guarding concerns). In these circumstances, we have a legal obligation to inform their doctor, family member or appropriate authority (see Chapter 12 for further discussion about managing risk). These restrictions to confidentiality need to be made clear at the initial meeting with the patient.

In private practice, it is best practice to write to the patient's doctor, notifying them that their patient has commenced psychotherapy with you, and that you will contact them should they require medical cover in future. The patient should be notified about this, including the rationale for doing so. It is helpful to feel there is another professional who shares responsibility for the patient's care, particularly were they to be in crisis and require additional containment. As with supervision, this allows for triangulation of care which is containing for the therapist. Some patients expressly don't want you to contact their doctor, perhaps saying they do not want it known that they are in therapy or expressing concern about mental health difficulties being on their patient record. Depending on the presentation, you may want to agree that the doctor will only be contacted should a medical need arise. In public health services, communicating with GPs and referrers about appointments, care plans and discharges is standard protocol, however, patient's rights under the General Data Protection Regulation (GDPR – data protection regulation introduced in the European Union in 2016) now means that patients can elect to opt out of these procedures. This leaves it up to the public health service to decide if they are able to manage the risks this may pose in offering treatment without the support of the patient's GP and the allied crisis networks. Increasingly, patients no longer have one GP whom they regularly see and who holds their personal and medical history. Other patients use apps like PushDoctor, Now GP and Babylon to see GPs using video link, phone or text message. As GPs become overloaded and virtual doctors replace face-to-face consultations with medical professionals, psychotherapists can't rely on this type of personalised support in the same way they used to. You may want to ask your patients for details of their next of kin, and establish the grounds under which you would make contact with that person in a state of emergency or extended absence, for example.

It must be kept in mind that we will need to hold confidential discussions about our patients with colleagues. All therapists are expected to have regular supervision of their clinical work and this is often a requirement of ongoing professional accreditation. This can be individual or group supervision, where case material is discussed. Such clinical material should always be anonymised as far as possible. If you have concerns that anyone in the supervision group has personal contact or knowledge of the patient, this should be flagged so they can absent themselves from the discussion. This allows us to protect the neutrality of the analytic setting, rather than allow us to be contaminated by external sources of information. It is important to notify our patients of this aspect of good professional practice (see how this is done in a 'terms and conditions' document in Appendix 1).

In the public health service, it is usual practice for essential patient information to be held on a central data base that is password protected. Patients may be discussed in team meetings and ward rounds, as appropriate. Patients should be informed about this and how their data will be used. Usually the therapist says something like, "I work here as a part of a team, and for us to be able to help you in the best way, we may need to think about your case as a team. What you say will be kept confidential within the team and the grounds under which we would have to break confidentiality are when you disclose thoughts of harming yourself or others". Trainees in particular need to discuss their work with supervisors on a regular basis, and this should be made clear to their patients. It can feel deskilling to trainees to disclose their trainee status. You can discuss with the service how best to express this to the patient so that you are both upfront and containing the patient's anxieties about being in safe hands. We have found it helpful to say that you have a professional qualification and are undertaking further training, if that is the case; you can also explain that you are receiving regular supervision of your clinical work. Therapists in public health services may be required to write letters to the referrer or other professionals about their work with the patient and to keep session notes on the data base. This should be discussed with the patient, and letters should ideally be copied to patients. You may want to read through the contents of any letters with the patient beforehand so as to ensure the letter is an accurate representation of their situation and there are no surprises. It is best to keep the content of such letters and process notes concise, with only the essential information provided. After all, the theoretical terms we use in psychodynamic psychotherapy are unlikely to make sense to professionals and individuals outside our profession, and can easily be misunderstood.

Another issue to consider in relation to confidentiality is the question of seeing patients who know each other. You may not always comprehend this on first meeting. It is helpful to enquire about the background to this referral, i.e. how did the patient find your details? Hopefully, this will alert you to any extra-therapy connections. It is best practice to avoid seeing two people in a close relationship to each other (e.g. partners, close friends, house-mates) as separate therapy patients in your practice. It can create problems where you find yourself in possession of information about one patient that has been provided by another patient, thereby contaminating the objectivity of the therapeutic space. The therapist would then have external knowledge about a patient that inevitably influences how they think about and respond to that patient. The patient may also be suspicious about what is being shared with the therapist by the other patient. This scenario has been used to comedic and dramatic effect in movies and TV. For example, in the movie *Prime,* the patient Rafi (played by Uma Thurman) is in a new relationship with David, her therapist's son, without knowing that they are related. Similarly, in the first season of *In Treatment* a male patient of the therapist Dr Paul Weston (played by Gabriel Byrne) starts a relationship with another patient of his, with both patients at first concealing their shared connection from him.

Fees

The issue of money and charging for therapy brings up all sorts of potential conflicts for patients and therapists alike. Those therapists working in public health services may never have dealt with issues around agreeing fees and taking payment. In the charity sector where a small charge is often levied, payment is often handled by central administrative staff rather than the therapist concerned. By contrast, for therapists in private practice payment usually represents their prime source of livelihood; it *is* a business, albeit a particular type of business.

Therapists have expenses to cover including room hire, professional registration and memberships, indemnity insurance, supervision and continuing professional development. While some people hold to the trope that behind every psychotherapist is a rich partner who subsidises them, many therapists are the primary breadwinners and need to be able support themselves and their dependents. Fees also signify that this is a professional, boundaried relationship, involving the *work* of therapy.

Many newly qualified therapists may feel uncomfortable dealing with issues around charging for sessions and the ensuing exchange of money. It may feel contrary to the notion of a warm, empathic therapist to be coldly charging someone for their services. Often this is an area that is not directly addressed in clinical trainings and therapists end up modelling their practice on the way their own therapist conducts themselves. A number of questions may arise around setting fees and how much to charge. Therapists' fees range widely and depend on a number of factors including the therapist's level of experience, expertise and location. The cost of room hire in central London, for example, is much higher than renting a room in the city outskirts or working from your home. It is advisable to search those therapists working in your area to establish the range of fees charged and then set your fees accordingly. Again, not all therapists will have websites with details of their fee structures and indeed, speaking openly about money and fees can be seen as taboo among colleagues. You may be tempted to set your fees lower when starting out and you may decide that you are not driven by financial concerns and would like to offer a more accessible service. Notwithstanding this, you should consider the message you may be conveying about your self-worth and confidence in your expertise. Many therapists in private practice have a standard fee for consultations as well as offering some reduced fee rates for those patients in need of therapy and with limited income. You can present your regular fee and then observe how the patient responds. In agreeing a fee, it is helpful to be able to have a frank discussion with the patient about what is affordable to them. We have been in situations where a low fee has been agreed, only to learn about your patient's other indulgences in taxi cabs and shopping blow outs. Agreeing the fee is not only about how you value yourself but also reflects the value the patient places on your services. For each patient, that is different. One of us worked in a child guidance clinic in Cape Town where patients were asked to contribute a nominal fee towards the service they were receiving. The young boy in the family being seen would count out the coins to pay for his session each week in a way that signified the enormous value the family placed on the help they were receiving. For some patients on reduced incomes, a reduced fee may still represent a sizeable chunk of their disposable income and the significance of this commitment should be respected alongside those who pay a full fee.

You should consider regularly reviewing your fees, whether this is annually or every two years, and this should be mentioned in the therapy contract. It may feel uncomfortable to increase fees even if by a few pounds each year. However, if you are seeing someone for long-term therapy, you can end up effectively working at a reduced fee after several years. Bear in mind that patients' circumstances change and the fee should be responsive to that, taking into account both when they are in a more fortunate financial position as well as situations of economic adversity. The amount of the increase can be negotiated with some patients while for others, you may want to present an amount to them. Therapists should be mindful not to commit to a fee arrangement (or appointment time) that will later become a source of resentment: this is problematic for both therapist and patient.

Another practicality that bears consideration here is how to invoice and receive payment. Some therapists regard the physical exchange of bills and payment in person at the start or end of sessions as an important signifier of the professional frame and the commitment between therapist as service provider and patient as service user. This often meant that therapists presented a handwritten bill at the beginning of the month for the preceding month while patients paid with a handwritten cheque the following session. Increasingly though, therapists are using online payments also known as BACS (Bankers' Automated Clearing Services) in the UK as this is how most people operate in daily life, with cheque books becoming obsolete. Of course, this means that the therapist has to have a system of checking that payment has been made and that it is the correct amount. Although the payment may not take place in the consulting room, the therapist would usually still give the bill in person, thereby bringing the issue of payment into the transference. Some therapists are using online accounting and billing packages that generate invoices to be emailed to patients. This seems to take the issues of money entirely outside the consulting room. We explore technological aspects of payment in Chapter 14.

When processing payments for patients with medical aid, do think about whether you want to bill the medical aid directly or ask the patient to settle the bill and claim back the payment themselves. The latter approach may result in more of a sense of ownership that the payment originates with the patient and would be more in keeping with the analytic setting we are aiming for. You should also factor in whether this will result in additional demands on your time, for example, are you required to write to the medical aid about the progress the patient is making or to request an extension of the allocated funding? These costs should be considered when arriving at your fee structure.

As with all aspects of therapy, fees and the payment of money have unconscious meaning for patients, which varies in relation to their own individual relationships to money and interpersonal dynamics. For some patients, being charged by the therapist for their time is a painful reminder of the therapist's separateness and relational distance. Others are reassured by the professional arrangements of a fee, distancing themselves from any sense of connection to the therapist by viewing the arrangement as purely professional. The amount of the fee may also elicit unconscious fantasies in the patient. Some may feel that a reduced fee (or no fee at all, in a charity or public health setting) means that the therapy is not as good, thereby fuelling feelings of deprivation and inadequacy. Others may feel guilty about taking up much needed resources, imagining other patients are in greater need than themselves. This can be prevalent in public health services, where some patients feel their difficulties are not serious enough to warrant publicly funded or reduced fee therapy. A reduced fee may raise questions in the patient's mind about whether or not they are valued by their therapist. How payments are made may also form part of the patient's transference towards their objects, as the following clinical example shows:

> *I once had a patient who insisted on paying in cash at the end of each session. He would stand up and peel away each note, counting and handing over the money in a manner that was suggestive of paying a sex worker for their services. I was left feeling demeaned (perhaps a disowned feeling of the patient's that was projected into me). The contemptuous manner in which he paid me allowed him to feel powerful and at the same time, communicated his anger and shame at needing my help. Paying at the end of each session gave him a sense of control, that if he wanted, he could leave unencumbered, without owing me anything. It represented an attempt to control the interpersonal contact whereby he could imagine each session could be the last.*

Paying in cash also invites the therapist to engage in a potentially dodgy exchange, whereby it can appear that the patient is inviting or testing the therapist to evade paying tax by pocketing the money without declaring it. To avoid this, you may want to give a numbered paper receipt that acknowledges these cash payments and that forms part of your income tax statement. Paying the final bill can be a difficult acknowledgement of ending, with some patients withholding payment, thereby (unconsciously) inviting the therapist to keep in contact with them around settling the bill.

It is worth establishing who holds financial responsibility for paying the bill. Sometimes it is a parent or partner who is funding the patient's therapy. This can complicate the way we understand the patient's attitude towards payment. If a session is missed, it may feel as if the patient is punishing their parent/partner by wasting their resources rather than feeling some sense of ownership and acknowledgment that it is actually the patient who is short-changed by not attending an appointment, In these situations, it is advisable to see if the patient can cover the cost of therapy themselves, perhaps obtaining financial help with other expenses, where necessary. We deal with the area of non-payment and other difficulties around fees in Chapter 12.

Holidays and cancellations

Therapists need to take holidays too. Of course, here the therapist would not charge for 'missed' sessions, as it is the therapist who is withdrawing their time. Therapists in private practice need to factor in holidays when structuring their fees since the job does not come with paid annual leave. It is commonplace for therapists to take leave over the summer (typically for the month of August in the northern hemisphere) as well as breaks that coincide with major festivities (such as Christmas and Easter). In the UK, some therapists may also take half term breaks (these are short school breaks in the middle of a term). Holiday breaks often coincide with school and university term times; however, you may choose to adjust your leave schedule and take alternative breaks. It is advisable to give patients advance notice of your planned leave so they can be prepared for the upcoming breaks and dovetail their holidays with yours to ensure continuity in the work.

Breaks may evoke unconscious fantasies in the patient, about where the therapist is going, who the therapist is spending time with and what they will be getting up to. While we are addressing holiday breaks, it is worth bearing in mind that similar feelings can be stirred up in the breaks between sessions and over weekends. Patients may feel annoyed or distressed that the therapist is off having fun when things feel particularly difficult for them. The break may evoke feelings of envy and jealousy. There may also be an understandable sense of respite at taking a break from the relentless 'work' of therapy. One of our patients often commented on feeling relief when the therapist was away, as if it were a holiday for them too. In exploring this, it became apparent that it was not a reflection of their dislike of the therapist, but rather that they experienced therapy as intensive, emotional and difficult. It was challenging for them to acknowledge these ambivalent feelings of relief at the break while also valuing the therapist's capacity to stay with their painful experiences. Other patients may find separations bring their feelings of abandonment to the fore. That is why time is needed to attend to these feelings in the lead up to breaks. This can be challenging when you approach the first break in treatment and the patient does not yet have a notion that the break may stir up more primitive feelings in them. Getting through the first break is often the first hurdle to overcome in establishing therapy as a viable enterprise. There are also those patients who don't appear to be too bothered about breaks, at least on the surface, saying that they appreciate that breaks are part of life.

Part of establishing the setting through the therapy contract entails explaining your policies around leave and cancellations, with a request that patients' holidays coincide with your own in order to ensure regularity of attendance. Of course, if therapists take leave outside the usual holiday periods or at unexpected times, this becomes more difficult to negotiate. The pattern of meeting regularly interspersed with breaks is an important part of the rhythm of psychotherapy. The breaks punctuate the work of therapy and allow patient and therapist to reflect on what has taken place. Sometimes it is during these caesuras that the patients will notice the internal changes that have taken place. One patient returned after a break with the realisation that she no longer felt angry and impatient with the world and was able to broach the subject of bringing treatment to a close. Another patient observed after a break that they were now aware of seasonal changes in their environment, something they had become inured to noticing up until then and which they put down to the internal changes that had taken place in the course of treatment.

Sometimes sessions need to be cancelled at reasonable or short notice by the therapist. This should be avoided as far as possible because as this chapter demonstrates, the therapist's consistency and reliability are core aspects of the analytic frame. Notwithstanding this, unforeseen events do occur. It is important to communicate any deviation to the patient ahead of the session about to be cancelled, and then to attend to any feelings this has evoked in the patient. In the case of an accident or emergency, where the therapist is hospitalised or has taken seriously ill for example, the therapist should rely on what is known as a 'living will'. A current list of your patients and their contact details should be entrusted to an experienced colleague or supervisor who will be notified by your family or partner and who can then contact your patients to inform them of your unexpected unavailability. Sometimes this entails offering holding sessions for the patients or even placing patients with other therapists should it be unlikely that you will return to work soon. Most professional bodies require this arrangement to be in place with their registered therapists. The therapist cannot expect their partner or a family member to contact patients directly as this would be a breach of professional confidentiality and would also potentially place them in a difficult position for which they are not professional trained to deal with.

Patients occasionally need to cancel sessions too. When this is unavoidable, the therapist can consider rearranging the cancelled session, where possible. You may want to distinguish between sessions cancelled for work meetings, significant medical appointments or funerals, for example, as opposed to planned holidays or discretionary events. We would be more inclined to offer an alternate time for the former than the latter. As your diary fills up, you may have decreasing capacity to offer alternate times. This area of patient cancellations gives rise to the somewhat controversial issue of therapists' charging for missed sessions. For some people, charging for a session that did not take place seems callous. However, what the patient is paying for is the therapist's time: the same time slot is reserved in the therapist's diary for the patient each week and it is unlikely that the therapist can fill that time with another patient or piece of work. The therapy contract recognises the patient's responsibilities, namely to attend sessions on time and pay for those sessions. Aside from the practical considerations, cancellations also need to be thought about as forms of unconscious communication. Cancelling a session because it was too cold and wet to leave the comfort of their bed may signal hidden aggression and resistance towards the therapy. The patient may be testing the therapist to see if it matters to them whether or not they show up.

Some therapists, particularly those working in time-limited therapy, offer a 24- or 48-hour cancellation clause, charging only for sessions cancelled at short notice or planned sessions that are not attended (DNA's or 'Did Not Attend'). In open-ended, long-term therapy, therapists typically charge for all missed or cancelled sessions and do not have this cancellation option. Of course, unforeseen events do happen. The patient may be in hospital and cannot attend their sessions. How this is handled really depends on a careful, case by case consideration that takes into account the history of the therapy up till then among other factors. Ultimately, it is at the discretion of the therapist whether to charge in full or part for these unattended sessions. Patients may have a planned extended break and it may be possible to negotiate a holding fee for the sessions at an agreed portion of the fee. Arrangements around charging for missed sessions and cancellations need to be made clear to the patient at the point of contracting for therapy, so that these are explicity understood from the beginning. It is difficult to suddenly introduce them into the therapy at the point when a cancellation has taken place. However clear you have been, it is also possible that the patient has not taken this piece of information on board. This is where having a signed contract or clear terms and conditions available on your website, for example, can be helpful (see Appendix 1).

Notwithstanding this area of therapist discretion and flexibility, it is important that the therapist does not shy away from acknowledging the implicit aggression that is often contained in these breaches of the analytic frame. After all, we are talking about the way the patient can get rid of sessions or drop knowledge of a regular therapy appointment from their mind in a way that 'kills off' the therapist at that moment. Winnicott (1949) writes in his ground breaking paper, 'Hate in the Counter-transference', about the ways the analyst has of objectively expressing hate to the patient, including: "Hate is expressed by the existence of the end of the 'hour'" (p. 71). He elaborates on this in his later writings, saying

> The analyst expressed love by the positive interest taken, and hate in the strict start and finish and in the matter of fees. Love and hate were honestly expressed, that is to say not denied by the analyst. (1955, p. 21)

If we consider this concept of hate in the countertransference in relation to the bills we give our patients alongside calling time on a session and taking a planned leave of absence, we can see that it is important that the therapist can sit with this, rather than feel a need to whitewash any imputed unkindness by being overly accommodating, particularly when this is at their own expense. The analytic frame provides a containing structure within which strong emotions can be explored by protecting both patient and therapist within the clear expectations and boundaries it provides.

Analytic attitude

All therapists have their own personal style. Some may be quieter than others. Some may be perceived as warmer and livelier than others. Some may be more formal, perhaps insisting on using formal greetings and surnames while others are more relaxed. Therapists vary in the way they demonstrate their curiosity. Patients often have a caricature of a therapist in their mind, perhaps based on what they have seen in the movies or on TV. Inevitably, patients may be surprised by the actual style of the therapist they see, whatever that may be. However, having a personal style does not give the therapist free licence to behave as they please. Lemma (2016) defines the core features of the analytic frame as involving: consistency, reliability, neutrality, anonymity and abstinence. Consistency and reliability are for the most part ensured through maintaining practices such as those outlined above, including providing a consistent and reliable setting and set of procedures. This extends to the therapist's internal setting, that is maintaining a reliable and consistent therapeutic attitude, which is "at the service of the patient" (Winnicott, 1955, p. 21) Winnicott (1955) describes how typically the therapist who is "reliably there, in time, alive, breathing [...] would keep awake and become preoccupied with the patient" (p. 21). He goes on to delineate how the therapist "is much more reliable than people are in ordinary life; on the whole punctual, free from temper tantrums, free from compulsive falling in love, etc.", and that the therapist can make a distinction between fantasy and fact, so that they are "not hurt by an aggressive dream" of the patient, who in turn, can count on an "absence of the talion reaction" (p. 21).

Winnicott reminds us of the purpose in providing this reliable container that allows the patient to express their innermost feelings without fear of retaliation (the talion reaction referred to above) and that in turn, facilitates the therapist's ability to interpret the meaning of the patient's material including their resistance to the process. In this section, we will look specifically at these guiding principles of neutrality, abstinence and anonymity

Neutrality

The therapist should maintain a neutral, non-judgemental stance. They should not bring their own views, opinions or experiences into the therapy room in the way that might happen with friends or work colleagues. In his list of the attributes of Freud's setting referred to above, Winnicott (1955) makes particular reference to the importance of neutrality, as follows:

> The analyst (as is well known) keeps moral judgement out of the relationship, has no wish to intrude with details of the analyst's personal life and ideas, and the analyst does not wish to take sides in the persecutory systems even when these appear in the form of real shared situations, local, political, etc. Naturally if there is a war or an earthquake or if the king dies the analyst is not unaware. (p. 21)

Taking sides would risk the therapist holding a suggestive influence over the patient's choices and becoming overly directive, thereby losing the emergent quality of psychodynamic psychotherapy. The therapist's primary role is to listen to the patient's unconscious communications and the meanings these hold in their internal and interpersonal world. Bion (1970) advocated that the therapist works without 'memory or desire', by which he meant that they should approach each session without an agenda or wish for what may occur. This is the ideal to strive towards. In reality, the therapist cannot avoid having some influence over the process of therapy, particularly in brief psychodynamic therapy. In an open-ended, intensive psychotherapy, there may be more opportunities for the therapist to hold back and let the patient explore freely during the session; in brief therapy, the therapist is more active, focusing on an agreed area of work and associated goals. Psychodynamic psychotherapy falls somewhere between these two extremes. Therapists inevitably bring with their own theoretical frameworks with inevitable assumptions such that it is impossible to remain completely neutral. However, it remains fundamentally important that the therapist both listens to, and attempts to understand, the clinical material in relation to the meaning it has for the patient at that time. Schafer (1983) states that the psychodynamic therapist's aim is to be helpful not through providing advice or reassurance, but rather through careful listening, attention and understanding.

While listening, the therapist monitors their own thoughts and counter-transference, thus attending to their own subjective affective states whilst maintaining an observing stance. This is a similar process to that which occurs externally in supervision, and it requires the therapist to find a separate position from which to reflect on their countertransference responses to the patient's material, something we elaborate on further in Chapter 9. Bateman and Holmes (1995) describe it as follows: the therapist "oscillates between empathic primary identification [...] with the patient and objectivity, perhaps representing maternal and paternal roles respectively" (p. 159). While listening and empathising with what is being said, the therapist's task is also to distinguish between different interventions, roles and responses, considering what is the most appropriate intervention for a specific patient at a particular time. Thus, in one situation, being alongside the patient in quiet may be important and containing while for another person, silence may feel abandoning and punitive, necessitating a different, more active response in moments of stillness to reach out and 'find' them.

Casement (1985) observes that holding an analytic stance necessitates the therapist being able to tolerate long periods of 'not knowing'. Therapists can feel a pressure to 'know' what is going on for the patient, which can lead to slipping into a non-neutral stance, drawing on preconceived assumptions or ideas. To listen effectively and understand the patient's experience, the therapist needs to be willing to tolerate 'not knowing' for some time, and, as Casement puts it, to "learn from the patient". He goes on to say that the patient's individuality needs to be respected, not "overlooked and intruded upon" (1985, p. 25). Through a process of learning from the patient, insight about a problem can be arrived at and offered to the patient, rather than imposed (Casement, 1985).

Therapists have to be aware of their potential biased assumptions, which may interfere with their understanding of their patient. Therapists are socialised into a particular context, and inevitably hold assumptions and prejudices about the state of the world and how it should operate. In Chapter 13, we consider issues of diversity, including biases and assumptions that can be found in psychoanalytic writing, such as blatant anti-homosexual attitudes. Supervision and personal therapy are important arenas for reflection on these unavoidable biases, allowing us to identify our blind spots so that they don't interfere with the work, and enabling us, as far as possible, to maintain a neutral stance.

In some instances, the therapist cannot, and should not, maintain neutrality. Destructive behaviours, for example, and other risk-related issues do need to be called out as such. However, this can be done in a non-judgemental manner, by naming the behaviour as problematic whilst still recognising the patient's motivations for engaging in them and what it means in terms of their subjective experience. We discussed the points at which neutrality needs to be set aside in the discussion around risk earlier in this chapter as well as in Chapter 5 on assessment.

Abstinence

A defining quality of the analytic stance is abstinence, by which we mean that the therapist should not satisfy the patient's wishes and desires. This not only includes the ethical requirement of not satisfying a patient's sexual desires, but extends to the patient's curiosities about and wishes towards the therapist. A patient may be inquisitive about the therapist's personal life. Is the therapist married? Do they have children? Are they familiar with the films, theatre and books the patient talks about? On the face of it, these may seem like reasonable questions to ask and be answered. However, in psychodynamic psychotherapy, we are concerned with what takes place intrapsychically and interpersonally, often at an unconscious level. So rather than immediately satisfying the questions by answering them, it is important to understand the motivation behind the question so that we can speak to that instead. The therapist should be asking themselves: why is the patient asking this question now? It may have to do with anxiety about not being understood, being too different, not being liked, or even about being too similar. Patients may ask if the therapist sees other patients who have similar problems: do other patients feel or experience the same as they do? It may seem therapeutically reassuring to answer, yet it is more important to understand the anxiety prompting the question. A simple intervention to such a question would be for the therapist to ask, "I wonder what prompted you to ask this?" Alternately, the therapist can reflect on the patient's curiosity: "You are curious to know something about me, perhaps it feels difficult to know how to talk and open up to someone you know little about".

Some therapists may feel that answering a 'harmless', minor question is of little importance. For example, if the patient is talking about a movie and asks if you have seen it, it may seem simpler to answer with "No, I haven't" or "Yes, I have". However, this may close down the opportunity to hear what the patient wanted to say about the movie, including how they chose to describe it. Saying 'yes' may imply a shared knowledge or understanding of the book while answering 'no' may suggest that the therapist is uninterested or won't understand. A more fruitful response would be for the therapist to say, "Why don't you tell me about it?", regardless of whether they have seen it or not. This is an occupational hazard, that you may often hear about films, theatre and books before you have had the chance to experience them yourselves, and without any spoiler alerts! We also don't want to prescribe always deflecting the questions posed by our patients because this may risk coming across as cold, distant and disengaged. Sometimes, acknowledging external reality is important, for example the therapist's illness or new hair style. It would be somewhat absurd for the therapist to avoid answering a question about their own health, when there is evidently something significantly wrong. In these instances, it is important to think about how much information you want to share with your patients, on a 'need to know' basis. This is relevant when cancelling a session, for example. We need to be mindful about the anxiety an unforeseen cancellation may give rise to and it can be helpful to say that this is for a routine medical procedure, for instance.

Questions often take place at the edges of the frame, at the start and end of sessions. Sometimes, the most difficult issues to raise or questions to ask are left until the last moment. These times are most likely to catch the therapist unaware. Particularly with threshold questions, it is easy to lose the analytic stance and fall into a more everyday way of relating, even disclosing your upcoming holiday destination. At such times, it is helpful to acknowledge the question (as well as the patient's curiosity) and say that there isn't any remaining time to attend to it and encourage the patient to bring the question or issue back to the next session.

Therapists must also abstain from satisfying their own needs, such as the need to be liked or the need to help and 'cure' problems. This does not mean we have to be unempathic and inhumane; a limited amount of gratification, help or reassurance may be needed but not at the expense of exploring and understanding the patient's predicament. Therapists need to be prepared to be hated and receive hateful projections in the transference in order to allow the patient to work through an internalised relationship with a 'bad' object. Lemma (2003) states:

> An important part of our role is to allow ourselves to become the receptacles for the patient's projections and his need to act out feelings that cannot be verbalised. However, it is also our responsibility to keep the boundaries and remind the patient of this if his behaviour threatens to undermine the therapy. Not retaliating does not mean passively accepting that the patient is abusive towards us because of what has happened to him. The therapeutic relationship may well be subjected to familiar patterns prominent in the patient's interpersonal repertoire, but it also has to be one with a difference, namely, one where these patterns, and their consequences for relating, are made explicit and can be thought about. (pp. 101–102)

Abstinence allows for a certain frustration of desires so that the patient regresses to earlier experiences of disappointments, wishes, hopes, losses and grievances, and reconnects with them. There may be a period of feeling disillusioned with therapy (Bateman and Holmes, 1995) by virtue of this process: the therapist abstains from gratifying the patient which leads to the re-emergence of repressed, painful feelings; the patient starts to feel worse and believes that therapy is not helping, in fact, it can feel it is making things worse. However, this process should be engaged with gradually and gently in a way that is containing and does not overwhelm the patient in a manner that is traumatic, and likely to lead to a rupture in therapy. It can be helpful to alert patients to the possibility that things can feel worse at the start of therapy before they start to improve.

Anonymity

Freud advocated for the therapist to act as a 'blank slate' onto which the patient could project their conflicts. This model of the anonymous therapist implies that the therapist should not be previously known to the patient, and that the patient should not know details about the therapist's interests, life and personhood, since this would interfere with the transference. The reality, certainly in contemporary society, is that therapists cannot be completely anonymous. Freud himself was certainly not anonymous as a prolific writer and well-known international figure; he was also known to blur boundaries between his personal and private life. Today, therapists may have an online presence setting out their areas of interests and expertise. There may be symbols that denote particular information to the patient (for example, the presence of a wedding band). Therapists have accents, individual dress styles, jewellery or even piercings and tattoos that all reveal personal information, inadvertently as well as deliberately. When it comes to maintaining anonymity, it is important for the therapist to keep their own life outside the frame as much as possible. This means refraining from recounting stories of their personal experiences as a way of empathising with the patient along the lines of, "Oh a similar thing happened to me too!"

We want to return to the therapist's dress style. Often new trainees ask what they should wear when they are starting work with their first patient. There is no set uniform, but you need to give thought as to how you want to present yourself, the possible message your outward appearance may convey, and the influence this could have on the therapeutic relationship. Nina Coltart (1993) observes an unspoken rule that therapists tend to dress more smartly for work than they would otherwise on weekends. Coltart would not hold with a 'casual Friday' dress code in our line of work and admits to preferences of her generation that we probably wouldn't agree with today, in particular that female therapists should not wear trousers. However, you should consider whether wearing a T-shirt, jeans and sneakers is appropriate professional attire. Clothing has an impact in creating an impression with your patients and so, it is important to reflect on what you may be communicating through your fashion choices. For example, it is advisable not to dress too provocatively, particularly when working with adolescents and young adults – you are more likely to be perceived in an overly sexualised way. If you are working in a deprived area, you may want to reflect on whether wearing designer clothing and expensive perfume or aftershave will communicate something unwelcome to the patient about your financial status. Consistency in dress as a therapist is another factor in providing a reliable setting. Sudden and dramatic changes in appearances (e.g. hair styles or colouring) may be alarming for patients with a poor sense of person permanence. They may perceive you as a different person altogether!

While we emphasise the importance of striving for neutrality, abstinence and anonymity, the goal is not to create a robotic, unengaged therapist with little of their own personality. These concepts become unhelpful when applied with great rigidity and indeed can be used defensively in iatrogenic ways. The core idea underpinning the analytic setting is to ensure the therapy session is a space for the exploration of the patient's feelings, thoughts, wishes, fantasies, anxieties and fears; and not a space for the therapist to intrude with their own issues. Casement (1985) helpfully reminds us to hold the following important question in mind as a way of monitoring ourselves: "Who is putting what into the analytic space, at this moment, and why?" (p. 25).

How to start and end a session

Trainee therapists that are just starting out will understandably have questions about how to 'run' a therapy session: how do I start and bring the session to a close? There tends to be no explicit guidance on this in training courses and textbooks, perhaps because it is something that is often learned experientially through the experience of being in personal therapy and learning first-hand how the analytic frame works. In CBT, there is an explicit structure to the session, with the therapist collaboratively setting an agenda with the client at the start and then actively managing the end of the session by summarising and setting home-work for the week ahead. In psychodynamic psychotherapy, the approach is very different in keeping with the analytic stance. The therapist wants to strike a bal-ance between allowing for whatever is on the patient's mind to freely emerge while still maintaining an awareness of the time frame of the session. How to start and end a session will also depend on whether this is brief or longer-term therapy.

It is advisable to begin the session by allowing the patients to start expressing whatever comes to their mind; this protects the emergent quality of psychody-namic psychotherapy. It is interesting to note how different patients start off the session. Some patients are able to start speaking straight off the bat by telling the therapist about their worries and concerns, including what has happened since the last session. Others may feel uncomfortable and resort to social niceties to manage the awkwardness of launching into their own narratives by asking the therapist how they are, saying hello or the like. Patients have been known to take charge of this lack of structure by bringing in a notebook or writing up their own process notes from the previous session to which they return in a business-like way, as if setting an agenda for the session. Some patients may be silent for a while, gathering their thoughts and finding their way into the session quietly. Impor-tantly, the therapist should not be the one to 'start' the session by introducing an agenda of topics for discussion since this interferes with the patient being able to express their concerns, consciously or unconsciously. In the case of brief therapy, the therapist does adopt a more active stance that would not be compatible with extended periods of silence, such that the therapist may give a prompt by asking open-ended questions such as "What's on your mind?" or "How are things?" or observing that it seems particularly difficult to start the session today.

It can be helpful for the start of the appointment to be seen as the business end of the session. Occasionally the therapist will have an issue they need to raise with the patient during the course of a session, for example a forthcoming cancellation, break or some other concern. Other therapists will prefer to provide an opportunity for the patient to start the session and allow time to explore this material, before making their announcement that may have an inhibitory effect on the patient at the start. However, the therapist should avoid raising an issue with the patient right at the end of the session, leaving no time for the patient to respond and for neces-sary discussion. There are no hard and fast rules here and it can depend on the particular dynamics with each patient. If you feel very distracted by the announcement you want to make, then it may be best to state it at the start and then look out for any associations to it as the session proceeds. Alternately, you can use a break in the session narrative should one arise, or indeed say to the patient something along the following lines: "As the end of the session is approaching, I need to let you know that …" This allows for a balance to be struck between allowing the patient to use the rest of the session freely while still making your announcement and having time to reflect on it.

In keeping with the boundaries and regularity of the session, ending on time is important. The therapist should have a clock in the room that is visible to them to allow them to keep an eye on the time. Managing the time is the therapist's responsibility in order to facilitate the patient relinquishing control over the setting and allowing them to be in touch with unconscious processes in which time is fluid. The therapist should have the end of the session in mind when weighing up whether to interpret something, ask a question or delve deeper into an issue raised. We want to avoid opening up something painful when there are only a couple of minutes left in the session and we have to cut off the patient. Inevitably the therapist may unconsciously communicate that the session is drawing to an end by becoming less active or indeed by glancing at the clock. The patient often picks up on these cues and has a sense of the session ending. After attending for a while, patients also build a sense of time, and will 'know' that the end of a session is approaching. There will also be times when patients will comment that a session went by very quickly or that the time is dragging, indicators of unconscious processes at play that influence our subjective experience of time passing. It may be that the therapist does need to stop the patient, by saying something like "Well, we do need to stop for today; we can come back to this next time if you wish" or "I can see there is much more to say but we will have to leave it there for today". Some patients may try to prolong the session with questions, saying something further or taking their time with gathering their possessions or putting on their coat. The therapist can simply say, "We do need to end, so let's discuss this next week". Your body language can help convey this by standing up and possibly moving towards the door.

Some patients may utter something important almost at the end of the session, disclose a traumatic memory, say something revealing or express something painful. This is what therapists may call 'a doorknob moment'. We can find ourselves in the painful position of having to end the session at a very challenging moment. It may be that the patient is unconsciously repeating an experience of feeling prematurely shut down and expelled by the Other in the transference, something you can come back to consider once you have observed this pattern between the two of you. It is important to acknowledge the importance of what has been uttered, and observe how it has been brought right at the end of the session when there is no time to consider it, by saying something along these lines: "This seems really important, but I note you have brought this up at the end of the session, leaving us no time to think further about it. You can bring it back for us to think about next time". It is rare for a crisis or emergency to be brought up at the end of the session; usually this would be addressed earlier in the session. Similarly, any assessment of ongoing risk should happen at the start of the session when there is time to address concerns.

Maintaining competences

Part of working within an analytic frame is to ensure that the therapist maintains and works within their level of competence. One way of ensuring this that is mandated by accrediting bodies, is through Continuing Professional Development (CPD). Most accrediting bodies and training institutions offer a variety of CPD events, such as workshops, conferences and short courses, aimed to enhance or develop new knowledge and skills post qualifying. CPD does not only involve training events. Keeping up to date with the literature and reading the latest relevant professional journals, is equally important. Therapists should not rest on the laurels of their years of experience: the world of psychotherapy shifts and changes over time, as new issues become salient. Take for example recent developments in thinking about gender diversity and trans identities. Most ethical guidelines explicitly state that therapists should practice within their level of competences and not take on work outside of these. For example, a non-medically trained therapist should not advise patients on psychiatric medication.

For those recently qualified and starting out in the field, there is often anxiety about not feeling competent, knowledgeable and skilled enough. It is easy to forget how much has been gained during training, particularly when you compare this to where you were at the start of the process. It is important to reflect on the specific knowledge and experience you have gained through discussions with your supervisors and tutors as well as reviewing the curriculum. This will allow you to assess your experience and strengths. Do not sell yourself short. Equally, the opposite should be avoided, whereby therapists – newly qualified or not – claims to have expertise in treating all sorts of difficulties. When you look online, invariably you will come across therapists' profiles with long lists of all sorts of psychological and psychiatric problems that they are purportedly able to work with. It is worth asking whether one person can indeed be an expert at working with everything!

Supervision, whether individual, group or peer supervision, is another important way of maintaining competences by providing the therapist a space to reflect on their work and understanding of their patients, as well as acknowledging the limits of their understanding, level of knowledge and skills. A psychodynamic therapist is usually expected to seek some form of supervision, typically with a senior psychotherapist, to help the therapist reflect on the powerful unconscious transference and countertransference dynamics that are evoked in this type of psychotherapy. Supervision provides the therapist with their own holding environment, whereby the container (therapist for the patient) can be contained (supervisor for the therapist) in turn. Casement (1985), while writing of the importance of supervision for these reasons, warns against the trainee and new therapist feeling overly directed by their supervisor, as if they are an extension of the supervisor rather than being encouraged to find their own style and voice. The therapist should use supervision for reflection, containment and learning; notwithstanding this, they are starting to shape and realise their own style as a therapist, something supervision should affirm. Supervision also provides some hindsight as to what has happened in the session as well as occasional foresight as to what might happen in a future session. Ultimately, the work of therapy requires the therapist to be able to reflect, think and have insight in the moment of therapy. Casement (1985) thus describes the importance of developing an *internal supervisor*; that is, to internalise the supervisor as a resource to be drawn on in the course of a therapy session.

As we move towards retirement age, a difficult and painful consideration is to assess your continuing competence to practice in terms of physical and mental health. There are many therapists who practice well into their 70s and beyond. Age in itself is not a barrier, particularly in this largely sedentary profession. However, it does require an honest assessment as to whether your cognitive functioning permits you to practice proficiently. Dementia in old age is a potential concern that all of us may have to face. Being healthy enough to continue practicing is an issue at any age, however. We do need to give thought as to what happens to our patients when we are suddenly ill, in an accident or in the event of our death. We referred to this earlier in the chapter in relation to the 'living will'. Many professional bodies require you to have one or two named clinical trustees, that is colleagues who hold an up-to-date list of your patients and their contact details and who can make contact with the patients, notify them of what has happened and where necessary, facilitate referrals to other therapists. As this entails sharing confidential information, you will need to ensure that this list is managed safely and securely by both therapist and clinical trustee. If you do share and regularly update the list by email, then we suggest using a password protected or encrypted file as a basic means of protection. Always send the password in a separate email to the locked file.

Self-care and preventing burnout

Coltart (1993) refers to 'survival' as a therapist alongside the importance of "survival-with-enjoyment" (p. 3) in her aptly titled book, *How to Survive as a Psychotherapist*. She uses the term 'survival' to highlight that work as a therapist is 'tough' work. As she and others (e.g. Kahr, 2019) have observed, psychotherapy can be a lonely occupation, in that you spend hours of the day alone in your consulting room with a patient engaged in demanding interactions while you adhere to the strictures of the analytic frame. You do not get to chat about yourself and have friendly conversations. The work involves listening to, empathising with and to some extent absorbing the emotional pain and distress of patients as part of their containment. As therapists, we are not able to come home at the end of a long day and 'complain' to our partners and family about the tough day at work or debrief about a difficult encounter; confidentiality precludes this unless they too are in the field. In the face of these challenges, Coltart stresses the importance of enjoyment; that is, to recognise the rich rewards that our work brings and the interesting lives that we may learn about along the way. Similarly, Kahr (2019) refers to the importance of thriving and flourishing as a therapist, embarking on a variety of activities, if one so wishes, to bring variety and interest to the work.

Where a therapist stops finding enjoyment in their work and becomes increasingly stressed, there is the risk of 'compassion fatigue' whereby your ability to empathise and have compassion is reduced and you face the possibility of burnout. You may notice signs of this if you start to feel that you have low energy and are dragging yourself off to work; you no longer start or end sessions on time; you don't feel present during sessions, perhaps distracted or sleepy; you find yourself giving advice or providing solutions to problems rather than exploring issues; you may notice that you are making formulaic interpretations with reduced personal meaning for the individual patient; and you feel reduced empathy for your patients. It is important to pick up on these signs as early as possible in order to address your stress.

Personal therapy is one way of relieving some of the personal stresses and difficulties that may be getting in the way of professional fulfilment, as well as being a space to reflect on the emotional impact of work. Trainings in psychodynamic counselling and psychotherapy require that the trainee is in personal therapy themselves, usually to the same degree of intensity as the frequency of therapy for which you are training. All too frequently, financial and time pressures mean that trainees stop personal therapy as they complete their trainings, often a time when even more support is required as people settle into this line of work. Some therapists choose to re-enter personal therapy at a later stage in their career, particularly at times of emotional strain.

Being a therapist is a sedentary occupation, with many hours spent sitting immobile. Over many years, this can be detrimental for your physical health, especially your back. Kahr (2019) humorously yet with all seriousness, advocates for ten-minute gym workouts between sessions – an opportunity to do some stretching exercises to energise and de-stress your body and muscles. Consider how you use your non-working days in order to counterbalance this inactivity. The advice often includes being active, engaging in your cultural life and community, having fun, doing yoga, eating healthily, sleeping well and so on. But as Kahr states: "burn-out can be staved off *not* by having fun outside working hours, but, rather, by doing our job as well as possible, so that we will derive the tremendous satisfaction of actually curing our patients" (Kahr, 2019, p. 90). While we may not consider the aim of psychodynamic psychotherapy is cure, it remains important to foster the very interest and enthusiasm that engaged you with pursuing a career in psychotherapy in the first place. Continued learning and development of new knowledge and skills is a good way to achieve this. Attending conferences and events where you can socialise with your peers helps alleviate the sense of isolation that can creep in. Diversifying your work is another useful way to alleviate the 'toughness' of the job. It is possible to combine therapy work with lecturing, teaching, writing, facilitating workshops or offering consultations. Some therapists have part-time roles in public health services or mental health charities where there is more team-based work and collegial support. Some therapists have completely parallel careers as musicians or artists; thought has to be given to potential conflicts that may arise.

Therapists need holidays and time to unwind. We often notice with trainees or newly qualified therapists that they are reluctant to take a proper holiday, carrying on working instead or allowing patients to take their leave as they need but always being available to see the patient throughout the year. This can give rise to burnout with therapists feeling overly responsible for the care of their patients.

It is important to remember that you cannot properly care for your patients if you are not in a healthy physical and mental state to do so. Remember the safety rule in the aeroplane – if the oxygen masks descend, put your own mask on first, then attend to anyone else who needs your help. Self-care is important and is increasingly recognised as essential in the caring professions.

Box 4.1 Useful resources

Readings

Roy Schafer's book *The Analytic Attitude* is an extensive and detailed text looking at the various aspects important for maintaining an analytic stance.

Patrick Casement's book, *On Learning from the Patient*, does not focus on the analytic attitude per se, but has many very useful thoughts, and clinical examples for how to maintain an analytic focus.

There is a useful paper by T. G. Gutheil and G. O. Gabbard, *The Concept of Boundaries in Clinical Practice: Theoretical and Risk-Management Dimensions* which is available online at this website https://kspope.com/ethics/boundaries.php

Online resources

For maintaining competences, the websites of the various UK professional bodies (BACP, BPC, BPS, UKCP) have regularly updated lists of different CPD courses and workshops. The website Psychotherapy Excellence – www.pesi.co.uk – has a large listing of various CPD opportunities offered by various training organisations.

Dr Elizabeth Cotton's useful blog, www.survivingwork.org and the associated website, www.thefutureoftherapy.org have helpful resources, podcasts, e-books and other material relating to research carried out in 2016 around conditions surrounding work in mental health across different professions in the UK. She flagged the question "Do you Have to Marry a Rich Person to Become a Psychotherapist in the UK?".

With regards self-care, the following website has useful tips about noticing and managing therapist stress and burnout: www.psychologytoday.com/us/blog/in-therapy/200811/therapist-burnout

5 Assessment and formulation

How do we know whether someone may be helped by psychodynamic psychotherapy? This is less a question about whether or not psychodynamic psychotherapy is effective, but whether the potential patient's difficulties are of a nature that can be helped with a course of psychodynamic psychotherapy – as opposed to another type of intervention – and indeed whether the patient would be able to work well within this approach. Alongside this, it is important for the therapist to consider their own capacity to employ a psychodynamic understanding of the potential patient's difficulties including arriving at a provisional psychodynamic formulation.

Before embarking on psychodynamic psychotherapy, it is customary to offer a consultation process in which we assess the prospective patient's difficulties they are seeking help with (the presenting problem), how that affects their current level of functioning and the links to their developmental history. The assessment should also consider how best to understand what is going on for the patient, namely, the formulation or working hypothesis. This will help us answer the question as to whether psychodynamic psychotherapy is best placed to address those difficulties. In this chapter, we examine both assessment and formulation: these are intricately linked and form the starting point of any course of psychodynamic psychotherapy. Assessment and formulation are key competences across all therapeutic modalities. For a psychodynamic approach, the required competence entails being able to assess whether a *psychodynamic* approach would be suitable for the patient. As we get to know the patient and their level of defensiveness, severity of their symptoms and level of support among other factors, we may decide not to recommend individual once weekly psychodynamic psychotherapy, but rather a referral to social services, CBT to tackle symptom reduction, bereavement counselling or even another form of psychoanalytic treatment such as group therapy or intensive analysis. Some prefer to call the assessment process a consultation because it has therapeutic value in its own right. It conveys a sense of what it is like to embark on psychodynamic psychotherapy and as such is part of establishing the contract and analytic setting. Often the therapist is able to get hold of the patient's difficulties and arrive at a formulation in a condensed and consolidated way, based on wide-ranging clinical material that includes past and present, areas of difficulty and areas of functioning. There are those who believe that only experienced clinicians should carry out psychotherapy assessments because it requires a breadth of knowledge and awareness that exceeds the task at hand. However, given that setting up your clinical practice from the start requires every clinician to assess their own patients, we feel this competence should form part of core trainings in psychodynamic psychotherapy.

What is a psychodynamic assessment?

Each initial encounter with a patient offers the therapist a privileged glimpse into someone's unique world. The challenge for the therapist carrying out the assessment is to get in touch with the patient's particular story and convey some of that understanding back to the patient, thereby deepening the emotional rapport between therapist and patient in the process. The assessment introduces the prospective patient to the model of psychodynamic psychotherapy and invites them to begin to think about their difficulties with an Other. An adjunct to this is the gatekeeping decision about whether the patient is suitable for this approach, and if not, suggesting an alternate way forward. Often, much of what the subsequent work of psychotherapy goes on to discover and unfold is distilled in the initial meeting. An assessment affords the therapist a compressed and succinct shorthand of the patient's difficulties that the ongoing work usually then loses sight of as more and more detail emerges: as we get to know more of the patient, we stop seeing the wood for the trees, so the expression goes, and insights are lost and re-gained. A good assessment will include a psychodynamic formulation, which we will discuss in more detail later in this chapter. Through our questions and stance, we can demonstrate to the patient that we are able to begin understanding and making sense of their difficulties. The patient's likely anxieties and shame at coming for help can be addressed and supplanted with some hope for their future.

The assessment process should allow for unconscious and transference material to emerge without too much hindrance. Excessive structuring and reassurance will interfere with the emergent quality of an initial consultation. At the same time, some structuring of the first encounter can be useful in orienting the patient. The more analytic end of the spectrum may start an initial consultation in silence. We feel that this can be overly challenging in an initial meeting where it is not always clear that someone can make use of an analytically informed approach and particularly where you are working in a health care setting and the assessor is usually not going to be the ongoing therapist. Referring to public health work, Milton (1997) argues that the purpose of an NHS assessment extends beyond suitability for psychodynamic psychotherapy and aims to get of the patient "as good a picture as possible in this limited time, of their inner world and the way it functions, and try to understand the nature of the distress they are presenting with" (p. 47). She argues for the role of the assessment in ruling out who is unsuited for psychotherapy rather than who is suited, namely those for whom psychotherapy would be harmful and/or ineffective (p. 52). This inevitably means considering a wider range of possible psychotherapeutic interventions, not just those you can offer.

You may want to consider whether to offer the assessment in the first place. Spurling (2003) makes a case for the therapeutic value of not offering consultations for psychotherapy and cites a referral where the patient had many years of psychotherapy without any clear benefit. The question then is what help would even more therapy offer? Deciding whether or not to assess for psychotherapy can be difficult to do without seeing the patient in person. However, there are times when it is evident from the referral process that the patient has been bounced from one department to the other, or has had several experiences of therapy all of which have ended badly. What would lead you to believe that this experience would be different? We have to withstand our own inclinations to omnipotence that lead us to imagine we would succeed where others haven't, and our pull to be 'helpful' when it may in fact be the opposite.

Another common reason to decline seeing a patient for treatment would be that the patient is in the process of meeting with another therapist or being assessed concurrently for treatment at another service. Most therapists would agree that multiple therapies at the same time are inadvisable and lend themselves to splitting and enactment (see Chapter 6 for a discussion of splitting). Occasionally the patient may have individual alongside couple therapy or there may be out-patient programs for both group and individual therapy. However, seeing two different individual therapists concurrently is contraindicated. You may consider offering some holding therapy while the person waits for a referral to another service, but this is likely to be more supportive than exploratory in nature.

The purpose of a psychodynamic assessment

An initial meeting serves the purpose of assessing not only the patient's presenting difficulties and needs, but also what the therapist is able to provide. Firstly, the assessment establishes the nature of the patient's difficulties by gathering a history of the patient's presenting problems together with their developmental history and current circumstances. The therapist may be asked to reach a diagnosis at this stage, particularly if working in a public health setting like the NHS and to make recommendations for alternate treatment provision should psychotherapy be considered inappropriate. In private practice, therapists would not be focused on providing a diagnosis, but certainly would need to develop an initial understanding of the problem and how it developed. All of this takes place in the context of establishing a reasonable therapeutic alliance with the patient to facilitate sufficient exploration of their issues during the consultation process.

Secondly, the assessor reflects on the patient's capacities to manage psychodynamic psychotherapy based on the severity of their difficulties, attachment history, current functioning, ego strengths, level of defences, capacity to relate to the therapist and speak in a free and appropriate way about their difficulties, any transference and countertransference observations, level of risk and external resources that may help or hinder the patient's engagement in treatment. All of this contributes to a psychodynamic formulation of the patient (we will explore these aspects further in this chapter).

Thirdly, the assessment conveys the contractual frame and realistic aims for psychotherapy while at the same time motivating the patient to engage in treatment, and conveying a sense of hope for the future. It is important to cover issues of confidentiality and consent as part of this. The patient's material is treated as confidential unless they disclose any risk to self or other, where the therapist then has a duty of care to notify someone else (often the patient's GP). The patient needs to give the therapist consent to write to their doctor about the outcome of the meeting. Consent may also be sought for other reasons, like selective sharing of information in supervision. Another aspect of the frame is agreeing to the terms of therapy including payment, frequency and policies around holidays and missed appointments. The assessment should give the patient a sense of what to expect in psychotherapy and set right any misconceptions about psychotherapy being overly supportive and warm, or psychoeducational and instructive, for example. Patients should be made aware of the unstructured nature of sessions and the rationale for this, including the therapist's interest in their dreams and free associations. The therapist should enquire about the patient's aims for treatment, both conscious and less explicitly stated. All these aspects of the psychotherapeutic frame and contract are discussed in more detail in Chapter 4.

Finally, there is also a need to assess the therapist's abilities, capacity and setting in relation to the particular difficulties the patient brings. You may feel there are certain difficulties that you enjoy working with while others are too provocative or challenging for you. A senior colleague who worked in the confronting area of sexual perversion proclaimed that he would never be able to work with patients who are diagnosed as anorexic because he found their preoccupation with death too painful to engage with. You may be at a point in your life where other demands or your stage of life dictate the type of work you can take on. For example, can you work with more disturbed patients if your consulting room is in your home? Do you have good links with other services that may be needed to sustain the patient in times of crisis? Do you have supervision and other support networks in place for your own mental health? Are you approaching retirement or are there health concerns that may make you want to think about taking on particular patients? Do you have a young family or are planning a child that may restrict your availability? You also need to reflect on your own competences in taking on particular patients. If you do not yet have the required competence, you would need to put in place appropriate support through regular supervision to facilitate developing the necessary skills.

It is important to assess the setting within which you will be seeing the patient. Will you be working alone or in the evening with someone that makes you feel uneasy? Has the patient given you permission to liaise with their doctor? If this is your last appointment of the day, will you have access to a supervisor or senior member of staff if you are left with concerns about the patient's safety? Do you know the location of your nearest Accident and Emergency department of a hospital should your patient present with acute risk? Does your therapy service have links to other departments or services that could provide alternate forms of treatment? We will return to issues around risk management in Chapter 12.

What works for whom?

When making an assessment, the therapist needs to hold in mind what type of psychotherapy is indicated, including whether psychodynamic psychotherapy is the right approach to take. Some of this involves attending to patient preferences: do they want a more structured intervention that helps alleviate symptoms, or do they want something more exploratory that offers a deeper understanding of themselves and their relationships? Psychodynamic psychotherapy is not suitable for everyone.

However, we want to dispel the notion that a psychodynamic assessment is strongly linked to research about what type of therapy is best for whom. In some respects, it is not the type of therapy, but rather the therapeutic relationships that matters most. In their comprehensive research of the evidence around therapy outcomes, Roth and Fonagy (2006) conclude that there is a moderate but consistent fit between therapeutic alliance and outcome, with therapeutic alliance being the most important factor alongside therapeutic technique. They go on to say that "it is most commonly accepted that alliance acts as a moderating variable – a catalytic mode of action that makes treatment more effective" (p. 464).

In Chapter 3, we discussed research into the efficacy of psychodynamic psychotherapy and concluded that chapter by outlining the distinctive features of psychodynamic psychotherapy. With these in mind, we want to consider what factors indicate that a psychodynamic psychotherapy may work for a particular patient. We will return to this question at different points in this chapter as we consider the question of suitability for psychodynamic psychotherapy.

Horowitz et al. (1988; 1993) report that patients who describe their problems in terms of interpersonal difficulties rather than symptoms, tend to have better outcomes in psychodynamic psychotherapy. As discussed in earlier chapters, psychodynamic approaches focus on a developmental and interpersonal understanding of mental health problems. There are other therapists who take the view that everyone should be considered suitable for a trial of psychotherapy and that suitability cannot be determined in advance (e.g. Rothstein, 1998). Wolberg (1995) provides a useful list of positive factors indicated for psychodynamic psychotherapy. These are listed in Box 5.1.

Box 5.1 Positive factors for psychodynamic psychotherapy

1   Strong motivation for therapy (including attending sessions, understanding oneself and willingness to change)
2   Existence of some past successes and positive achievements
3   Presence of at least one good relationship in the past
4   Personality that has permitted adequate coping in the past
5   Symptomatic discomfort related more to anxiety and depression than to somatic complaints
6   Ability to feel and express emotions

7   Capacity for reflection and curiosity
8   Desire for self-understanding
9   Adequate preparation for therapy prior to the referral
10   Belief system that accords with the therapist's theories

Adapted from Wolberg (1995, p. 49)

The referral route

For therapists working in public health services, there are more established referral routes for assessment, usually by the GP or mental health professional in contact with the patient. For those therapists working in private practice, the patient could have been referred to you by a colleague or perhaps they contacted you directly by email, text or phone to request an initial consultation. In today's world, patients will often use google to search for a therapist and may approach you through a search engine or online platform for psychotherapy services. It is always worth enquiring about the way the patient found your details. Were they focused on finding a convenient location or did they research it more carefully? Was there a personal recommendation and if so, are there any boundary issues that may prevent you from seeing this patient if, for example, they know another patient in your practice? Has the patient come across you in a different setting, perhaps hearing you lecture or teach somewhere? More frequently, it seems that patients 'shop around', trying to sort out logistical details like costs, availability and timings before having an initial meeting, or even meeting several therapists before deciding which one to see. One such prospective patient likened the process to going on a series of 'first dates'!

Coltart (1993) points out that in her experience, patients referred for psychotherapy by ex-patients tend to be highly motivated and suitable for psychotherapy. Those who are obligated to have therapy can prove to be trickier patients. Sometimes psychology trainees seek psychotherapy because they think it would be a good idea to know 'what it feels like to be a patient'. This is not motivation enough to commence the often-demanding business of psychotherapy. Others may be obliged to attend by the courts, their partners or families (perhaps as the scapegoat or designated problem) as well as by psychotherapy trainings that require trainees to undertake personal therapy. We feel it is crucial to establish a personal basis for embarking on psychotherapy so that the prospective patient can take ownership of this decision in their own right. Otherwise, therapy can become a tick-box, 'as if' experiment, rather than a genuine endeavour motivated by personal need.

Throughout the assessment process, it is important to retain the space to decide whether we want to work with the patient or not, as well as whether we think psychotherapy would be suited for them. It is all too easy to get caught up in marketing ourselves to a prospective 'customer', particularly as you are establishing your practice. Some patients convey a huge sense of urgency at finding help and this in itself should be a warning sign about the suitability of psychodynamic psychotherapy. It may suggest a preoccupation with symptom relief rather than a capacity to stay with difficult feelings without being prone to acting out between sessions.

When you have had no prior information about a patient, it is advisable to have a brief screening phone call before offering a face-to-face appointment. We would suggest giving the patient a sense of the timeframe for the call, which should usually be no more than ten to fifteen minutes. The phone call allows you to find out what is prompting the patient to seek psychotherapy, whether they have seen other therapists in the past, as well as agreeing a mutually suitable time for an initial meeting should you feel this is indicated. It can be easier to do this 'live' rather than send emails back and forth while you both try to find a suitable time. We would suggest leaving any negotiating of fees to the meeting in person, although you should give an indication of your usual fee. This information can be helpfully held on a professional website (see Chapter 14). You may want to make use of a referral or pre-assessment preparatory questionnaire which you can send the prospective patient by email ahead of meeting, something that is routinely carried out in public health and charity settings as well as reduced fee therapy schemes. This serves the purpose of helping the patient focus their thoughts, and also provides you with some preliminary information to hold in mind when it comes to conducting the assessment. We have provided a pro forma questionnaire in Appendix 2.

It is important to keep an open mind when you do find out information about the patient prior to seeing them. We have had experiences of hearing biographical information that fills us with worry and concern yet being met by someone who elicits a very different response in person. It is critical to pay attention to your countertransference throughout the consultation process. Are you feeling seduced by a flattering patient? Are you pulled to reject a patient and thereby repeat the pattern of interpersonal relating they have been describing throughout their lives? Are you feeling overly maternal and protective towards a patient? We have described the therapist's role responsiveness and countertransference in Chapter 9, which is often at play from the start.

The different roles of assessor and therapist in organisational settings

In the public health service or training institution, the assessor is usually a different person to the therapist they will go on to see for treatment. If you are the assessor, you should tell the patient that they will be allocated to another therapist. Despite brochures, emails and letters communicating this, often patients arrive at the consultation after a considerable wait and feel as if they are starting treatment. Patients should be made aware of this being a consultation since it may inform how deeply they explore issues with you. It also avoids a potentially difficult reaction when this emerges towards the end of the consultation. Schachter (1997) describes how this gatekeeper function during assessment steered her central aim away from exploring the transference relationship and towards engaging "the patient in talking about their inner world of unconscious feelings, conflicts and anxieties, to the extent that these can be deduced from the material available" (p. 58). She warns that too exclusive a focus on the transference during the assessment may be at the expense of exploring other areas of the patient's life and could jeopardise the safety of the patient and efficacy of treatment. The exception is where there is an overtly negative transference that would need to be interpreted in order to avoid a rupture that would prevent engaging in treatment altogether.

Spurling (2003) writes about the responsibilities incumbent in carrying out NHS assessments that include considering the various expectations and needs of patients, referrers and an overstretched waiting list, as follows: "The gatekeeper functions as a kind of immigration officer patrolling the borders of the psychotherapy department and deciding who will be granted admission" (pp. 3–4). To this, we can add the pressure of assessments for training therapists, where patients who drop out of treatment or are unsuitable in other ways, end up impacting adversely on the difficult road towards qualifying as a psychotherapist. There are pressures when your assessment report will be shared with a training organisation and another professional then decides on the basis of your report whether the patient is suitable for a training therapist, exposing our assessment and evaluation to peer scrutiny.

When working in an organisational setting, it is always worth asking yourself whether you would be willing to see the patient for psychotherapy rather than putting someone on the waiting list because you think they deserve a chance at getting help. If you and the patient had a tricky engagement during the assessment, you may want to consider the possibility of the patient being assessed by another person in your team, so that these particular dynamics don't cloud your decision to offer treatment or not. Similarly, when a patient has to wait for an extended period of time, it is useful to offer them regular review sessions so as to keep abreast of their state of mind and any changes in their circumstances, including managing any risk issues.

Conducting an assessment

An assessment is not a therapy session. We outlined above the purpose of the assessment, which requires a focused conversation in order to gather the necessary information alongside more emergent processes that give the patient a taster of psychodynamic psychotherapy. We focus on this section on how an assessment can be conducted, including how many sessions to offer, how to start and end the assessment and the necessary topics to cover.

How many sessions to offer?

Some therapists offer a one-off extended assessment of up to two hours (e.g. Coltart, 1993) while others prefer to offer several 50-minute appointments over a period of several weeks, where the patient and therapist have a chance to go away and think about what happened in the encounter and explore any emotional impact stirred up by the process (Garelick, 1994; Schachter, 1997). The Tavistock Clinic in the UK offers an extended consultation service for young adults, and this four-session model has been found to have therapeutic benefits in its own right (Searle et al., 2011). The downside of the extended assessment model is that the patient is likely to form a deepening attachment and transference to the therapist and/or clinic. This can make it trickier either to refer the patient on to another therapist or decline psychotherapy altogether. You may want to see what works best for your practice and setting. In our experience, seeing patients for two assessments, no more than a few weeks apart, is a useful compromise between these two approaches. If you do feel that the person is unsuited to work with you in this approach, you have some time to explore alternate options that you can then discuss with the patient.

You may want to keep a regular assessment slot open in your diary, where you have access to a longer period of time within which to see prospective new patients. An assessment is time-consuming beyond the time of the meeting because you then have to write up your report of the encounter, inform the referrer of the outcome (where applicable) and possibly refer the patient on to a suitable therapist or service. If you are working in an NHS setting, you will also have to do a range of mandatory reports that include inputting and scoring departmental outcome measures, completing risk assessments, evaluating clinical severity and assigning psychiatric diagnoses. You may find that while you are unable to place a patient in your practice, you can recommend a colleague with a vacancy at an appropriate time and fee for the patient. In this way, you can develop a helpful network of contacts and support infrastructure in the isolated world of the sole practitioner.

How to start an assessment

This initial encounter can be confusing and challenging for prospective patients and can throw up doubts about someone's ability to survive, let alone thrive in psychodynamic psychotherapy. A psychodynamic assessment is very different to a psychiatric assessment that is more structured, where the expert doctor takes the lead and writes down notes during the meeting. We would not expect the assessor to write anything down while the assessment is unfolding because this sets up the clinician as the expert and means the patient may start to pay attention to what is deemed worthy of being written down and what is not, thereby colouring the experience and compromising the neutrality of the setting.

Coltart (1993) described her practice of shaking hands with the patient, saying their name and then introducing herself by name to establish the frame of the assessment as well as orienting the patient to the consultation frame. This includes pointing out where the bathroom is, where they should sit and how long the consultation will last. We recommend a minimal amount of orientation to the purpose of the meeting by starting in an open-ended way by saying, "What brought you to seek psychotherapy?" We may invite the patient by asking, "Where would you like to start?" (see Box 5.2 for a list of some useful questions that could be asked in an assessment). This more organic approach requires the therapist to follow the patient at the point where they choose to begin their narrative. Alternately, we may say to a prospective patient that we know something about them from the referral or their earlier conversation with us and that this is an opportunity to explore their current difficulties that have brought them to seek therapy now. At this point, we would sit back and see what the person does with our invitation. If the patient is unable to respond to this open-ended question, you can then prompt the patient. However, we are trying to see whether the patient can make use of a more open-ended space to express and explore their difficulties. If the patient keeps looking for direction from us, it can suggest that they would be better suited to a more structured and/or supportive type of intervention. Initial awkwardness or self-conscious inhibition may settle down, allowing a rapport to develop between therapist and patient.

When we listen to the narratives the person relates during the assessment, we are listening not only to what they are telling us but also what is omitted. It is important for the therapist to consider what is being left out by the patient in their account. For example, does the patient focus on their work to the exclusion of their intimate relationships, or vice versa? Do they focus only on themselves and not on others? Do they present an overly cognitive version of events and neglect their affects, or vice versa? We would want to explore those topics and areas that we sense the patient is avoiding. We may choose not to confront the patient with these discrepancies but instead, to carry them in our minds. This fluid structure of the assessment gives us a sense of where the person's defences are operating as well as where their preoccupations lie.

This open-ended conversation would probably weave back and forth from the presenting problem to early and recent history as well as other key relationships. Holmes (1995) likens the psychotherapy assessment to a friendly chess game in which there are an infinite number of moves that he divides into opening gambits, middle and end games:

> In opening the interview I proceed in a fairly standard way with each patient; the middle game includes attempts at interpretation and observation of their affective impact; and the end consists of a gathering up of the threads and coming to a decision about what it to happen next. (p. 28)

Let's turn to some clinical material to illustrate what we have been saying:

> *Alicia was referred to me by her GP for chronic depression. The GP gave a sketchy history of Alicia as the youngest daughter of four children. She had lived with her mother until her death four years ago and never recovered from her loss that coincided with the end of her only serious romantic relationship. She had no children and was socially isolated. She had worked in the past as a social worker but took a leave of absence to care for her mother and had been unable to return to employment since. I was aware that there was no mention of her father in this account. The GP said Alicia was ashamed about needing help yet unable to overcome her own difficulties. He had prescribed anti-depressants, but these were not*

helping shift her unresolved grief. Alicia was now open to considering a psychotherapy referral because nothing else had been helpful.

Alicia arrived on time. She was a Caucasian woman in her early forties, with a beehive hairstyle and a lined face yet she was dressed like a teenage girl in a denim pinafore with bright green leggings and candy-striped T-shirt. This created a confusing first impression of her as operating across two different ages. It also didn't match the depressed woman I was expecting to find. After discussing the referral and confidentiality, I explained that this appointment was a chance to think together about her difficulties and whether psychotherapy is the right way forward.

Alicia said: Yes, I'm quite nervous being here and what the outcome will be, to be honest. I didn't sleep very well last night. I've had quite a few closed doors.

[I was aware of several possible lines of enquiry at this point: who had closed doors to this patient in the past when she sought therapy? What had kept her up last night? I also wanted to address the anxiety about an assessment today with me and felt under pressure to already agree to offer her therapy given she had raised the outcome of the consultation from the outset. I chose to acknowledge her anxiety and open up discussion about why she was looking for therapy at this point. There are alternative directions that other therapists may have followed, like taking up her anxiety and/or transference more directly.]

I said: It sounds like you've come desperately wanting psychotherapy and aware there is no guarantee that you will be offered it. I know a little bit about your difficulties from your referral and it would be useful to get an idea of what brings you here today.

Alicia responded: I guess at the moment, I'm really depressed and struggling to get through each day, to be honest. I can't find a purpose to my life and it's an effort most mornings to get out of bed. That's the most difficult time of day for me. As soon as I wake up, I don't have any energy. I am tired all the time. Even after I've slept, I can't face the day ahead. (She laughs). I don't really understand my life. I am lost and it seems a struggle to keep existing, finding the energy to keep going. Then there's the judgmental side of me saying, people are worse off than you. Refugees are camped in tents risking their lives to get to Europe. So, this feels indulgent (She sighs). What reason do I have to be depressed? A lot has happened to me in the last five years. Every episode feels like I am pushed and punched and it's a fight to get up, like being in the boxing ring. When will I get the knock-out blow? I'm against the ropes (more laughter), trying to clamber up.

[I was aware of her conveying a vivid description of her desperation with oblique suicidal references to not being able to continue with her life while at the same time inviting me to minimise her distress (e.g. comparing herself to refugees). I made a mental note to assess her risk later in the consultation. I also wondered if at some unconscious level, she felt like a refugee in her own life. I decided to underline the distress she was bringing, thereby indicating my interest in her acute emotional states and I linked it to her fear of another knock-out blow from the consultation (the emerging transference)].

I said: I'm hearing what a real struggle the past five years has been and your worry that I won't take your distress seriously and another door will be closed…

Alicia interrupted me, saying: It's been one thing after another over this time. First my mum died after a year of battling breast cancer and I had to take time off work to take her to chemotherapy, because none of my siblings were able to do it and that wasn't surprising actually because I always was left caring for mum. I ended up leaving my social work job before I was fired. Then my partner of six years walked out on me. I had a couple of brief relationships after that, but they also ended badly. The last straw was two close friends in the past year decided they no longer wanted to see me. It feels there are less and less people in my life.

[Again, here are several lines of enquiry that I could follow, depending on which direction I want to go in: past or present, outside or inside the consulting room. What did the loss of her mother mean to her? She has hinted at difficult sibling relationships and I was curious about why she as the youngest child had assumed the caregiving role in this family. Did this tally with her working as a social worker? What area of social work had she been involved with? I noticed that her father was absent from the account. A pattern was emerging of someone who felt abandoned and this formed a cautionary tale of how she might feel entering into psychotherapy and her expectations of this repeating in the therapeutic relationship. In my countertransference, I felt overwhelmed by too many losses and so, I elected to focus on the most recent loss of the friendship, which she had signalled was the last straw that brought her to seek help].

I said: You've described a lot of painful losses and how the loss of your friendships was the last straw. How do you understand these friends breaking off contact?

Alicia replied: Well, one was a misunderstanding. She just thinks I'm not caring ... (she tailed off).

I waited to see if she would come back to say more, but after several minutes of silence, I prompted her: Can you tell me what happened?

[Here I am aware that the patient holds back and pulls me into a position of having to come and find her, to push and prompt her to continue. Again, I am hypothesizing about what this might say about her early experience of her caregivers. Was there a depressed mother who disengaged from Alicia, leaving her dropped from her mind? In this way, we can see how an experience of here-and-now relationships contains clues about the early then-and-there relationships of her past as well as hinting at the transference relationship with the therapist].

Alicia went on to give an account of how her friend was going through her own depression following a family bereavement and a misunderstanding that emerged where Alicia was not aware of how affected her friend was. This led to an email exchange in which Alicia felt told off for not being understanding enough of her friend's low mood, which she experienced as an unfair and critical attack. She felt accused of not caring about her friend and withdrew from any contact.

It is not possible to replicate the entire consultation here, but we hope that this excerpt from the start of the process conveys a sense of the various choices the therapist has, and how each thread may lead to different information being uncovered. It is impossible in the process of a consultation to elucidate all the patient's history; however, we are working with the hypotheses we construct in our mind, based on observation of the process as well as the content of the interview and we then test these out by evaluating the way the patient responds to our interventions and trial interpretations. In this way, we can obtain a picture of the patient's psychodynamics and thereby reach an informed decision about the way forward, whether that is to offer another consultation or move to contracting around the start of treatment.

We need to balance unstructured exploration with obtaining essential information in order to carry out this assessment of the patient's needs and treatment recommendations. We turn to these now.

What key information needs to be covered in an initial assessment?

The therapist needs to balance supportive containment with exploration, in the knowledge that an assessment may not necessarily be followed by treatment and indeed, in a public health service, there is often a wait to be seen by a therapist. We recommend that this wait is kept to a minimum where possible, out of respect to the patient and to keep alive the hope for help that the assessment has introduced. In an assessment, the assessor has an opportunity to ask questions and be curious in a way that would be considered overly intrusive during subsequent psychotherapy, including obtaining a detailed history of the patient. As Coltart (1993) writes: "my feeling about getting a good history is: 'Now's your chance!'" (p. 79). If the therapist is also the assessor, it is still relevant to take a few sessions to gather this information and conduct a thorough assessment which forms the foundation of the ongoing work. This avoids making spurious interpretations down the line that are not based on details of the patient's history but on generalisations and over-reliance on the transference.

1 Why now?

The starting point of an assessment is the presenting problem and how the patient makes sense of their current difficulties. There is usually a gap between the referral letter and the time of the assessment in the NHS. It is helpful to acknowledge any waiting period and be mindful of how the patient may be feeling about coming for help. Sometimes, we can forget that the act of coming forward to put into words what is troubling a person can be experienced as so exposing, even dangerous, that it leaves patients feeling very stirred up. Something has usually broken down in a patient to make them seek help now. This can be related to the age or stage of life they are at, and there may be links with other significant events or people in their life. It is important to answer the question 'Why now?' in order to understand why the patient has come for help at this juncture. Has there been an exacerbation in their difficulties and what has contributed to this? Has therapy been prompted by someone else laying down an ultimatum or recent changes? Sometimes, a crisis is triggered upon reaching a particular stage in life that chimes with parallel events in significant others' lives (like turning 40 which was the age their father was when he abandoned his marriage and family; or having a small child of the same age they were when they were put into care). Patients can also present for help at developmental stages in life where life is not progressing as expected or they are facing challenges like difficulties posed by infertility, parental challenges, an empty nest, significant illness or bereavement. We are curious about whether the patient can connect key life events with an exacerbation in their difficulties and resultant wish to get help. Long gaps between these events may raise questions about the patient's resistance to treatment.

A later event in the patient's life can trigger earlier traumas and reawaken an unresolved conflict or issue. Freud spoke about the concept of 'nachträglichkeit', which Strachey translated as 'deferred action' and which the French analysts termed 'après coup'; it has also been described by the neologism, 'afterwardsness' to synthesise the deferral and retroaction of Freud's term (Laplanche, 1999). The concept refers to the way in which a later event reactivates an early trauma that has been repressed from memory. The earlier trauma becomes accessible again and can be reworked and integrated after this protective delay. The following clinical example is provided to illustrate this:

> *Jamal arrived at his initial appointment complaining of panic attacks that filled him with dread. These began after he was made redundant from his job after a bruising relationship with his demanding and critical female manager. All his earlier confidence had leached away. He felt unable to face job interviews, convinced he would never be able to work again. In exploring other events in his life that contributed to his heightened state of panic, it emerged that his partner was putting pressure on him to start a family and he felt trapped at the thought of what this would mean. Links were made to his own childhood, where he was acutely aware of the financial strain his parents were under as emigrants to this country and their expectations that he would make the most of their sacrifices by excelling at school in order to secure a well-paid job after university. He became aware of his own anger at finding himself in a familiar situation at work and imagining that he would repeat this in turn with his partner. As he made these connections, his motivation to address these dynamics increased because he did not want to repeat the same patterns with his own children.*

To adopt the language of clinical psychology for a moment, we want to identify the precipitating factors for the current difficulties and link these to the predisposing factors. In assessing suitability for psychodynamic psychotherapy, we would like to identify clear motivations for seeking help that are more ego syntonic (in keeping with the conscious goals and needs of the ego) since this bodes well for the patient's future engagement in psychotherapy. As Thomä and Kächele (1987) put it, the patient needs to be "sick enough to need it [i.e. psychotherapy] and healthy enough to stand it" (p. 184).

2 Current circumstances

We want to form a view of the patient's relationship to external reality by asking about their current level of functioning and living arrangements. What is their housing situation? Do they have a support and/or social network? Are they working? Have they been able to hold down a job for a sustained period of time? How do they spend their leisure time? Do they find their relationships with others pleasurable or satisfying? We would be concerned about isolated and disconnected individuals with impoverished social connections. Instability in the workplace may foreshadow difficulties in settling into psychotherapy and raise the likelihood of a therapeutic rupture. We would also be on the alert for individuals lacking stability around their basic human needs for physiological safety and security, as represented by the lower rungs of Maslow's (1943) hierarchy of needs. It is impossible – indeed counterproductive – for someone to explore their internal and interpersonal world in psychotherapy if they have no safety and stability in their lives. States of homelessness, domestic violence, substance abuse, unemployment and extreme insomnia need to be attended to as a matter of priority. This is often part of the assessment process: to evaluate whether the person has the external and internal resources to begin psychotherapy. In such cases, it is often prudent to suggest that practical help and support is put in place first before starting therapy. In the UK, the NHS is a useful starting point to link patients into local support services and there may be specialist provision for particular groups of the population such as shelters, employment support or substance abuse programs.

3 Developmental and attachment/relationship history

Schachter points out that "implicit in history-taking is the idea that the present problems are rooted in the past" (1997, p. 63). In taking a history, we are conveying the premise of psychodynamic psychotherapy to the prospective patient. We want to map the key interpersonal relationships across different areas and times of the person's life. How do they experience romantic relationships? How do they relate to authority figures? We particularly want to ask about the person's previous experiences of help, whether this was psychotherapy, counselling or other forms of treatment. These can provide useful pointers towards the likely transference towards starting therapy with us. We want to get a picture of early relationships to parental and key figures in their lives. Families are not always straightforward with reconstituted families, half siblings, step-parents, same sex couples and so on, confronting us with our assumptions about tidy nuclear families of mum, dad and two children.

While exploring the patient's history and relationships, it is essential to observe the patient's emotional responses. We would be concerned where the patient's affects are very disconnected from the content of what they are describing. Some patients smile or laugh while describing awful trauma or abuse. Such a disconnect of content from affect suggests the operation of defences such as denial and splitting and would inform our thoughts about the challenges psychodynamic psychotherapy may pose for the patient. Garelick (1994) describes the particular way we explore the history in a psychodynamic assessment:

> The history-taking is from the psychoanalytic perspective: the assessor tunes himself into the affective qualities of the people described, rather than focusing on the factual information; this can be known but quite split off in terms of emotional meaning. Idealisation, for example, often reveals itself in the manner and the way a parent is spoken about. Similarly, it is of note when important family-members are not mentioned; or are mentioned, but colourlessly, in a way that makes it impossible for the assessor to form a picture of them in his own mind. (p. 107)

By mapping key relationships and understanding the aetiology of the patient's difficulties, we can start to identify repeated patterns of interaction that allow us to formulate the patient's struggles and conflicts, both external and internal. This is worked on transparently and collaboratively with the patient in brief psychotherapy in order to agree a focus for the work, something we elaborate in Chapter 11 on brief psychotherapy.

The developmental history will give you a picture of key stages of change in the patient's life and how these were managed, as well as any evident points of delay or fixation. We would explore any early signs of difficulties around feeding, sleeping, toilet training, managing separations, peer relationships and school life that can then be mapped on to later problems in adulthood. For example, early separations from caregivers may link with later depression and an insecure attachment style, while struggles around sleeping as a child may connect with clingy interpersonal relationships in later life.

It is important to get a clear history of the patient's reaction to losses and separations in life since this gives you an indication of how the patient may respond to breaks in therapy and ultimately to ending treatment. There can be a pattern of 'not-enough-ness' as well as 'too-much-ness'. We need to be alert to those patients who form adhesive attachments early on, where there is more likelihood for difficulties around separations and endings. This links with Ogden's (1992) notion of the cautionary tale, a glimpse of the unfolding transference to the therapist (see Chapter 9 for further discussion of this). We may be able to pre-empt the patient's characteristic way of dealing with conflict or disappointments in relationships (for example, by cutting and running), by flagging this with the patient during the assessment process so as to avoid this being repeated yet again with us.

We may want to borrow the following approach of the adult attachment interview (George et al., 1996), whereby we ask the patient for five adjectives that characterise their relationship with each parent, following which we ask for anecdotal elaborations of those descriptors. This approach gives you a better sense of the quality of their attachments. Too often, patients say, "I had a happy childhood" yet they cannot give any substantiating examples, or their anecdotes relate to the perfunctory aspects of family life, like being fed, clothed and housed.

> *I asked Megan during an initial assessment to describe her relationship with her mother. She seemed flummoxed at this seemingly straightforward question, shrugged her shoulders and said that she was her mother, what more could she say about it? She was evidently uncomfortable at her inability to reflect on her relationships; indeed, she struggled to reflect on her own experiences. Yet it was possible to embark on therapy despite these limitations.*

We are not engaged in a search for the 'perfect patient', as if that ever existed. Rather, we are using the process to flag any concerns we have. This alerts us to areas in the work that will need careful attention and care; at times, this may lead to the difficult decision of declining to offer treatment.

Box 5.2 Examples of useful exploratory questions for an assessment

At the start of an assessment

- How do you understand your current difficulties?
- What brought you to seek psychotherapy?
- Where would you like to start?
- I know a bit about you, but it would be helpful if you could tell me in your own words what brought you here today/why you are looking for help?
- What was on your mind as you thought about today's appointment?
- What was going through your mind as you were sitting in the waiting area?

When asking about a developmental and relationship history

- Who is significant in your life?
- Tell me about your family of origin and the nature of those relationships?
- With whom are you closest and most distance?
- How would you describe your mother/father? Then, ask for examples to illustrate these adjectives.
- What is your earliest memory?
- Have you suffered from any significant losses/illnesses/separations in your life?
- Which interpersonal relationships help you feel better or worse?
- Can you tell me about a recent dream you have had?
- What do you daydream about?
- What are your secret/private ambitions?

Asking about symptoms

- What situations do you find stressful?
- Do you feel better or worse when you are alone or with others?
- Who has a calming, soothing effect on you?
- Who do you feel better being with?
- Who is affected by your difficulties?
- Do your difficulties spill over into all areas of your life or does it affect one area more than others?
- What do you think about just before falling asleep at night?

4 Psychiatric and medical history

In a psychodynamic assessment, we are not carrying out a formal psychiatric interview with a mental state examination and diagnosis. However, we should familiarise ourselves with signs and symptoms of major psychiatric and medical illnesses so that we can be alert to any indications of syndromes or conditions that may require specialist attention. It is critical to get a good sense of possible psychiatric symptoms around depression and anxiety, including suicidal thoughts and intent, flashbacks and other signs of trauma, psychotic processes, organic disturbances, severe personality disorders, eating and substance disorders. If you feel concerned about the significance of someone's symptoms, then it is helpful to get clinical supervision and potentially refer the patient to a psychiatrist or their GP for further investigation. Blood deficiencies like hypothyroidism and anaemia can mimic psychological symptoms of depression, for example. If you have doubts about the meaning of the person's presentation, then it is important to have colleagues with whom you can consult to consider the significance of the clinical material.

> *Roberto was sent to see me for a psychotherapy consultation after having had a difficult time on holiday with his girlfriend. He described a period of hearing voices and seeing visual hallucinations that he put down to taking a drug several days earlier. The two experiences did not add up in my mind and I thought it was important to rule out a psychotic illness. I referred him for a psychiatric evaluation to ensure this was fully investigated.*

Seeing someone with a poor grip on reality is a poor prognostic indicator for psychodynamic psychotherapy, in our view. As mentioned earlier, you can choose to use a screening questionnaire or referral questionnaire (we have included one in Appendix 2) as a way of preparing the patient for the assessment process and to ensure you have covered the key areas of information. Given that the more structure we introduce to the assessment process and analytic frame, the less emergent it becomes and the more aware the patient becomes of our 'agenda', we leave it up to you as to whether you use such forms in your own private practice.

We want to ask about any medication the patient routinely takes, including prescribed and recreational drugs. It is not enough to ask whether someone drinks alcohol, for example. It is important to understand the frequency and amount that is consumed. It is commonly accepted that most people underestimate how much they drink, wanting to present as more prudent than they are, whether consciously or unconsciously. There are different patterns of problematic substance abuse that include addictive patterns of regular, sustained and increasing levels of consumption as well as patterns of bingeing that alternate with times of abstinence or low use. A useful question is to ask patients if anyone in their lives has ever complained about their use of substances. It is also be useful to ask if their substance use has interfered with their personal lives or their ability to function at work. We would be curious about the function of the substance use. Often people self-medicate with alcohol and drugs when they have underlying psychological or psychiatric conditions. For example, people with social phobia may turn to alcohol to gain 'Dutch courage' in intimidating social situations while patients with bipolar mood disorder are known to use substances to slow themselves down or speed up.

5 Risk

It is important to assess risk directly with the patient. If you are in a service that uses outcome measures and questionnaires, then you should pay attention to the questions related to risk since these form part of the patient's communication to you, albeit indirect. A raised score on items around risk of harm to self or others should be explored further to establish the severity of the risk. A distinction is drawn between suicidal *ideation* and *intent*. Many patients can have passive thoughts that they would be better off dead or that they can't see the point to their lives (suicidal ideation) and we would want to know whether these ever progress into planning ways of acting on those thoughts (suicidal intent). Part of the risk assessment includes establishing the protective factors that inhibit the patient from making any suicidal gestures: who or what in your life stops you acting on those feelings or thoughts? It is important to ask whether the person has ever made any suicide attempts in the past and how these were dealt with. Details of past suicide attempts provide important information about times of crisis and allow us to ascertain the risks going forward.

It is important to elaborate on any family history of suicide, since this is a known predictor of risk. The more people in the person's life who have killed themselves, the more seriously we would take their own suicidality. In assessing risks, we enquire about past breakdowns while also anticipating the nature of a possible breakdown were the patient to enter psychodynamic treatment and ascertaining what support systems the patient has in place. We can expect that their worst form of breakdown is likely to recur at some point during the course of extended psychotherapy (Milton, 1997). These considerations will inform the assessor's thinking about the frequency and form of psychotherapy.

We know that often it is those patients who say nothing about their suicidal thoughts that pose the greatest risk. Asking someone if they feel suicidal or have any plans to kill themselves is no guarantee of full risk disclosure. Yet, being able to speak about this openly with patients and show that you are able to bear knowing about how awful things can be for them, can assist with bringing these issues to awareness and allowing the risk to be managed in a more transparent way. Risky behaviour that occurs impulsively or in the context of states of intoxication is more challenging to manage. Evaluating risk is a dynamic process that will change from moment to moment, requiring ongoing assessment beyond the initial consultation.

You may want to consider using specific contracts around risk with patients who present with a greater suicide risk, along the lines suggested by Yeoman et al. (2015). This was developed for Kernberg's Transference Focused Psychotherapy model for Borderline Personality Disorder where patients often grapple with suicidal states of mind. The contract is arrived at jointly with the patient and usually considers three scenarios, as follows:

1   The patient has suicidal ideation and feels they can control their behaviour
2   The patient waits to discuss the impulse in the subsequent session.

3   The patient feels they cannot control the suicidal impulse
4   The patient manages the risk by using external supports or going to A&E where they will be assessed. If they are discharged, they would return to therapy; or they may be hospitalised and would return to treatment after the admission. The therapist will only engage with the patient if they use the wider system to safeguard themselves; if they refuse to engage with A&E or hospitalisation, they are discharged.
5   The patient has taken suicidal action
6   The patient goes to hospital where they are evaluated, and the decision is taken to either discharge them back to therapy or admit them to hospital.

(Yeomans et al., 2015, p. 125)

The therapist contracts explicitly with the patient to retain therapeutic neutrality and keep active involvement in the patient's suicidal impulses and actions outside the therapeutic relationship by asking the patient to be in charge of evaluating when they feel unable to contain their suicidality and to engage with the agreed emergency procedures, thereby safeguarding themselves. The steps to safeguard themselves could include calling family or friends, a crisis line or going to the Accident & Emergency department of a nearby hospital. In this way, the therapist remains outside the "decision-making and action-taking 'loop'" (Yeomans et al, 2015, p. 127). The patient also agrees to accept the recommendations that arise from this evaluation. Ongoing therapy is contingent on the patient going along with this process. The guiding principle is that therapy needs to feel safe to explore what is on the patient's mind and that safety is compromised when the risks are too great.

The realistic limits of the therapeutic situation are made explicit. For example, Yeomans et al. (2015) would say something along these lines to the risky patient:

> your life is ultimately in your hands; although I can try to help you gain more mastery over your self-destructiveness, I cannot guarantee your safety – only you can do that. If you have taken suicidal actions, such as an overdose, and then decide to try and save your life, your responsibility would be to get to an emergency room for a medical evaluation and subsequent psychiatric evaluation. (p. 127)

Yeomans et al. (2015) argue that it is important that the therapist establishes these boundaries in relation to the patient's suicidality and their feelings of omnipotence that often underpin their risky behaviour. They state that these boundaries are intended to contain the patient's anxiety and increase autonomy. Understandably, it is helpful to work with a supportive team so that the therapist feels contained and able to hold this position.

A meta-competence for psychodynamic psychotherapy is to be able to establish an appropriate balance between supportive and interpretative work. With a suicidal patient, more supportive work is usually required. The more suicidal the patient, the more we may question the value of interpretive psychotherapy for the patient at this time. Psychotherapy is demanding in its own right, and the patient needs to have sufficient ego resources to manage these demands. We would try not to overload an already stretched system and may think about more supportive or specialised interventions as a first line of treatment. Mentalisation Based Therapy, Dialectical Behavioural Therapy and Transference Focused Psychotherapy are designed to deal explicitly with emotional dysregulation and ensuing risk issues.

There are other forms of risky behaviour that need to be explored during the consultation process, like self-harm, eating disorders, substance abuse, sexual promiscuity, unprotected sex, stepping into the traffic without looking, taking risks while driving and so on. We previously touched on the use of substances for self-medication; substance abuse usually increases levels of risk, including driving under the influence or being vulnerable to sexual assault.

> *Rihanna, a young female patient once told me about going to a party in the countryside in the middle of winter and getting so drunk, she passed out in the snow and almost died of hypothermia. This may not have been understood by her as a suicide attempt, but it felt extremely troubling to me as the assessor.*

We would be particularly concerned about any memory lapses that relate to substance misuse, particularly alcohol-induced black outs. This suggests a more dangerous and sustained level of substance abuse. Some of this may be contextualised by the person's age and circumstances. We probably think differently about a university student who reports drinking copiously when socialising with friends over the weekend and an elderly person who drinks heavily alone in the evenings. We would be alert to the person's response to the account they are giving us. Do they feel any remorse over what they are saying or is it presented in an underplayed or defiant way? Many therapists will not work with patients with a primary substance abuse and require the patient to demonstrate at least six months of abstinence before commencing psychodynamic psychotherapy.

When to consider the role for psychotropic medication

Many patients have already been prescribed a course of anti-depressants by their GP before or concurrent with starting psychotherapy. Research has shown that nearly half of depressed patients have discontinued their anti-depressant medication within the first month (Powell, 2001). Often, there is a poor or partial response to medication that leads the patient to seek psychotherapy (Fonagy et al., 2015). Similarly, some patients reach the decision to come off their medication once their psychotherapy is established. It can be an important step to feel that the benefits they are experiencing belong to the work they are doing in therapy rather than attributable to drugs. It is important to explore the meaning of the wish for medication and the transference implications around the timing of this. Is the request to go on to medication cropping up just as the therapist is about to go on an extended summer holiday? Is the patient wishing to be self-reliant and reduce their growing dependency on the therapist in a healthy or defensive way? Is a patient letting you know via their wish to start medication that the 'dose' of therapy is insufficient? Does the patient feel too much for you and is trying to lessen the perceived burden they perceive themselves to be through medication? Does the patient believe that medication represents a quick way of alleviating their pain, as opposed to the slow, often painful work of psychotherapy? And yet, we know that while medication may help with the neuro-vegetative symptoms of depression (like insomnia, poor appetite, decreased appetite), it does not address its causes, which is why it is used in combination with therapy, as stated by NHS England (www.nhs.uk/conditions/antidepressants).

There may be times when it is appropriate for a patient to explore the adjunct of medication and dismissing this altogether can be understood as a show of the therapist's omnipotence. This may apply particularly when the patient is stirred up by a recent change or loss. It may also be based on the patient's past psychiatric history of break downs, where the assessor insists on a full psychiatric evaluation as a precondition of treatment. It is helpful to have contact with the patient's GP so that you can raise these concerns with a third person. However, Powell (2001) cautions around a split transference whereby important information is missed when discussions around medication take place outside the consulting room with different practitioners. In the past, it was seen as unhelpful for the treating psychiatrist to also prescribe medication for their patients because it represented a shift into the directive role of caregiver doctor and a likely defence from feelings of helplessness in the face of the patient's difficulties. Medication can become the language for talking about particular aspects of the patient's difficulties and may hold the negative transference towards the therapist (Powell, 2001).

Powell (2001) considers that the patient's 'medication life' can hold rich and significant meaning, in much the same way we think about their sex life, dream life, working life and so on: "When we allow ourselves to listen for unconscious meanings, the possibilities for discovery involving medication are boundless" (p. 219). She advocates paying attention to the latent content of the patient's responses to medication, including the transference and countertransference:

> Questions about the medications, side effect presentation, request for refills, handling of pills, choice of time when pills are taken, storing of tablets, sharing of medication information with other people, and relationship with the pharmacist provide bountiful detail about our patients. These details highlight the patient's level of ego functioning, ability to connect with others, self-advocacy, and favoured defenses. (p. 219)

The act of prescribing is just that, an enactment, yet this may not mean that it is off-limits. There may be times when we have great concern about the level of symptomatology the patient displays at assessment or during the course of therapy. It is likely that overly high levels of anxiety suggest likely difficulty in tolerating psychotherapy, where the patient may become even more stirred up. Interestingly, the converse situation of no evident anxiety in the patient is also concerning to the assessor, leaving us to wonder about the level of repression, denial or disavowal at play.

Bringing the assessment to a close

As the end of the consultation session approaches, it is important to set time aside to summarise what has been covered and focus on recommendations and next steps. This may be something you are ready to do in the moment or you may want to take time to reflect on the assessment and discuss it with your supervisor or team. You may want to obtain the patient's permission to speak to their previous psychotherapist, psychiatrist or doctor to obtain collateral history or access to their records. You may also want to schedule a follow up appointment to continue the assessment process.

It is useful to allow time for the patient to ask any questions they may have about therapy, your qualifications and so on, as well as to ask them if there is anything significant in their lives that they have not told you about during the course of the consultation. This can bring to light important information that would otherwise have been omitted. Towards the end of the consultation, it is helpful to ask the patient to reflect on this experience and how it compared to their expectations. Sometimes patients will say they expected to feel judged and criticised, or that the therapist would be a blank screen and say very little. Sometimes patients comment on how surprised they are that they were able to speak about a particular issue with you and that they had not expected to share this much at an initial meeting. All of this feedback is helpful in gaining insight into the patient's internal object world and detecting possible cautionary tales in relation to starting treatment. It also lays down 'transference tracers' (Allen et al., 2008, p. 189), indicating to the patient that we consider the therapeutic relationship a significant part of this way of working.

It is possible to discuss other treatment modalities or areas the patient needs to address as part of their commitment to therapy. These may include protecting their busy schedules by making a regular time to attend sessions, pointing to a possible increase in session frequency going forward, highlighting likely challenges for the patient in therapy and when the assessor is not the therapist, suggesting they address this in therapy as far as possible. There may be a need to tackle particular defences or difficulties in order to support psychotherapy, such as reducing or abstaining from alcohol and drugs, addressing defensive and destructive behaviours, finding paid work or volunteering, structuring their week and time as well as considering medication or other medical investigations.

The end of the assessment process also introduces the analytic contract. You should allow time to discuss the arrangements for fees as well as your own policies around payment, holidays and so on. This is covered in detail in Chapter 4.

Developing a psychodynamic formulation

We now turn our attention to the psychodynamic formulation, which is often written up as an assessment report and includes your countertransference and experience of being with the patient. As such, it is a confidential document and should not be shared with those outside the profession who may not understand the framework and language used in such reports. You should also bear in mind data protection considerations when writing these reports (see Chapter 14).

The formulation is concerned with making sense of the patient's difficulties and history in light of psychoanalytic theory, rather than apportioning diagnostic labels. We arrive at a formulation as a working hypothesis of the difficulties facing the patient, condensing the mass of information we have gathered during the consultation process into a coherent, meaningful and sensitive account of the patient's core difficulties. Hinshelwood (1991) describes the "special clarity of thought" required to reach a formulation in the initial meeting with the time pressures and inevitable high levels of patient anxiety.

The formulation informs the choice of psychotherapy for the patient, whether this is open-ended or short-term therapy, the frequency of sessions, length of treatment, therapeutic modality, face-to-face or on the couch, and so on. A good formulation will allow the reader to make sense of why this particular patient is presenting for help now and how their difficulties are located in their early history and life circumstances. The formulation is usually held in the therapist's mind as a way of informing the intervention that is offered. It is shared more explicitly with the patient in brief psychotherapy, like Dynamic Interpersonal Therapy (DIT, as discussed in Chapter 11), where the patient agrees the focus for the work collaboratively with the therapist. Nonetheless, in a psychodynamic assessment, the therapist has listened carefully to the patient's interpersonal narratives and arrived at some initial thoughts about recurring patterns in the patient's object relationships. In DIT, the interpersonal and affective focus is offered as an initial starting formulation that is refined during the course of treatment, where it shifts and deepens as more material emerges. A similar process applies during longer term work. The therapist's initial working hypothesis similarly will change over the course of treatment as new information comes to light.

A psychodynamic formulation is informed by the therapist's particular theoretical framework. A Freudian formulation typically focuses on drives and resulting conflict between id, ego and superego within the structural model of the patient's internal world. A Kleinian formulation usually focuses on internal object relationships in the patient's world, looking at the way the patient shifts from the paranoid-schizoid to depressive position; typically there is a focus on defences of splitting and projective identification with particular attention paid to the transference and the way early object relationships are played out with the therapist. An Object Relations Independent formulation tends to concentrate on the patient's external object relationships, past and present, and the way these have been internalised, alongside the resulting defences of false self and the patient's capacity to make use of transitional objects as well as the therapist in more benign ways.

Hinshelwood's seminal 1991 paper on psychodynamic formulation sets out his thoughts about how formulation – and indeed psychotherapy itself – is predicated on

> the intuitive production of hypotheses – they are for trying out with the patient.... Our evidence comes from watching the fate of our hypotheses.

The response to an interpretation is then the criterion for deciding whether to retain the hypothesis or abandon it. (pp. 166–167)

He describes thinking about the clinical material as "pictures of relationships with objects" (p. 167) and the formulation we arrive at "forms a baseline on which the future work can be grounded and guided" (p. 171). As we will see in Chapter 9, sometimes these refinements in formulation can emerge in the lived transference experience in the room.

The hypotheses we form about our patients start taking shape before we meet them in person, as does the transference and countertransference. Hinshelwood (1991) describes this as another source of information about the patient's object relationships where the referrer has possibly been caught up in acting something out by the way the referral has been made. He gives examples of the ways we can start to hypothesise about the patient through the referral process, including the qualities and information the referrer has chosen to focus on.

I was encouraged by a supervisor of mine to write up my initial hypotheses before seeing the patient for the initial consultation. Not only did it allow me a chance to integrate my thoughts and gather together the information I had obtained about the patient, but it also flagged for me those areas that were neglected by the referring letter and that required further investigation. Questions arose in my mind about areas that felt significant to understand and this provided me with an internal map for the consultation. However, in true analytic fashion, my supervisor then advised me to set this aside during the meeting with the patient, in order to protect the emergent quality of a psychodynamic session and the analytic stance. This allowed me to meet the patient anew, without being overly coloured by pre-existing assumptions.

If we have too determined and rigid a perception of a patient, then we will foreclose the opportunity to explore freely and openly during the consultation process. We have read heart-sinking histories of patients with traumatic lives and then met them in person where we are struck by their resilience and engaging warmth that could not be transmitted in a referral letter. We find ourselves reading between the lines of the doctor's referral letter, for example. When the GP writes, "I would be grateful if you could see this delightful patient", how do we decode their message? These formalities can signify identifications, challenges, antipathies and rejections. As scientists test out hypotheses in search of truth, so we need to be willing to give up our understandings in the light of unfolding and contradictory information. This is where supervision is helpful in providing tri-angulated thinking around formulating our patients. Occasionally, the supervisor or members of the supervision group will be in touch with aspects of the patient's disturbance, of which we have become oblivious. This is referred to as a *parallel process*, whereby the patient's dynamics are transferred across and re-experienced in the supervisory setting. It offers another helpful avenue towards understanding the patient's unconscious communications.

In order to arriving at an object relations formulation in psychotherapy, we map out the patient's recurring experience of others in relation to their sense of self, the affects that link this repeated, internalised experience and the patient's defences in the face of these patterns. Meaningful patterns will be evident across different relationships and times and will take account of early relationships, current relationship patterns and the transference relationship with the therapist. Does the patient expect others will abandon them? Criticise them? Humiliate them? Does this leave them feeling worthless? Unwanted? Small? And what are the feelings that link this – do they feel angry, afraid, ashamed and so on? There will be affects that are more – and less – conscious. We will also think about the patient's defensive strategies as well as the overall defensive function of this pattern. Hinshelwood uses the concept of the "point of maximum pain" (1991, p. 171), by which he means the particular core of pain generated by the patient's object relationships. This tends to lead to a different constellation of object relationships that are used defensively to avoid that pain. Here, we may think about the development of a false self, for example, or idealised object relationships that then switch to denigration based on the underpinning defence of splitting.

Another, similar model for formulating the patient's difficulties relies on Menninger's (1958) triangle of insight as well as Malan's (2001) triangle of person, with "a tripartite formulation bringing together the current difficulty, the transferential situation and the infantile or childhood constellation of conflict or deficit" (Holmes, 1995, p. 34). Alongside this, the formulation would comment on the triangle of conflict, where underlying the presenting anxiety is a defence and hidden impulse. These triangles draw on classical analytic theories of intra-psychic conflict and link them to interpersonal relationships. It can be argued that working with these two triangles of person and conflict forms the basis of all psychodynamic work. We will discuss these in greater detail in Chapters 6 and 9.

Hinshelwood (1991) gives helpful clinical examples to illustrate how information from all three corners of the triangle is carefully explored in an assessment and how this leads to forming hypotheses as the basis of the psychodynamic formulation. This is similar to the way we formulate the Interpersonal and Affective Focus in DIT (see Chapter 11). By attending to these different aspects of past and present, including the transference relationship, we can get closest to an internal object relationship that keeps playing out in a meaningful way across the patient's life. As mentioned earlier, Hinshelwood (1991) directs the assessment towards identifying "the point of maximum pain". In finding the particular pain of that object relationship, we are also looking at the way the patient defends against that pain, including in the way they establish other object relationships to avoid facing that pain again.

The type of psychodynamic formulation you write will depend on both its function and target audience. Highly analytic formulations are best kept out of public records because they require the reader to have a particular level of understanding when reading them, without which they are likely to be more iatrogenic than helpful. The formulation can be useful starting point for a therapist with a new patient. Where should the key focus of the work lie? What is the patient's capacity to hear certain interventions and what impact is psychotherapy likely to have on the patient's external life as well as their internal world of dreams and fantasy life? This is never a static picture and requires frequent updating. As we have said earlier, a psychodynamic formulation differs from a psychiatric report in that it is not designed to arrive at a diagnosis. In psychodynamic formulations, we would see the patient's difficulties as overdetermined, namely there are many contributing factors that could all explain the patient's difficulties, but we cannot isolate a particular variable:

> In analytic therapy, it is the unravelling of many different strands of causation that eventually permits patients to get mastery over patterns they seek to change. Therefore, when trying to come to an understanding of a complex human being and his or her complex difficulties, a therapist is silently pondering several related questions while drawing out and listening to the client. (McWilliams, 1999, p. 27)

Structuring a psychodynamic formulation

Here are some proposed structures for writing a psychodynamic formulation that can be helpful starting points. You can write under particular headings, such as those suggested below.

1   Why now? What have been the predisposing, precipitating and maintaining factors in the patient's presentation
2   Developmental and family history
3   Defences and unconscious conflicts
4   Risks and protective factors
5   Suitability for psychotherapy and possible challenges this may pose in treatment

In formulating the patient's difficulties and why they have come for help now, it is important to focus on the dominant narrative in their account of their story. This is the issue causing the most difficulty at the moment and most related to why the patient is seeking help now. It may not be the most long-standing difficulty. We are looking for the dominant representation of a self-other dynamic. We also want to identify the affects aroused between the patient and the key people in their lives as a result of the activation of this relational pattern. Some affects are more conscious and easier for patients to be aware of while others are less conscious and more defended against by patients. What defensive strategies does the patient employ and at what cost does this come? For example, the patient may be very compliant and people-pleasing, but this comes at the cost of having their own needs met; or if they are dismissive and denigrating of others, the cost is that they push others away and make it difficult for others to like them.

It is helpful to integrate the formulation with the patient's attachment style and early indications of the transference, both negative and positive as well as the reason for entering treatment now. We can hypothesise about the patient's likely attachment style, whether it is anxious avoidant, preoccupied or dismissive (see

Chapter 2 for elaboration on attachment styles). We can expect that the therapy situation will evoke the patient's attachment style. Although you enter this profession with benign motives (we hope!), the patient may feel otherwise, particularly if their attachment style leads them to expect others to respond in negative, critical and rejecting ways. When patients present with conflicting attachment styles by presenting with both avoidant and preoccupied attachment styles, this suggests a more complex presentation with claustrophobic- agoraphobic anxieties regarding interpersonal relationships, something Glasser (1986) identified as the Core Complex (see Chapter 6). The patient is likely to both feel overwhelmed by closeness in relationships and then want to pull away becoming overly distant, but then feeling alone. Neither position is comfortable. If the person has a disturbed attachment history, they often struggle to give a coherent account of their life. This in itself is important information – does the patient have a clear timeline about when things happened in their life and does their account of their difficulties add up in your mind? As we have pointed out, those patients who have no memory of their early childhood and who can't give any detail beyond saying they had a happy childhood, often have had traumatic or disruptive early lives. This poses a greater challenge to engaging in psychotherapy. It will also have a bearing on recommendations about the frequency and length of treatment.

In writing up your psychodynamic formulation, it is helpful to include your countertransference and any observations about what it was like to be with the patient during the consultation. This can include the patient's appearance, how they entered the room, their body language and tone of voice, their talkativeness or silence, any lateness, enactments, and how the contact developed over the course of the meeting.

> *Jo arrived at the consultation dressed in a striking manner as if about to go trick-or-treating for Halloween. Her attire demanded my attention and captivated my gaze, yet she very quickly rebuked me for staring at her. I suddenly felt an extreme awkwardness about where to look. In this way, I felt I had the experience of being pinned to the spot in much the same way I imagined this patient had felt in her life. As we were just getting started, it felt too confronting to take up the mixed message I was receiving of her both wanting to be noticed and concealed. I noted to myself that there was an intensity to the consultation that was uncomfortable for the patient and withdrew my gaze, focusing instead on building an alliance with the patient. Towards the end of the interview, I returned to the way we had begun and explored with her how it had felt, recognising her ambivalence around wanting to be seen as well as finding that overly intrusive. The countertransference I had in the consultation informed the outcome of the consultation alongside other considerations: I recommended group psychotherapy. It felt to me that the intensity of the therapeutic dyad may overwhelm both patient and therapist.*

An observation of a patient's behaviour also gives important clues as to their internal world. For example, one of us had a patient who conveyed her mental state very powerfully by entering the room with so many parcels and bags that spread out across the space, displaying her fragmentation and dislocation in this evocative manner.

An illustrative psychodynamic formulation

We have given this clinical example of a patient, Zara, in order to illustrate a psychodynamic formulation. We provide a brief summary of her history (rather than an extensive detailed assessment) and use this condensed information to develop the start of a formulation.

Zara was the youngest of three daughters, born to her mother just as the parental relation-ship was disintegrating. There was a larger age gap between Zara and her two older sisters, with Zara's birth a last-ditch attempt to save the relationship. Her father left the family when Zara was a few months old and mother reportedly told her it was because he was disappointed at not having a son. Zara was put into a nursery from a young age to allow mother to return to work in order to support the family. Zara was aware of how over-stretched and exhausted her mother was and did her best to impact her as little as possible. She learned to anticipate her mother's bad moods and would stay out of her way. Her oldest sister was often left in charge of her but preferred to hang out with her friends and resented being left with baby Zara. As a result, Zara was often left to entertain herself. She experienced herself as an unwanted burden on the periphery of her family.

At school, Zara had one close friend who then moved away with her family and she never recovered socially from this loss. When she became a teenager, she attracted attention from boys in her school and gained some popularity as the person other people confided in about their problems. She was praised by her teachers for being sensible and helpful. She found herself on her own at home once her older sisters moved away to pursue their own lives. Her mother would offload her difficulties on to Zara yet compared her unfavourably to her older sisters, describing them as leading more successful and colourful lives. She felt unable to open up to her mother about any of her problems and swallowed her resentment at her mother's continued criticisms and disappointments. She was reluctant to get involved in a steady relationship because she was convinced that she would end up being rejected. Zara had a few casual sexual encounters in her late teens and early twenties which left her feeling used and discarded. She took comfort in food where she could give herself what she needed. She remained dissatisfied with her body shape and believed that if only she were slimmer like her sisters, then she would have no difficulties in finding a boyfriend.

Zara studied social work because she was drawn to the helping professions. She worked with Looked After Children and advocated for their rights. She kept herself very busy with work and caring for her mother, tending to neglect her own needs. She met her partner through a work colleague when she was in her late thirties and was acutely aware that this may be her last attempt to have a family of her own. However, her partner already had two children with whom he had intermittent contact, and he was opposed to settling down with her, let alone having another child. She felt he demanded her full attention and care, which gave her a sense of feeling important and valuable. She had to put aside her wish to fall pregnant. However, when her mother fell ill and required her care, he became jealous and eventually announced he was leaving her for a younger woman that he had met on the internet.

Zara brought a dream after the first consultation that she was leaving her workplace and trying to get home, but everything went wrong. The lift cable dropped, and she fell down the four floors but managed to exit unharmed. There was a mass panic in her environment, and she became afraid of being trampled underfoot. She tried to speak but her mouth was full of sticky toffee and she couldn't form any words. She worried that she was going to have such bad tooth decay she would end up toothless. She woke up at that point and had to check her mouth to make sure all her teeth were still intact.

Formulation:

Zara's history presents a picture of repeated abandonments that have led to an internalised sense of being a disappointment to her objects. She was unable to express her anger and resentment because of her experience of her objects' emotional fragility and unavailability and in turn, she was afraid that her needs would be too much of a burden for others to bear. Her conviction of herself as unwanted has led her to neglect her own needs and focus on the needs of others in a defensive attempt to hold on to her attachments. Her anger has been turned inwards as low self-esteem and is concealed in symptoms of tiredness, anxiety and depression. Zara has also used food as a way of symbolically addressing her unmet needs, yet this also serves a defensive purpose by creating a barrier that keeps her away from men and conceals her sexual, female body. Zara's belief that she has the ability to address her difficulties through cycles of overeating and dieting offers her an omnipotent sense of being in control of her life, yet paradoxically, it ends up controlling her, by taking over her thoughts and keeping her distant from others, particularly romantic partners.

   Her father's abandonment of the family was located in the family narrative as something Zara had no control over. She was scapegoated as the reason for the parental relationship breaking down. Her father's disappointment in her has been repeated in later life when her partner abandoned her for another woman. Zara also felt her sisters rejected her for being 'the baby', feeling burdened by having to care for her. She did not feel her mother could see her in her own right and felt she had no space for Zara's difficulties. Zara learned to become a carer and helper, as if this moral defence (Fairbairn, 1944; see Chapter 6) would demonstrate to others the care and support she so desperately needed. In her professional career, Zara became identified with the Looked After Children, who carried her projected sense of vulnerability and abandonment. At its most benign, we can see this as a form of sublimation of her own infantile needs in a constructive way. Yet, there are signs that Zara neglects herself through these identification with her early attachment figures, thereby repeating painful, early experiences of feeling unwanted and burdensome.

   Zara's early dream can be understood as a gift to the therapist, given I had explained to her that I was interested in all aspects of her mind, including her dreams. She could be seen as overly compliant in responding to my invitation, perhaps wanting to keep me sweet (hence the reference to the toffee). This is something I will bear in mind over the course of treatment. The dream did not allow her anxieties to be contained; instead they broke through and interrupted her sleep, leaving her in a state of confusion about fantasy and reality. We can think about the dream as some anxiety at what will happen to her once she starts to explore her internal states of mind. She may end up toothless, without any bite or aggression, and we may think that the dream expresses a wish to shut this down. We can also see elements of her feeling dropped, unable to speak her mind and feeling trampled that echo aspects of her early history and interpersonal relationships. There is a possible warning about the transferential implications for therapy. Will she drop out of treatment if she feels too disturbed? Perhaps the dream alludes to her silencing of me and any dangerous interpretations.

*In the transference, I noticed from her appearance and pleasant demeanour that it was diffi-
cult for her to take this referral for psychotherapy seriously. She invited me to consider her as less
worthy of treatment. I became aware this would be an ongoing pressure on me, as her the
therapist, to respond in dismissive ways that are in keeping with the patterns of object relating
identified above. I could be experienced in the transference as the self-absorbed mother who was
seen to be using Zara for her own needs. The ending of psychotherapy is likely to be problematic
with this type of history, since it is likely to bring a painful repetition of Zara's early and recent
losses. There are likely to be fantasies about a better, more worthy patient who will take her
place. I may feel pressure to prove to Zara that she is cared for, particularly when she is likely to
dismiss the care she is receiving as a financial transaction based on her paying a professional for their services. One possible way Zara might manage the inevitable dependency that entering into therapy will bring is to employ an intellectual defence of
consulting another professional rather than being a patient in treatment. I may be lulled
into a false sense of therapy progressing well if Zara's defensive false self is not tack-
led. There would be a wish to please me and possibly deny her understandable hostility
around endings of sessions as well as breaks in treatment. At these times, I may be
experienced by Zara as abandoning her, activating this early object relationship pattern.*

*In offering Zara psychotherapy, my hope is that this would allow her to occupy a more
active position in her relationships, including beginning to harness her anger in a productive
way. Zara would be encouraged to focus on her authentic needs and take ownership of the
way she arranges her life. She could find ways of negotiating her needs in her relationships
more adequately and begin to have more satisfactory relationships. The pain of not having
entered therapy sooner including the loss of her own fertility are further areas that she will
need to work through the many losses in her life.*

A psychodynamic formulation helps the therapist keep in mind pertinent
background information that informs the patient's presentation and it fore-
shadows areas of the work that may prove challenging. It is useful to keep
revisiting the formulation, updating it as new information and key themes
emerge in the therapy. Writing up a formulation gives us an avenue to reflect
on our work and articulate the theoretical assumptions that inform our approach
with a particular patient. Given the solitary nature of psychotherapy, this ability
to formulate and communicate our clinical work is an important part of ensuring
competent and ethical practice.

Assessing suitability for psychodynamic psychotherapy

Psychotherapy is not helpful for everyone: it has the capacity to harm as well as
help. This is something very few people consider when coming for an assessment
consultation. There are some patients who have managed to reach a point of
equilibrium in their lives, perhaps having overcome huge adversity and starting
to unpick this may threaten the delicate balance they have achieved. As mentioned earlier, the patient has to be ill enough to need psychotherapy yet well
enough to withstand it (Thomä and Kächele, 1987). It is up to us to ascertain
what type of intervention would best suit the patient. In arriving at a decision as

to whether you (or your service) will not offer treatment to a patient, it is helpful to balance this against a recommendation about other forms of treatment the patient could benefit from and how these can be accessed. Coltart (1993), in her experience over several decades of conducting assessments, suggests that about 5% of people fall into the category of being unsuitable for psychotherapy. In some instances, she will arrive at the decision with the patient about "the possibility of abandoning the notion of any sort of treatment, and carrying on from there without help" (1993, p. 55). She elaborates:

> If one is not prescribing anything at all, an essential piece of work is to establish a conviction of the rightness of this in and for the patient. It requires considerable skill to reinforce the often-hidden wish in the patient to be 'let off', and to strengthen his resolve and his ability to take full responsibility for himself. This emphasises a need for authentic conviction in the assessor that for this person to commit himself to the expensive, dependent process of therapy would be disadvantageous, would be a brake rather than an accelerator on his progress through his life. (Ibid., p. 56)

In our experience, those patients who focus on their illness and symptom reduction rather than showing curiosity into their part in their difficulties, tend to do better with a more structured, symptom-focused intervention, such as Cognitive Behaviour Therapy, Acceptance and Commitment Therapy, Interpersonal Therapy, Mindfulness Based Cognitive Therapy and Mindfulness Based Stress Reduction (for people living with chronic health conditions). If a patient presents with severe and enduring mental health difficulties, including greater levels of disturbance and struggling to structure their time as well as care for themselves, possibly suicidal and isolated, then an acute day service would be considered appropriate. This allows the patient to be seen daily in a supportive setting, to have access to a key worker who can help with the likely practical difficulties they would be facing in their lives and to gain psychiatric help. If there is a suicidal risk, then additional support can be added by engaging a crisis team in the patient's local NHS service or working closely with their GP. At their best, these types of collaborative relationships with other parts of the health service can be relied upon over breaks and times of crisis, yet we are cognisant that, as the health service becomes increasingly overstretched, these valuable connections are being axed.

Key areas around suitability for psychodynamic psychotherapy

These areas are offered as points of consideration, bearing in mind that this is a subjective process. It would be reductive to offer a list of inclusion and exclusion criteria, however helpful that may seem to be. Each patient is different, as is each therapist's capacity to work with that patient. We offer these questions to help you with your thinking process in assessing whether to offer this person individual psychodynamic psychotherapy.

1 Does the patient have sufficient ego strength to manage psychodynamic psychotherapy?

In making an assessment of ego strength, we are considering a range of factors, including whether the patient has sufficient freedom of intellectual thought to listen to the therapist, lower their defences, manage to try new things out and handle breaks and frustrations inherent in psychodynamic psychotherapy. As outlined in Chapter 2, Freud described the ego as that part of the patient's personality that is in touch with external reality, and that balances the demands of the id for gratification against the constrictions and prescriptions of the superego. The ego is ruled by the reality principle. When we talk about assessing the patient's ego strength, we want to consider the way the patient is oriented to external reality, and whether they can differentiate between internal and external realities. Can the patient tolerate the necessary in-built frustrations of psychotherapy, which require waiting and forgoing instant gratification without acting out?

We would explore how the patient manages the demands of life: can they get to appointments on time and meet their deadlines? Are they relying on substances to get through their lives and to what extent? Are they engaging in other self-destructive acts? Poor impulse control is likely to manifest around breaks in therapy and can lead to escalations in demands for contact with the therapist, including presenting at a hospital's Accident & Emergencies department in a crisis, suicide attempts, sexualised or aggressive behaviour, relapses in eating disorders, substance abuse and self-harm. It can be helpful to think with the patient about the possibility of ruptures in the therapeutic relationship and encourage them to return to address this with the therapist. While we can try our best to prepare patients for the impact of a break in therapy, it can be difficult for someone to anticipate how they will respond at first, particularly if they have developed a powerful transference to the therapist. However, it is essential that we keep in mind how a break can replicate earlier separations and traumas, leaving patients at risk of dropping out of treatment prematurely in an effort to protect themselves from what feels like yet another experience of abandonment.

Ego strength can be evaluated by asking about the patient's external life, most notably their vocational/employment and relationship history. Can they work or study independently and see things through to completion? Are they able to sustain interpersonal relationships over time? In the Tavistock Adult Depression Study (Fonagy et al., 2015), one of the factors that predicted a positive outcome to therapy was whether patients had a university degree. Given that all the participants had treatment resistant depression, this factor seemed to distinguish whether certain individuals had the resilience to persevere with a long-term goal as well as the ability to take information from someone and make use of it. We are interested in whether the patient can both take and give back to their environment and interpersonal network.

Another indicator of ego strength is how the person treats their body and responds to advice from their doctors. We would understand the way they relate to their own body as an indication of their internal object world, that includes internalised early caregiver relationships. Can they make use of medical advice or do they continue to engage in self-destructive or neglectful behaviours? We consider here attacks on their own body as well as possible attacks on others. Domestic violence and other acts of aggression would suggest someone with poor internal controls who easily becomes overwhelmed and stops thinking, resorting to action. Can they protect the mental and physical health of any children in their household? We have a legal obligation to explore and report any emotional and physical neglect and abuse of children as well as vulnerable adults. A very disturbed patient may not always recognise the impact their mental health has on their children. Mental health problems in parents and siblings, including depression, obsessive compulsive disorder and other forms of anxiety, often have a huge impact on the rest of the household. In individual psychotherapy, we would try to encourage the patient to make space for their therapy by organising childcare to allow them to attend reliably, including over school breaks. We would also assess the impact of their difficulties on other key relationships in their lives, including parents, spouses, siblings and so on, paying particular attention to vulnerable adults.

> *At one assessment I carried out, Jane was so disturbed by the ticking clock in the consulting room and the acute anxiety it aroused in her, she became unable to think. She had concrete associations to the location and address where she was being seen that had a psychotic flavour, having lost the "as if" quality, she was psychically transported back to that earlier space. She hinted at the bad things that happened to her in that space and it felt as if she was afraid harmful and intrusive experiences would repeat themselves in this space with me. Jane told me she was looking after her elderly father as well as three small children. I was unable to assure myself that she could manage these responsibilities, having experienced her loose grip on reality and paranoid thinking. After discussing it with my supervisor, I made the difficult decision to alert her GP and Social Services to the concerns I had, aware that they required further investigation including collateral reports from her children's school and a home visit.*

If you do have safeguarding concerns, your membership organisation or workplace should have a contact person with whom you can discuss these. This can allow you to ascertain whether you should take further steps and alert the authorities to your concerns. Clearly doing this will have implications for the therapeutic relationship. It may mean that trust is breached to such an extent that the therapeutic alliance can never recover. However, on balance it is better to ensure safety by allowing a relevant professional to make an independent evaluation. We are acutely aware that the information our patients report to us is a subjective account of their worlds and is coloured by their own filters, unconscious fantasies and defences. When carrying out a consultation, we look out for inconsistencies, false reassurances that have no substantiation when explored further as well as monitoring our own countertransference and paying attention to feeling alarmed as well as the opposite experience of being lulled into a false sense of reassurance. Nina Coltart (1993) reminds us of the importance of "trusting that whole apparatus, conscious and unconscious, which we bring to our work, and which is called 'intuition'" (p. 66).

During the assessment process, we are evaluating how the patient responds to our questions and to the setting. Can they receive your interpretations without becoming overly defensive? Can they apprehend, consider and expand on what you have said? Are they able to make links to the transference situation and be willing to consider how you as their therapist may become part of their pattern of object relating? The more defended or vulnerable a patient is, the more stirred up they are likely to become when asked to consider the relationship to the therapist. This is often assessed by making a '*trial interpretation*', which can be an interpretation of an aspect of the patient's functioning or dynamics, or more specifically, an interpretation of the transference. We convey through an interpretation that we are listening in particular ways to the patient's narratives, looking for links and possible meaning in this material as well as conveying that there are connections to the live therapeutic relationship. As an assessing therapist who has just met the patient for the first time, we do need to be wary about not conveying a transference interpretation with great certainty. Patients are probably afraid of being misunderstood or even being treated with contempt. It is better to couch a trial interpretation as a hypothesis rather than an absolute truth, for example: "I am wondering if …", "It seems that …" or "I have noticed that this seems to keep happening, am I on the right track?" The examples of interpreting a cautionary tale (Ogden, 1992, see Chapter 9) show the way in which a trial interpretation can be used to deepen the therapeutic alliance. Hinshelwood (1995) comments on the use of the trial interpretation during an assessment, as follows:

> The kind of response, unconscious as well as conscious, to an interpretation is, in my view, extraordinarily productive as a way of (a) assessing the suitability and psychological mindedness of the patient, and (b) the best form of preparation for psychotherapy since it is giving a taste of the real thing. (p. 165)

He counters the argument that the trial interpretation deepens the patient's connection to the assessor who may not continue to work with the patient by reminding us that this connection begins by virtue of the patient entering into the consultation with us. These interpretations can help restore a more balanced connection to the assessor by taking up the more challenging and uncomfortable aspects of the patient's personality, thereby making an idealised transference less likely.

2 Is the patient psychologically minded?

We ask questions in the initial consultation to explore the prospective patient's curiosity in their internal world and the world of others, and whether they can make links with you in the session. We are invited to let our curiosity flow, to look for repeated experiences and invite the patient's reflections. For example, we may ask whether the patient understands why they responded in a particular way to someone? Do they see any similarity between one situation and another? We may ask what thoughts they have as to why this situation keeps recurring in their lives.

Coltart (1993) sets out nine qualities that add up to psychological mindedness which we have reproduced below:

1 An acknowledgement, tacit or explicit, by the patient that he has an unconscious mental life, and that it affects his thoughts and behaviour.
2 The capacity to give a self-aware history, not necessarily in chronological order.
3 The capacity to give this history without prompting from the assessor, and with some sense of the patient's emotional relatedness to the events of his own life and their meaning for him.
4 The capacity to recall memories, with their appropriate affects.
5 Some capacity to take the occasional step back from his own story and to reflect upon it, often with the help of a brief discussion with the assessor.
6 Signs of a willingness to take responsibility for himself and his own personal evolution.
7 Imagination, as expressed in imagery, metaphors, dreams, identifications with other people, empathy, and so on.
8 Some signs of hope and realistic self-esteem. This may be faint, especially if the patient is depressed, but it is nevertheless important.
9 The overall impression of the development of the relationship with the assessor.
(Coltart, 1993, p. 72. Reproduced here with permission)

Coltart goes on to point out that to engage in psychodynamic psychotherapy, prospective patients should demonstrate at least three to four of these qualities, while to engage in a full psychoanalysis, most of these qualities should be present together with other necessary requirements such as motivation and resources, financial and time.

We do need to take account of variations in the cultural backdrop when working with patients from different ethnic groups and how this impacts our curiosity, for example some cultures are more likely to attribute motivation to external reasons or the karma of earlier lives than internal motivations (Kakar, 1985). We will discuss these aspects further in Chapter 13 on working with difference.

3 Can we establish trust and the start of a therapeutic alliance with the patient?

The ability to form a therapeutic alliance and engagement in therapy depends in part on the practicalities of therapy (fees, availability etc), which should be discussed with the patient when establishing the contract. An important consideration, however, is to assess whether it is possible to establish a trusting relationship. An initial meeting both conveys to the patient a taste of working psychodynamically as well as giving them a realistic sense of hope in the journey they are contemplating undertaking. Wille (2012) describes his approach to the initial meeting as more encounter than examination, in which the therapist strives to give the patient an experience of working analytically in an emotionally charged way:

If the analyst is truly capable of listening on several levels to emotional meanings, and can find the nonverbal attitude and words to convey this to the patient in such a way that the patient is emotionally touched, moments of connectedness can arise. (p. 890)

Wille links this sense of connectedness to Ellman's (2007) term, 'affective interpenetration', whereby the experience leads to a deepening of the therapeutic relationship as well as enhancing the patient's trust, motivation and engagement. We can see how this aligns with the concept of epistemic trust (described in Chapter 7) and is central to the question of whether the patient can engage in psychodynamic psychotherapy.

The therapist's attitude towards treatment plays an important part in establishing a working alliance and is underpinned by our own convictions and trust in the model of psychodynamic psychotherapy, something we can unconsciously undermine or feel ashamed of. Perhaps at some level, we harbour beliefs that this approach is old-fashioned and out-of-date, or that we are financially exploiting our patients by offering them open-ended work, or perhaps that we are using the patient to meet our own training needs. This will need to be openly acknowledged and worked with in supervision and/or personal therapy so as to prevent it undermining our clinical work. Danielle Quinodoz (2002) writes that:

the patient should discover during the preliminary interviews that the analyst is suggesting an encounter that is *not* educational, *not* psychological and *not* psychiatric, and that this situation is different; the important thing for the patient is to *feel* what a psychoanalysis is. (p. 121)

Realistic aims for psychotherapy

Psychotherapy aims to develop greater insight into the patient's difficulties, to increase a sense of agency, solidify a cohesive sense of identity and ego strength, develop a healthy degree of self-esteem, improve affect regulation, enhance the capacity to love and work including feeling securely attached to others, improve interpersonal relationships, facilitate greater sense of enjoyment in life as well as help with symptom relief (although symptoms are not directly targeted unlike other therapies such as CBT) (McWilliams, 1999, p. 12). Psychodynamic psychotherapy aims to transform "infantile dependency into mature adult dependency" (p. 24).

Freud spoke about psychoanalytic treatment aiming to transform "hysterical misery into common unhappiness. With a mental life that has been restored to health [the individual] will be better armed against that unhappiness" (Breuer and Freud, 1895, p. 305). There is evidence of other benefits of psychotherapy including reduced hospitalisations, improved physical health and increased stress tolerance (Gabbard et al., 1997).

Part of the assessment process involves imparting a sense of hope to the patient that positive change and growth may be possible. The assessment needs to pace itself so that it doesn't leave an already vulnerable person feeling traumatised by the end of the process. We may want to think about where the patient is going at the end of the consultation and what they plan on doing to take care of themselves if they are emotionally shaken by the consultation. They may need encouragement to take a little time to consolidate the experience before rushing into work, for example.

The type of orienting information that can be useful to share with patients during the consultation process includes the following:

> *People coming to see a therapist for the first time sometimes want to be asked questions because that is what they are used to, but it is important that sessions are led by you, rather than by the therapist because what you are feeling and thinking is the focus of the work. Psychotherapy does not provide quick solutions and therapists do not give advice. It is common to feel that the therapist says very little, but it is important to realise that psychotherapy is a specialised conversation. This means talking freely and therapists realise this is not always easy. The therapist will listen carefully to – and comment on – what you are saying about your feelings and how you deal with them, as well as focusing on what happens in the sessions and your relationship with the therapist. Psychotherapy can be a highly charged experience and while this can offer relief, it can also stir up difficult feelings.*
>
> *In regular sessions, you will be encouraged to explore freely what is in your mind, including early and current relationships, feelings, thoughts, wishes, fears, memories and dreams. The relationship with the therapist in the room is an important part of this. The assumption behind this treatment is that new understandings of yourself may offer greater choice about how to alter your life situation. Regular attendance is an important part of treatment.*

Box 5.3 Useful resources

Readings

The following journal papers provide important considerations for assessment and formulation in psychodynamic psychotherapy:

Coltart, N. (1987). Diagnosis and assessment for suitability for psycho-analytical psychotherapy. *British Journal of Psychotherapy, 4*(2), 127–134.
Hinshelwood, R. D. (1991). Psychodynamic formulation in assessment for psychotherapy. *British Journal of Psychotherapy, 8*(2), 166–174.
Milton, J. (1997) Why assess? Psychoanalytical assessment in the NHS. *Psychoanalytic Psychotherapy, 11*, 47–58.
The following book chapters are also useful, and provide clinical examples:
Coltart, N. (1993). *How to survive as a psychotherapist*. London: Sheldon Press – Chapter 5, The Pleasures of Assessment and Chapter 6, The Art of Assessment.
Lemma, A. (2016). *Introduction to the practice of psychoanalytic psychotherapy* (2nd edition). Chichester: John Wiley & Sons – Chapter 4, Assessment and Formulation.

Online Resources

The American Journal of Psychiatry has a Clinical Case Conference with a helpful transcript of the case discussion of a psychodynamic assessment and formulation with Glen Gabbard and Kristin Kassaw: https://ajp.psy chiatryonline.org/doi/full/10.1176/appi.ajp.159.5.721

An online copy of a chapter written by Ruth Berkowitz, entitled "Assessment for psychoanalytic psychotherapy: An overview of the literature", is available on YouTube: https://youtu.be/CWRhB2IQvbc

6   Anxiety and defences

"Why are you being so defensive?" We are all familiar with the idea that someone is behaving defensively. This psychoanalytic concept has seeped into everyday nomenclature. Psychoanalytic theories propose that we all experience psychic conflict and psychic pain that fall under the collective umbrella of *anxiety*. Anxiety is an inevitable part of the human condition. It is hard-wired into our brains for both phylogenetic and ontogenetic survival. The flight–fight response is designed to allow us to respond adaptively to danger. Anxiety is an essential part of the attachment system, designed to keep babies and toddlers safe during this vulnerable time in their development (Fonagy et al., 2002). By remaining close to their key attachment figures, the young child can explore their world from the security offered by the parental safe base. Yet in today's age, we are plagued with chronic anxieties that overload our natural stress responses. Sapolsky (2004) writes that zebras don't get ulcers because they only have to deal with acute stressors that are short-lived, like being attacked by a lion at the watering hole. By contrast, humans become stressed by their own often anticipatory worries, that lead to a range of emotional and physical consequences. Being in a state of stress is unpleasurable and we are driven to find ways of reducing and coping with it.

In psychoanalytic theory, the way we learn to cope with anxiety from an early age underpins the development of defence mechanisms. It has become part of everyday language to describe the ways we use defence mechanisms to protect ourselves from uncomfortable realities. We may describe a colleague as defensive when they struggle to receive negative feedback or we may tell our partner not to take out their bad day at work on us (*displacement*). We talk about someone being in *denial*, ('having their head in the sand') or *rationalising* their position ('talking the hind leg off a donkey'). We all have our preferred defence mechanisms that we use to cope with difficult experiences. These may not always be healthy and adaptive responses, but rather defences that we have learned to employ or rely on time and again such that they become automatic and unconscious. The more defences a person use, the more calcified and rigid their personality structure has become. Thus, psychic defences form a type of character armour. While our defences are intended to protect us from harm, real or imagined, paradoxically they often end up entrapping and restricting us.

A basic competence for all therapeutic work is to be able to address the emotional content of a session. A key competence for psychodynamic psychotherapy is the ability to recognise and work with defences, which result from painful affects. The competence extends to making dynamic interpretations of the patient's anxiety and defence. Typically, interpretations begin with the defence which is closest to the patient's conscious awareness, before interpreting the underlying conflict. In this chapter, we will outline some of the theoretical foundations for understanding anxiety and defences, including identifying different types of defences. We will focus in greater detail on defences that crop up more frequently, as well as touching on more complex defence mechanisms that patients utilise. Finally, we will discuss ways of interpreting defensive behaviours in psychodynamic psychotherapy as well as how to work with the affects that defences attempt to deflect.

Understanding anxiety and defences

Freud posited that anxiety arose out of unconscious conflicts related to the death and life instincts as well as the competing demands of the id, ego and superego. At first, Freud (1923a) theorised anxiety in terms of his drive model, where anxiety was represented by the state of 'unpleasure' that results from the build-up of instinctual sexual or aggressive energy. Freud's theory of the pleasure principle implies that we have an inherent drive towards discharging this unpleasure. Later, Freud (1926) understood anxiety in relation to his structural model of the id, ego and superego. This gives rise to a variety of anxieties, depending on which structure is involved. Anxiety can signal a real or imagined threat or danger to the ego, warning of a trauma that is putting the ego in danger. Superego anxiety is experienced around fear of punishment for unacceptable aggressive or sexual desires. Id anxiety involves a fear of losing control of one's sexual and aggressive instincts.

Anna Freud (1954), in her seminal work *The Ego and The Mechanisms of Defence*, writes evocatively about the intrapsychic conflicts that give rise to anxiety by using the metaphor of war. The two neighbouring powers of the id and the superego make aggressive incursions into the 'territory' of the ego. She describes how the ego (governed by the reality principle) has to navigate between the conflicting demands from the id for gratification on the one hand (driven by the pleasure principle), and the superego's demand that these impulses conform with ethical and moral laws, on the other. She writes that

> In favourable cases the ego does not object to the intruder but puts its own energies at the other's disposal and confines itself to perceiving; it notes the onset of the instinctual impulse, the heightening of tension and the feelings of 'pain' by which this is accompanied and, finally, the relief from tension when gratification is experienced. (Freud, 1954, p. 6).

In such cases, the ego is a neutral observer that does not need to enter into battle. However, Anna Freud points out that where there is a conflict between the instinctual demands of the id and the moralistic demands of the superego, the instinctual drives will pursue the wish for gratification with:

> tenacity and energy, and they make hostile incursions into the ego, in the hope of overthrowing it by a surprise-attack. The ego on its side becomes suspicious; it proceeds to counter-attack and to invade the territory of the id. Its purpose is to put the instincts permanently out of action by means of appropriate defensive measures, designed to secure its own boundaries. (Freud, 1954, p. 7)

The challenge for the therapist is to tease out the structural layers of anxiety, as exemplified in the diagram below (Figure 6.1). Of course, all of this usually takes place outside conscious awareness. The therapist as an observer after the fact often becomes aware of the operation of defences by what is absent or lacking from the patient's narratives as well as through careful attention to countertransference. This allows us to infer the operation of defences such as repression, denial, disavowal, reaction formation, sublimation and so on (see Table 6.1 for a description of these defence mechanisms). We may also become aware of a concealed conflict when the defence mechanisms break down, leading to a *return of the repressed* (through the repetition compulsion) with the original anxiety intruding.

Klein (1932) developed this further, arguing that anxiety is present from the start of life, and is essential to the process of development. While Freud posited that we develop an ego in the first years of life, Klein argued that we are born with a basic ego structure, and so from birth, we experience anxiety in relation to real or imagined threats to the ego. A baby is born with an inherent terror of ceasing to exist. These early primitive anxieties are related to the fear and anticipation of being annihilated. Anyone who has observed a small baby will recognise the incredibly vulnerable state of the infant after leaving the safety of the womb with its continual companionship of sound, warmth, containment and instant feeding only to have to face the external world with experiences of delayed gratification, isolation, coldness and hunger. The unswaddled newborn's limbs flail as if they are falling apart. When the mother is unable to contain and make sense of these anxieties, the infant becomes

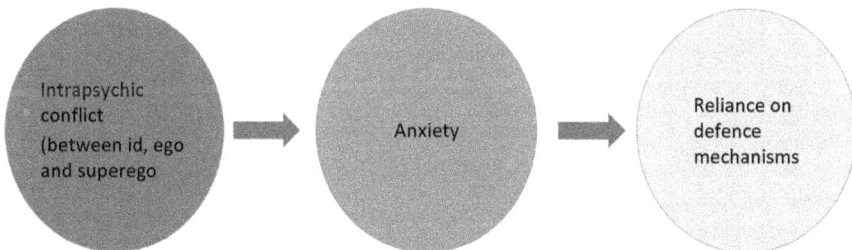

Figure 6.1 A diagrammatic representation of Freud's model of anxiety and defence

Table 6.1 Different types of defences

Primitive defences	
Primitive withdrawal	A psychological withdrawal from reality or consciousness. In adults, the individual may withdraw from social life, or may alter their consciousness (e.g. through the use of drugs) to withdraw from reality. The withdrawal is into one's internal fantasy life, rather than the unpleasant or unsatisfying realities of external life. This can happen in states of trauma (see also derealisation and depersonalisation).
Denial	The refusal to accept an unpleasant reality. Denial may be a temporary way of coping with something painful which can then be felt and processed later; or as a way of avoiding a reality, such as avoiding medical procedures like having an HIV test or getting a lump examined. Denial may also involve the refusal to acknowledge a problem; e.g. alcoholics who deny they have any dependency.
Splitting	Where two opposing feelings or thoughts are kept apart from each other (and thus, ambivalence is not tolerated). Usually objects are perceived to be good (or idealised) and are kept apart (split off) in the mind from those deemed to be bad.
Projection	When one attributes one's own state of mind or feeling to another. For example, we may attribute our own failures and shortcomings to the mistakes of others, whom we can then blame.
Projective identification	When one attributes one's own states of mind to another and then behaves as if that person is taken over by that state. For example, assuming that someone is hostile and dangerous, then experiencing paranoid anxiety when around them.
Dissociation	When one is cut off from all feeling or consciousness about an event. Sometimes patients describe this as if they are seeing the world behind a pane of glass, leaving them feeling cut off from what is going on. In trauma, we understand this as depersonalisation and derealisation. In depersonalisation, there is a dissociation from oneself whereas in derealisation, there is a disconnect from what is happening in one's life. For example, a trauma victim who cannot access any affect or detail about the traumatic event.
Omnipotence	The sense that one has unlimited power and influence over the world. What is being defended against is any form of vulnerability and dependency. The person compensates for powerlessness by imagining themselves to be all-powerful. Adults who experience themselves as omnipotent and powerful in the world may have anti-social personality traits, whereby they may enjoy being manipulative, winning over others and exercising their power. This is also a feature in narcissistic personalities as well as an aspect of mania (see below).

(Continued)

Table 6.1 (Cont.)

Primitive defences	
Idealisation	Attributing omnipotence and benevolence to another person, to whom we then feel attached. A sense of safety is felt when merged with this powerful Other. The opposite of idealisation is devaluation, whereby the Other is denigrated; these represent two sides of the same coin and one often follows the other. Narcissistic persons may seek idealised others (e.g. someone wealthy, attractive or powerful) as a reflection of their own sought-after perfection. Therapists can be idealised only to suddenly fall from the pedestal when the patient is inevitably disappointed. However tempting it may be to collude with this defence, it is not in the service of therapy and it does need to be taken up (see Chapter 9 on transference).
Manic defences	This is a group of defences marked by activity and mental states where one believes the self to be all-powerful, invulnerable, cut off from depression and any sense of guilt. There is a denial here of depression, with the person feeling triumphant over others and over any sense of vulnerability. Typical 'every-day' manic defences include going on a shopping spree as a way to deny depression (colloquially referred to as retail therapy). We sometimes speak about a manic flight to health as the ending of therapy approaches. This is something we discuss in greater detail in Chapter 10 on Endings.

Neurotic defences	
Repression	Where unacceptable wishes or fantasies, thoughts, feelings or memories are pushed out of the conscious mind into the unconscious. This is different to denial in that reality is not negated; rather it is acknowledged first and then repressed. These repressed memories are subject to 'the return of the repressed' when they break through this defence.
Regression	Where a person reverts to an earlier, more child-like state of functioning, in order to avoid the conflicts of the (mature) present.
Undoing	These are actions or verbalisations that neutralise the affect or meaning of something that was said or done. For example, talking sympathetically about a person immediately after criticising them.
Displacement	When unpleasant feelings towards one person are displaced and directed onto another. For example, a child upset with their teacher, returns home and is angry with their mother. In adulthood, there may be hostility towards all authority figures as a displacement of aggression towards the parents.
Reversal	This involves switching position from passive to active or vice versa. For example, switching from being dependent on others, to making others dependent on them.
Isolation	When feelings are separated from knowledge about something. The person may be aware of something and able to talk about it, but its emotional meaning is excluded. For example, being able to talk about an unpleasant thing that happened in a flat way, without any affect. This differs from dissociation, in that part of the self is removed from consciousness in dissociation whereas here it is the affective part of the experience that has been isolated.

(Continued)

Table 6.1 (Cont.)

Neurotic defences	
Conversion	When a psychic conflict is transformed into a physical symptom. For example, experiencing a stomach pain as a symptom of an underlying anxiety or fear.
Acting out	An action (behaviour) used to discharge a disturbing feeling that can't be thought about. For example, the man who has been rejected by his partner becomes very drunk and starts a fight. We talk further about the operation of this defence in the transference in Chapter 9 and distinguish it from 'acting in'.
Rationalisation	Finding reasons to justify an unacceptable act, thus making it acceptable. For example, not achieving success in getting a job, and then deciding that you did not want the job anyway.
Intellectualisation	This is a particular version of isolation, namely being able to talk about feelings in an intellectualised, emotional disconnected way. For example, talking about feeling depressed and lonely, but as concepts, with no actual emotion. This is what is referred to as pseudo-mentalising in Chapter 7.
Reaction formation	When one turns a disturbing idea into its opposite. For example, the man who fears he is homosexual becomes vehemently homophobic.
Sublimation	Modifying and diverting sexual impulses by divesting them of their sexual aims and turning them into other constructive and adaptive channels that often include cultural activities. This is considered a more mature form of defence. For example, playing rugby as a way to discharge one's aggressiveness; or redirecting romantic energy into hard work and productivity.
Humour	Where painful or difficult issues are dealt with by making light of them. Humour may also be considered a mature form of defence.

overtaken by "nameless dread" (Bion, 1962b, p. 309). This is such an extreme state of anxiety that it strips out meaning, thereby returning the infant's terror with the force of a psychic black hole.

The infant develops primitive defences against this persecutory anxiety. It is persecutory because it represents fear of the threatening nature of the world outside of the self. This is characteristic of Klein's *paranoid-schizoid position* whereby the baby learns to split good and bad experiences in an attempt to preserve and protect positive experiences (the prototype 'good breast') from attacking, negative ones (the prototype 'bad breast'). As the baby develops and moves into the *depressive position*, the nature of anxiety changes as the infant becomes able to integrate these split-off part-objects into ambivalent feelings towards the same object (the 'bad' and 'good' object are one and the same person). Alongside this, the baby develops the capacity for guilt as a consequence for having hated the 'bad' object as well as growing concern for the good object and fear of its loss (resulting from earlier impulses to attack the 'bad' object) and the wish to make reparation for the perceived damage.

Sigmund Freud, Melanie Klein, Anna Freud and other classical psychoanalysts viewed anxiety and defence mechanisms as intrapsychic phenomena. Subsequent theorists understood anxiety and defences in interpersonal terms, as coping strategies we develop in response to others. Object relations theorists like Fairbairn and Winnicott elaborated particular ways in which defences develop in relation to others, including the *moral defence* and the *false self* respectively. We will elaborate on both of these later in the chapter. Bowlby's (1969; 1973) work around attachment and that of Fonagy and colleagues (2002) around mentalisation demonstrate that our ability to regulate our affective states, including anxiety, develops through early relationships to our primary attachment figures. A disturbance in the parent's capacity to represent the infant's inner states leads the baby to distort the self-experience defensively in order to protect their tie to the parent, thereby resulting in particular internal working models or internalised procedures for being with others (Fonagy, 2002; see also Chapter 7). This chapter will explore both intrapsychic and interpersonal approaches to conceptualising and tackling anxiety in psychodynamic psychotherapy.

Patients may come to the therapist with different types of core anxieties (see Box 6.1). As mentioned earlier, a key competence of psychodynamic psychotherapy is to recognise, elaborate and interpret the patient's conscious and unconscious anxieties, and the associated defences they commonly use. We need to pay attention to what is being said as well as what is being omitted during sessions, by carefully observing and attending to unconscious communication (see Chapter 8) as well as transference and countertransference phenomena (see Chapter 9).

Box 6.1 What makes us anxious?

In the consulting room, many patients' struggles and interpersonal difficulties revolve around these common types of anxiety:

- Anxiety about separation, loss, and abandonment (separation anxiety)
- Anxiety about feelings of inadequacy or humiliation
- Anxiety about being overwhelmed or taken over, or losing a sense of oneself (annihilation anxiety)
- Anxiety about one's own potential for destructiveness
- Anxiety about being attacked (persecutory anxiety)
- Anxiety about the intactness of the body (castration anxiety)

A psychodynamic interpretation involves working from the surface to depth, starting with interpreting the patient's use of defences, and then addressing the underlying anxieties which they are defending against. Kernberg (2016) details the sequence of interpretations as follows:

In general, interpretation of a defense or a defensive relationship initiates the interpretative process, followed by the interpretation of the context, or the impulsive relationship against which the defense was erected, and the analysis of the motivation for this defensive process. (p. 287)

Before we discuss how to interpret anxiety and defences, we need to help you with recognising the different types of defences that patients typically employ. Bear in mind that the more defences the patient uses, and the more primitive those defences are, the greater the likelihood of early trauma and/or sensitivity of the patient to environmental impingements; and the more challenging psychotherapy is likely to be.

Are defences necessary?

Given that we all experience anxiety, conflict and potential threats to the self, we all need and employ defences. Defences work at an unconscious level such that we are typically unaware of what defence mechanism we are deploying in the moment. We may reflect on things 'after the fact' when the heat of strong feelings has subsided and then realise that we were using a particular defence to protect ourselves. Defences can be adaptive, particularly given that they result from a wish to protect the self from threats, real or imagined. However, they can quickly become maladaptive and pathological, particularly when these protective ways of responding become procedural and happen instinctively in the absence of a real threat. Defences can also become overly fixed and rigid, thereby restricting the interpersonal experiences of the individual. In these instances, the cost of the defence becomes too great and outweighs any benefit it once served. In order to be motivated to change dysfunctional patterns, the patient needs help with understanding those costs. For example, the person who frequently makes use of humour as a defence may experience others becoming distant with him as they tire of their excessive jokes and inability to take things seriously, and this may lead to having fewer relationships with depth and intimacy. Patients who are very avoidant of close relationships so as not to be hurt again will find themselves isolated and lonely, the price they have to pay for this emotional safety.

Patients tend to enter psychotherapy because their current defence mechanisms are not working for them, and they feel overwhelmed by feelings of anxiety, despair, anger and so on. Alternately, their defences have become so inflexible that they have become isolated from the world and others. Let us take the example of a patient with a diagnosis of Obsessive-Compulsive Disorder. The compulsion to repeatedly wash their hands was first set up to keep the person safe from germs, however, over time this action reinforces the belief that there are harmful bacteria in the world and the person eventually ends up spending more and more time washing their hands in the bathroom, until their skin is cracked and bleeding and they are unable to function in their daily life.

The aim of psychotherapy is not to strip the individual of all their defences, but rather to help them become more conscious of the defences they deploy, to understand why they use them and appreciate the cost of those defences so they can make more conscious decisions moving forward. This may result in making use of fewer or 'healthier' defences, in a more flexible manner. The less intensively the therapist works with a patient, the more respect should be shown for the patient's defences. Monitoring how the patient responds to therapy will include paying close attention to their defences and whether these intensify as therapy gets underway. For example, a patient might relapse with their abstinence from drinking at the start of therapy, and this may alert the therapist to their vulnerability, requiring a more supportive approach at first, focusing on supporting ego strengths. In Chapter 5, we touched on the need to consider defences when assessing suitability for psychotherapy.

Types of defences

In psychoanalytic theory, defence mechanisms are differentiated by the stage of development in which they develop and then come to be utilised. At each of Freud's psychosexual stages of development, the child can develop different points of fixation, with associated defences. Defences are usually categorised as *primitive* or *neurotic* (see Table 6.1). Primitive defences are those that are most prominent in the pre-Oedipal stage of development, where the infant and young child have unsophisticated psychic mechanisms at their disposal to defend themselves against threat and anxiety. Post-Oedipal, neurotic defences are regarded as more mature and adaptive ways of managing internal conflicts. Primitive (or primary) defences have been understood as those involving the boundary between the self and the outside world, what is 'me' and 'not me'. By comparison, mature (or secondary) defences are those involving intrapsychic boundaries, such as conflicts between the id, ego and superego (McWilliams, 2011). An adult who is still reliant on those primitive defences characteristic of early childhood is considered to have more disturbed psychological functioning than an adult who uses neurotic defences in a more flexible manner. However, we need to be circumspect when applying this since we all operate with primitive defences at times, for example, when we revert to the paranoid-schizoid position.

Defences can also be ranked by the degree to which they are adapted to reality. Primitive defences have the quality of lacking some connection with reality and the appreciation of the separateness between self and other, that is, an inability to see the object as separate. For example, the primitive defence of *denial* is maladaptive in that individual negates reality by behaving as if the painful reality is simply not happening. Sometimes we refer to this as putting your head in the sand or being blinkered. *Intellectualisation*, on the other hand, is a more mature defence whereby the individual is engaged with reality but only at a level of cognition and at the expense of any emotions. Notwithstanding this, even denial can be considered adaptive if an individual makes use of it temporarily and flexibly at times of acute stress. For example, someone may be in denial about impending death when they receive an initial diagnosis of a terminal illness. In this instance, denial probably helps manage their fear and anxiety as the reality of the stark diagnosis starts to sink in. Many of us use denial, albeit briefly, in the face of bad news, often responding initially by saying, "No, it's not true!" Thus, some defences can encompass both 'primitive' and mature aspects. For example, *idealisation* can refer to putting someone unrealistically on a pedestal by seeing them as perfect or supreme at one end, while a more mature form of this defence would be admiring someone as superior while also being aware of their limitations, such as with heroes and role models.

Three significant primitive defence mechanisms and clinical concepts that are central to Klein's formulation of the paranoid-schizoid position are *projection, splitting* and *projective identification*. They are included in Table 6.1, but it is worth discussing them in more detail here, since they are likely to feature frequently when working with patients. Although these are primitive defence mechanisms, they are not merely seen as defences that we outgrow. Remember that Klein referred to the paranoid-schizoid and depressive *positions*, rather than developmental stages, because she saw these as iterative mental and emotional states that babies, children, adolescents and adults shift in and out of throughout life. The defence mechanisms of the paranoid-schizoid position are disturbing and unsettling because they involve un-integrated experiences whereby parts of the self are disavowed and denied.

Projection

Let us consider the process of projecting an image onto a surface, as in the case of a slide projector: an image in the form of a slide is inserted inside the projector, and by means of lights and lenses, the image is then magnified and projected onto an outside surface like a wall or screen. Thus, projection involves moving the location of a representation from inside to outside. In psychoanalysis, the term *projection* refers to a defence mechanism whereby an internal experience is expelled and projected onto an outside object (Hinshelwood, 1989). Typically, this involves getting rid of unpleasurable bodily experiences or internal conflicts by attributing them to outside sources, rather than locating them internally. Thus, projection aims to reduce internal anxiety and conflict, by locating the threat or danger as coming from outside where it is attributed to an object that can then be attacked or fought. So, for example, aggression and hatred can be purged by projecting these qualities onto others, who then are experienced as aggressive and hateful. In this way the self is protected as 'good' (I am not hateful; you are). Sometimes it is positive qualities that are projected outwards in order to protect them, although this can leave the Self depleted. Let's consider a clinical example:

> *Helen sought therapy in her mid-thirties because she felt unable to maintain intimate rela-*
> *tionships, leaving her depressed. She had various brief relationships where she expected to be*
> *disappointed and rejected by her partners. On the face of it, she protested that she was*
> *searching for a close relationship, however what became clear was that she had a tendency to*
> *avoid closeness by maintaining a cautious distance, thus projecting her own dismissiveness*
> *onto others. As we explored her avoidance of getting into the romantic relationship she so*
> *wanted (on a conscious level), what emerged was her fear of losing her identity and*

becoming subsumed by being in a couple. She didn't focus on wanting children and when I asked whether this was something she wished for herself, she responded as if she had all the time in the world. I was aware of how preoccupied other female patients of this age can be with their biological clocks, with some women electing to freeze their eggs in order to keep their options open, yet for Helen this did not seem to be on her horizon. I became aware that there were powerful defences of denial in operation.

Freud and Klein regarded projection as the basis for paranoia, whereby the outside world comes to be feared because of what has been projected onto it. We can see that there is a strong connection between anxiety and aggression, with anxiety often being the feared consequence of projected aggression. Freud and Klein also described how parts of the self could be projected out (not just feelings and conflicts). For example, we can think about racism in terms of projection, in that what is disowned in the self (e.g. 'primitiveness', 'animality'), is projected onto others, who are then denigrated, hated and feared. In the Victorian era, for example, it was not uncommon for white Europeans to refer to black Africans as "primitive" and "animalistic", thus ridding the white racist of their own animality (Fanon, 1967). Similarly, notions of the body as vulnerable and mortal may be projected onto people with disabilities, who are then feared and denigrated (Watermeyer, 2012). We will return to some of these ideas in Chapter 13 when considering psychodynamic approaches to diversity and difference.

Splitting

Freud (1938) acknowledged that the integrity of the mind could be compromised by a splitting of the ego, whereby two separate, conflicting ideas are held in mind in a segregated way. Klein later developed this idea to include both splitting the ego and/or the object, leading to un-integrated and fragmented object relational experiences (Hinshelwood, 1989). The object is split so that it can be separately perceived as either a 'good' or a 'bad' object (this is the *raison d'etre* for the paranoid-schizoid position). In relationships, we can see this defence of splitting when the object is idealised (loved) at some times, and another version of the object that is denigrated (hated) yet kept apart. Individuals who resort to splitting in their relationships may experience intense love and idealisation for their partner one day, only to hate and denigrate them the next day (without being able to hold on to an enduring, balanced feeling of love of a whole object).

At the start of therapy, Sam complained freely about his father's aggressive, bullying treatment of him, which he contrasted against his mother's. He idealised her as a saint who could do no wrong. As the work progressed, he began to get in touch with, and work through, his repressed anger towards his mother. It became evident that his mother had not protected him from his father's bullying. So, the split allowed Sam to keep some sense of his mother as a good object, by splitting off and locating all the bad experiences entirely in his father. The work of therapy allowed him to reconcile this split and integrate his objects, thereby facilitating his movement from the paranoid-schizoid to the depressive position.

Klein described splitting of the ego, whereby aspects of the self are split off and projected. We see how patients can create an idealised version of themselves as hard-working, caring and considerate, which is kept separate from a more troubling version of themselves as unwanted, worthless and bad. Although the split occurs to protect some sense of self-worth, it remains precarious at being undermined by discordant responses from others. The self is also weakened by this split. Thus, we can see that the defence of splitting is not wholly successful, because what is split off is projected outwards and constantly threatens to return. Experiences of splitting are often linked to feelings of paranoia. It is also evident that splitting and projection go hand-in-hand.

Projective identification

One of Klein's defining contributions is her formulation of the defence of projective identification, a complex object relational matrix. As the name suggests, this includes the defence mechanism of projection which has led to difficulties in differentiating projection from projective identification; sometimes the two terms are thought to refer to the same process (Hinshelwood, 1989). However, whereas projection refers solely to the process of projecting something from the inside out, projective identification also includes the process of *introjection* as part of this object relations dynamic. Introjection is the opposite of projection: it is the process of incorporating an external object into oneself from the outside-in. Introjection can operate as a defence mechanism where a good external part-object is introjected and incorporated into the self, thereby defusing an internal conflict or anxiety. However, 'bad' part-objects can also be introjected.

In projective identification, what is split off is not just projected *onto* the object, but rather *into* the object. What is split off (e.g. the 'bad', aggressive self) is split off and projected into the object, who in turn introjects this projection (i.e. takes it in), and in so doing, unconsciously takes on the role of the 'bad' and aggressive object. Through this process, the self then attempts to control this split off part through trying to control the object. The self projects fantasies about others in relation to the self; those fantasies are then located *in* others who are co-opted to respond unconsciously in concordant ways. As you can see, this is a primitive form of communication of internal states that are often unbearable for the self to know about. Let's look at a clinical example of projective identification:

In my work with Leroy, I became curious when I found myself increasingly enraged with detailed accounts of his neglectful and manipulative parents. By contrast, my patient seemed very tolerant, even defending their actions. When I attempted to interpret his negative experience with his parents, he insinuated that I was being uncharitable and nasty for having such thoughts. And yet more material emerged of his parents' ill-treatment of him. In one session, Leroy described how his partner was angered by something his parents had done. Having become aware of this dynamic between us, I offered the following interpretation. I said that he seemed to need others, including me, to feel the anger towards his parents on his behalf, and that he could not bear to get in touch with his anger for fear of destroying the good aspects of his relationship with them. He reluctantly acknowledged that this was probably the case, and this allowed him to express some of his past hurt and frustration with his parents.

The first step in arriving at this interpretation of the projective identification at play, was to notice my powerful response, and how I was being inducted a very Cartesian view of Leroy's family as all bad. Prior to this, I had been drawn into this response without being aware that the anger may not belong to me. This allowed me to consider what psychological function my anger (ultimately, his split off anger) was serving him. In this case, he found his anger so distressing he was convinced he would not survive the imagined retaliatory attacks from his parents, thereby destroying any fragile goodness there was in his relationship with his parents. Leroy disowned his anger and projected it into me. In this way, he felt he was able to control and have mastery over it, turning me into the judgmental and critical therapist. In this way, Leroy protects his parents as well as himself, by keeping the goodness intact and split off from awareness.

Klein (1957) concentrated on the pathological, destructive aspects of projective identification. For example, she introduced the way envy is involved in projective identification, whereby the projected 'badness' is forced into the object in an attempt to spoil or destroy its good attributes. Bion (1959) recognised a more benign form of projective identification in which emotional states are projected into the object as a form of communication about those emotional states. This is implicated in Bion's notion of containment. We can see that this communicative type of projective identification was at play in the clinical example above of Leroy and his therapist. Hinshelwood (1989) summarises these two different aims of projective identification:

(i) one is to evacuate violently a painful state of mind leading to forcibly entering an object, in phantasy, for immediate relief, and often with the aim of an intimidating control of the object [while] (ii) the other is to introduce into the object a state of mind, as a means of communicating with it about this mental state. (p. 184)

Table 6.1 sets out some of the commonly found defences in psychotherapy. Anna Freud (1954) listed nine (neurotic) defences in her book *The Ego and The Mechanisms of Defence* (namely, repression, regression, reaction formation, isolation of affect and intellectualisation; undoing, projection, introjection, turning against the self and reversal into the opposite). She later added sublimation, which was supposedly less of a defence than a normal mechanism (Akhtar, 2009a). Akhtar (2009a) goes on to point out that in an interview Anna Freud gave to Joseph Sandler in 1983, decades after writing her monograph, she noted that one does not really count such things (as defence mechanisms). We should also bear in mind Charles Brenner's (1981) observation, "Modes of defence are as diverse as psychic life itself" (p. 561). He points out that "Any aspect of ego functioning may be used for defence" (p. 586) and as such, there are no special defence mechanisms. He goes on to say that "Every defence denies or negates something" (p. 568).

Destructive defensive behaviour

As we said earlier, any aspect of ego functioning can be used as a defence, which includes how we act in the world. Anna Freud noted how a patient of hers resorted to behaviours like falling asleep and arriving late in order to defend against his aggression (Sandler and Freud, 1981, p. 18). Some people may resort to behaviours that often have destructive consequences as a form of defence against painful feelings, including drug and alcohol misuse, compulsive sex and addiction to pornography, gambling, extreme sports and so on. While some of these behaviours may be mental health problems in their own right (e.g. alcohol dependency), they can also be understood as manic defences or forms of acting out against painful emotions (see Table 6.1). For example, taking part in extreme sports can sometimes function as a manic defence against feelings of vulnerability and mortality. Binge drinking or taking drugs may be a way to act out feelings of anger, with some describing the moment of starting to get drunk or deciding to snort a line of cocaine as prompted by a defiant and hedonistic attitude of "Fuck it!" The focus of psychodynamic psychotherapy is to think about what prompts these behaviours, and what is being defended against by partaking in them. With alcohol and drugs, we can also see this as an attempt to drown out or obliterate painful feelings. We need to weigh up the power of these addictions against the willingness of the patient to tolerate the inevitable painful feelings that will arise when entering psychotherapy treatment: will we be able to compete with the thrall of tranquilisers or alcohol?

Sex can also be used defensively, particularly when it becomes compulsive sex. For example, in the movie *Shame* directed by Steve McQueen, we witness the main character, Brandon (played by the actor Michael Fassbender) and his defensive use of sex. The film depicts Brandon as someone who often masturbates to porn, has sex with women he hooks up with in bars, and frequents sex workers. We could initially describe Brandon as someone who enjoys sex, but we soon witness a downward spiral into anonymous, compulsive, potentially destructive sexual activity, following a surprise visit from his sister. As the narrative unfolds, we come to understand that the two siblings hide a traumatic childhood history, probably involving abuse, which is alluded to but never explicitly described (his sister tells him "We are not bad people; we just come from a bad place"). We start to understand Brandon's compulsive use of sex as a means of defending himself against unbearable feelings of shame: an orgasm provides temporary but ineffective relief, leaving his underlying conflict and difficulties unaddressed.

Defences and attachment styles

While defences are commonly understood as an unconscious mechanism for protecting the self against internal conflict and anxiety, many defences operate in the context of interpersonal dynamics. As we have discussed earlier, the defences of splitting, projection and projective identification are key defences operating in Klein's object relations model of moving from paranoid-schizoid to depressive position functioning, where the individual becomes able to tolerate ambivalent feelings towards the whole object.

We can also conceptualise defences in relation to attachment styles. The primary defensive strategy in the face of an attachment threat is seeking security from a trusted figure (Shaver and Mikulincer, 2007). However, individuals will also develop defensive secondary attachment strategies of hyperactivation and deactivation of the attachment system. Hyperactivating attachment strategies involve upregulating emotions in response to the perceived unavailability of the object, in an effort to get greater emotional closeness and the reassurance that brings. Typically, this involves a lot of 'protest behaviour', as Bowlby (1969) termed it. In babies and small children, this takes the form of crying and calling for the loved parent, as seen in the Strange Situation experiment (described in detail in Chapter 2). In adults, this can manifest in demanding and clingy behaviour, overwhelming affect (at the expense of cognition), actions designed to signal distress like suicide threats and attempts, self-harm, aggressive outbursts, taking unnecessary risks, eating disorders, harmful substance abuse and so on. A hyperactivating attachment strategy is linked to the preoccupied attachment style. There is a push for clinging and closeness in the face of feared rejection and abandonment by others. In this strategy, there is an over-focus on others at the expense of the self. These patients are overly sensitive to rejection and experience anaclitic depression, a fear of being abandoned and feeling unloved (Blatt, 1974).

By contrast, the deactivating attachment strategy is linked to the fearful avoidant and dismissive attachment styles. These people downplay affect and relationships, focusing exclusively on cognition. They may even be alexithymic, that is, without a vocabulary for expressing their emotions. Although these patients seem to be calm in the face of stress, when their galvanic skin response and cortisol levels are measured, they are in fact raised (Mikiluncer et al., 2009). There is a disconnect between the internal distress and the outward manifestation of calm. We can see that this split has developed defensively to keep the individual safe from further threat, keeping any vulnerability under wraps.

In the case of more significant environmental trauma or abuse, more complex defensive structures are at play. We have found the following two psychoanalytic theories – the core complex (Glasser, 1986) and the moral defence (Fairbairn, 1952) – useful when thinking about defences and attachment in the context of trauma and abuse.

Core complex

Glasser (1986) wrote about the 'core complex', which he identified as a key feature of 'perverse' patients as well as a feature of development. In the core complex, the individual fears both separation from the object on the one hand, and complete merger with the object on the other. This creates an ever-present conflict of feeling either too close, or too distant from the object. When the object is perceived as moving emotionally closer, this activates fears of engulfment including being taken over and even annihilated by the object. The individual's aggressive defence is then to push away by negating the importance of the object. When there is emotional distance between self and object, the individual fears separation and abandonment and longs for merger with the object, and so becomes needy for the object. Glasser usefully summarises the core complex structure as:

> a basic, central, coherent structure established in early infancy and made up of the inter-related ingredients of the longing for intimate gratification and security, the anxieties of annihilation and abandonment, with the attendant depression, and the aggression and sado-masochism. (1986, p. 10)

While Glasser wrote about the core complex in relation to 'perversions', sadism and masochism, it has become a useful concept to understand troubling relationship dynamics in patients whom we might not label as 'perverse'. Many patients have some difficulty with elements of separation and merger between self and object. Blatt and Luyten (2009) describe two developmental trajectories that we all have in our lives, namely a wish for attachment and closeness to others on the one hand, and a wish for self-definition and separateness on the other hand. These two developmental lines come together in the core complex in a defensive way, where there is a movement from one extreme to the other. The fear of merger leads the individual to pull back from any closeness, favouring self-sufficiency. However, this withdrawal leaves the person isolated and alone. It is difficult for the person to find the right distance from their objects. This brings to mind Schopenhauer's parable about the dilemma facing porcupines on a cold night who struggled to find the right distance: when they were too far apart, they were too cold but when they were too close, their quills pricked one another (Luepnitz, 2002).

Moral defence

In cases of severe abuse or emotional deprivation, Fairbairn (1952) observed what he termed the 'moral defence'. This is where the abused child, feeling loyalty towards their abusive parent, would blame *themselves* for their maltreatment, rather than their parents. Here, the child would prefer to feel that they were treated as such because *they* were 'bad' rather than the parents. In this defence, the child maintains some sense of omnipotence (in fantasy) that if they became good, the abuse would stop, and the parents will be good parents. In this way, there is some sense of control in a situation where they are actually helpless. In adults, we can sometimes observe this defence in abusive relationships, where the victim of abuse may blame themselves for what is happening, thereby protecting the abuser.

The false self

In Chapter 2, we introduced Winnicott's key theories including his formulation of the false self and authentic, or true self. We are reintroducing the concept of the false self here because it serves a form of character defence. You will recall that Winnicott described how the young child in the face of environmental impingements from key figures, learns to protect the authentic self by developing a false self. In this way, a split develops within the ego, whereby an external shell is constructed to engage with the world without exposing any vulnerable internal experiences. Over time, this can lead to a disconnection with the internal self and an increasingly empty and unsatisfying experience of being in the world. Although we may feel that it is good to be authentic and bad to be false, this would be an oversimplification. We all have to moderate what we would like to express as part of the process of socialisation through childhood and into adolescence. We may want to swear at our teacher but doing so will not serve us well. Hiding our 'authentic' response is adaptive in this instance. However, where the young child learns to repress their own wishes and desires because they do not believe these will be received warmly or even safely, this leads to a false adaptation to others that is restrictive rather than adaptive. This may include taking the blame back on to the self, as seen in Fairbairn's moral defence. It may also manifest in over-compliance, self-denigration, perfectionism, an inflated sense of self-worth, and so on. Here is a clinical example to illustrate this:

Mary described growing up in a family where she was always on edge, afraid of her dad's drunken rages and her mum's inconsistent responses to her. She became finely attuned to any shifts in their mood and learned to adjust herself to their behaviour, anticipating it, for example, by waking up to ensure her father had dinner when he came home intoxicated late at night. She spoke about how she was able to attend to his needs better than her mother; this gave her a sense of being appreciated and indispensable. With her mother, she tried to gain her approval by being the type of daughter she thought she wanted, demure and well-behaved. She learned not to argue with her and to swallow any anger she had. Over time, she found that she turned to food to manage her unexpressed feelings, often bingeing on sweets and chocolates that she then purged. She felt a sense of shame around this behaviour but hid it from everyone. In her relationships, she tried to please her partners often at her own expense. In one relationship with a much older man, she found herself alternately neglected and debased by him. In another relationship, she was willing to change her religion and appearance in order to gain his approval.

When Mary entered therapy, she often took her cues from what I said, subtly altering how she presented herself. She was acutely sensitive to any interest I showed in her. Mary struggled to share her distress in sessions, tending to laugh and play down her difficulties. She was surprised to learn that I was interested in times when she may inevitably feel let down or misunderstood by me. We came to see how she had learned over time to develop a mask behind which she hid her true feelings. The façade she presented to the world covered up aspects of herself that she believed were unacceptable to others and inhibited her ability to express herself freely. She always felt she was a worthless outsider in relation to others, a situation that cropped up repeatedly in her work, family, friendships, intimate relationships and in the transference. When she arrived in tears having been dumped by her boyfriend, she was unable to edit herself as carefully as before and this allowed our work together to deepen. We often returned to this moment in which she took a risk and dropped her usual coping strategies yet did not receive the judgemental response she expected from me.

Working with defences in therapy

Patients usually come for therapy wanting help in understanding a certain pattern of behaviour or why they feel so intensely about something that has happened to them. In relating their predominant narrative, we listen for the manifest content, that is, the factual story and sequence of events of who did what to whom, yet as we have seen, there is usually another, latent level of meaning with unconscious dynamics at play (see also Chapter 8 on unconscious communications). A key competence in psychodynamic work is the ability to recognise and work with defences. When we encounter problematic behaviour, we need to uncover the underlying conflict and how the patient makes use of different defence mechanisms in an attempt to cope with it by keeping the conflict outside of conscious awareness, as far as possible. However, these attempts are not wholly successful. Freud (1914a) posited a dynamic unconscious in which repressed contents return to conscious awareness. The material the patient is attempting to repress, threatens to erupt into consciousness, usually in a disguised form, such as a physical symptom, feeling, dream, slip of the tongue or other manifestation of latent content.

How to interpret the patient's use of defences

Malan (2001), building on Menninger's (1958) work, has usefully conceptualised a heuristic for working with defences and anxiety in psychotherapy, namely the 'triangle of conflict' as shown in Figure 6.2. The triangle represents the relationship between the three core elements involved in working with defences: defence, anxiety and the underlying hidden feeling. The triangle is placed upside down on its apex to indicate that there is an underlying element to the other two sides of the triangle, in this case the concealed or repressed affect. Malan linked this triangle with a second triangle, the *triangle of person*, reflecting the transference dynamics between the therapist, other current or recent relationships, and the parent or

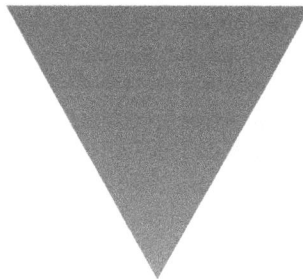

DEFENCE   ANXIETY

HIDDEN FEELING
(Often an impulse)

Figure 6.2 Adapted from Malan's triangle of conflict
Source: Malan, 2001, p. 90

sibling. It can be considered that the tasks of the psychodynamic therapist are summarised within these two heuristics. We will discuss further the relationship between the triangle of person and the triangle of conflict in Chapter 9.

When making interpretations about the patient's anxiety and defence, it is advisable for the therapist to work from left to right, starting with naming and observing the defence before moving on to linking it to the expressed anxiety. Only once this has been understood, can we move towards making links with the hidden feeling. By then, the patient has become more conscious of their behaviour and we have a foundation on which to begin to hypothesise about the less apparent, repressed feelings.

By way of example, let us return to Zara, whose history and psychodynamic formulation we introduced in Chapter 5. One of her defences was her tendency to minimise her distress and be superficially cheerful and helpful to others, even if at her own expense. The therapist may make an observation such as, "I noticed that you just made light of something, feeling it is indulgent to complain", thus observing the defence of *reaction formation*. The therapist can then link the defence to Zara's anxiety by saying, for example, "I can see that this is a way you try to protect yourself from the painful realities". This allows space to explore further those painful realities and the feared responses. The therapist can then go on to link this to the hidden feeling, by adding, "You fear being a burden to others, and so minimise your distress, but this takes you away from knowing about the needy part of you who wants to be close to others, but fears abandonment".

It is important to stress that the therapist can only proceed to explore these hidden feelings when the patient indicates their willingness to engage at this level. So, while this example proceeds from defence to anxiety to hidden feeling, this series of interpretations may take place over a series of sessions, depending on the individual dynamics of the patient. Malan (2001) describes how the therapist needs to be engaged in an internal reflective process when considering when and how to make an interpretation with a patient. He reminds us that an interpretation is not a mechanical technique that can be learnt as a formula; rather it is "essentially intuitive and subconscious" (p. 84). The therapist has to reflect on what is communicated in the room verbally and non-verbally, as well as their theoretical knowledge and understanding, together with self-awareness of their own mental states in order to offer an interpretation to the patient. This involves reflective engagement with the following aspects of the session (Malan, 2001, p. 84):

- The depth of rapport between the patient and therapist and the extent to which the patient seems in touch with their feelings
- The possible nature of the hidden feeling or impulse
- How accessible these feelings may be (i.e. are they bubbling just below the surface?)
- The intensity of anxiety or emotional pain that is invested in them, and
- Whether the patient may be able to bear hearing it at that moment in time.

The therapist may need to sit with a period of not knowing before moving to interpret. Some gradual exploration is needed, with the therapist learning from the feedback that the patient gives them. This may be observable through changes in the depth of rapport or further emotional engagement of the patient. If a tentative interpretation is well-received, it usually leads to a deepening of rapport and this indicates that the therapist may well be on the right track. We pay careful attention to the direction of the patient's response to the interpretation to sense whether what we have said has facilitated the patient's ability to explore further and gain additional insight themselves. If on the other hand, rapport falls off, this may indicate that the therapist may be on the wrong track, or they may be intervening with an interpretation too soon. Interpretations can't be rushed or forced because they will create the opposite effect, resulting in an even more defended patient and reducing epistemic trust.

Resistance in psychotherapy

Resistance refers to the operation of defences in the therapeutic setting and can appear clinically in both obvious and unobtrusive ways (Glover, 1927). Some forms of resistance are overt like getting on to a train going in the opposite direction to the therapist's consulting room or forgetting to pay a bill on time. Others are less clear, like quietly complying with what the therapist says without expressing any conflicting reactions the patient may have or the realisation that therapy has ground to a standstill, with the same material being recycled over and over again. Even relentless punctuality can be understood as a hidden resistance, protecting the patient from ever disrupting the frame of therapy and the feared reaction of the therapist. Glover (1927) points out that "the mind will exercise a defensive function" (p. 486) throughout the course of psychotherapy and that all the defence mechanisms can function as resistance. He highlights that

> The most successful resistances are silent, and it might be said that the sign of their existence is our unawareness of them; in other words, resistances exist which we are able to detect most often in retrospect, and of which we first become cognizant either on account of a slowing of progress or because of some more or less explosive break-through in obvious forms. (p. 486)

Resistance finds expression in many different ways in therapy, including falling silent, speaking inaudibly, chattering on, acting out by missing sessions, forgetting what has been discussed in previous sessions, feeling drowsy or even ending therapy when things start to feel too uncomfortable. We will explore particular aspects of resistance in greater detail in Chapter 9 on transference and countertransference, Chapter 10 on endings and Chapter 12 on challenging situations and clinical dilemmas.

A more challenging expression of resistance is the continuous use of defence mechanisms during therapy sessions that serve to keep the patient at a distance from making emotional contact with their underlying issues and the therapist. For example, some patients resort to intellectualisation in therapy where insight is maintained at a superficial, cognitive level, with little emotional engagement in their underlying feelings and conflicts. They may employ psychoanalytic terms as part of this rationalising defence and this can be particularly evident at the beginnings and endings of sessions. We may be invited to join with the patient as if they were a colleague, even being drawn into discussing someone in their lives who is presented to us as the 'identified patient' in their own place. One patient regularly began sessions by questioning why they were in therapy after all and what was the purpose of dredging up the events of the week and their past. It would take them much of the session to feel reconnected to the therapist. Another patient would disengage as the ending of the session approached, asking the therapist what they would do with the material that had been shared and feeling unsafe and suspicious as the time to part ways drew close.

Much of the work of psychodynamic psychotherapy, particularly in the early stages of building a therapeutic alliance, involves recognising the patient's resistance and addressing this. Resistance is an integral part of the transference relationship. Careful thought is needed about how and when to interpret this. As stated earlier, we do not want to strip the patient of their defences entirely, particularly when working in more short-term and focused ways. We need to respect that patients progress at their own rate of change. In brief psychotherapy, we do become more active with patients, for example by flagging the number of sessions and encouraging some change in relation to the agreed goals. This is slightly different in longer term psychotherapy where we don't work with a circumscribed focus for the work. Whatever the length of time, it is important to take up with the patient the way they avoid facing certain topics. This fits with one of the basic psychodynamic competences of helping patients become aware of unexpressed or unconscious feelings. We pay attention to what is not being said and what is being skirted, as well as what is being said. It is possible to work with the effect of resistance and the underlying fear it defends against in a similar fashion to the way we would work with the cost of keeping a secret rather than allowing the truth to come out.

Often there is a countertransference response to resistance that may represent the therapist's complementary role response to the patient's struggles (see Chapter 9). For example, some therapists may stay away from interpreting the patient's aggression because they are afraid of conflict, hurting the patient or rupturing the relationship, particularly if this is their training patient. We need to keep monitoring this in order to avoid being drawn into interpreting too quickly, for example, or moving to discharge a patient prematurely.

Box 6.2 Useful resources

Readings

You may want to read Anna Freud's (1954) slim volume, *The ego and the mechanisms of defence* (first published in 1936).

Alessandra Lemma has written a book on humour, entitled *Humour on the couch: Exploring humour in psychotherapy and everyday life* (2000).

As mentioned in Chapter 2, Bartholomew and Horowitz (1991) have developed an adult attachment questionnaire that match on to the four different attachment styles that can be observed in childhood. This questionnaire, available at the end of their paper can be used as a useful tool with patients during an assessment to think about the possible defences they may be drawing on in their interpersonal contexts.

Bartholomew, K. and Horowitz, L. M. (1991). Attachment styles among young adults: A test of a four-category model. *Journal of Personality and Social Psychology, 61*(2), 226–244.

Online resources

There is an amusing clip of various film excerpts chosen to illustrate eight of the defence mechanisms that you can find at this website: https://youtu.be/FnRBAU6Yg2A

Patricia Coughlin is an Intensive Short-term Dynamic Psychotherapy (ISTDP) practitioner who uses Malan's triangle of defence in her work and you can see her talking about how she works with defences in a clinical example in her YouTube clip https://youtu.be/eVOgXhq49ek; she also has a post on defences and countertransference https://youtu.be/72GfT-uHE0o and a post on anxiety https://youtu.be/_BFHSKcax08

You can also watch Alan Abbas, an ISTDP practitioner, talking about resistance at https://youtu.be/0LFP4fvGgOU and he focuses particularly on the somatic experience of defences and resistance

The School of Life have a useful clip on Anna Freud and Defence Mechanisms https://youtu.be/v80Nd8w1uts

7 Mentalising

Imagine a patient sitting quietly in the session when suddenly they begin to cry and clench their fists. As you picture the patient in this scene, you are probably imagining the person's emotional states and their likely back story. You are probably wondering what thoughts were in their mind to prompt this emotional outburst. You may be comparing yourself to the imagined patient, at some level. All of this mental activity falls under the banner of mentalising. You are mentalising whenever you are attempting to make sense of what goes on in the mind, whether this is your own mind or the mind of others.

Mentalisation is an elusive concept, familiar yet confounding. This chapter will locate mentalising within psychodynamic theory as well as link it to existing concepts with which you may be familiar. We will focus on how the capacity to mentalise develops, how to recognise poor mentalising in our patients and most importantly, how to restore mentalising to maximise the effectiveness of our interventions as therapists.

Mentalising tends not to be included in texts on psychodynamic psychotherapy nor explicitly taught in psychodynamic and analytic psychotherapy trainings. Mentalising does not appear in its own right in the UCL list of competences for psychodynamic/analytic psychotherapy. However, as we outlined in Chapter 2, Fonagy and colleagues' mentalising model of development draws substantially on psychoanalytic theories to understand the development and capacity for emotional regulation as well as mental states. As we will come to see in this chapter, some of the generic psychotherapy competences can be subsumed under the banner of mentalising, including the ability to engage the patient; the ability to foster and maintain a good therapeutic alliance; the capacity to grasp the patient's perspective and 'world view'; as well as the ability to deal with emotional content of sessions. We also feel that the following basic analytic/dynamic competences can be considered as aspects of mentalising, namely the ability to work with both the patient's internal and external reality; as well as the ability to identify and respond to difficulties in the therapeutic relationship. Finally, we consider the following meta-competences also fall within the concept of mentalisation, namely the capacity to adapt interventions in response to patient feedback; the ability to make use of the therapeutic relationship as a vehicle for change (both generic competences); the ability to apply the model flexibly in response to the patient's individual needs and context; the ability to establish an appropriate balance between interpretative and supportive work; as well as the ability to identify and skilfully apply the most appropriate analytic/dynamic approach (all analytic-specific meta-competences). This should already give you some sense of mentalising as an overarching concept.

Although mentalising has its roots in psychodynamic theories, it is fair to say that psychoanalysis as a profession has seen it as more of a threat than an ally, in a similar way that Bowlby's attachment theory was considered an analytic outlier. Perhaps this is because the techniques proposed by mentalisation-informed therapies differ radically from traditional analytic techniques that emphasise interpretation and insight, most notably the mentalising stance of not knowing, being curious and asking questions. Perhaps the antipathy is related to research findings that showed Mentalisation-Based Therapy (MBT) can treat patients diagnosed with Borderline Personality Disorder more efficiently than psychoanalytic/dynamic psychotherapy, and that classical psychoanalysis may even be considered contra-indicated for this patient group (Bateman and Fonagy, 2006), particularly where working in the transference activates the patient's already hyperactive attachment system, thereby further inhibiting their capacity to mentalise.

It is possible to situate mentalising as a bridge across cognitive and analytic techniques. We are including it in this book because it represents an important development in technique that empowers therapists to work with their patients more effectively by recognising when patients are mentalising poorly and improving their capacity to mentalise, thereby increasing the effectiveness of therapeutic interventions. It also equips therapists with ways of dealing with breakdowns in the therapeutic relationship at times when we often defensively retreat into theoretical certainty about what is going on and we thus lose our own mentalising capacity and become less effective as therapists. It is also one of the techniques used in Dynamic Interpersonal Therapy with depressed and anxious patients who typically have compromised mentalising capacities.

In writing this chapter, we are hugely indebted to Peter Fonagy, Mary Hepworth (formerly Target) and Anthony Bateman for their work in this area. There may be times when key concepts related to mentalising appear not to be referenced, however, the entire chapter contains ideas emanating from their body of work and it would be cumbersome to keep making reference to this without interrupting the narrative flow of the chapter.

What is mentalisation?

We gave a brief introduction to the mentalisation model of development in Chapter 2. Mentalising involves a creative mental activity of holding several possibilities in mind at the same time, allowing us to represent the same situation in many ways and adopt multiple perspectives. Another way of putting it is that mentalising is the ability to see yourself from the outside and others from the inside. It is mostly a preconscious, imaginative mental activity in which we

envision what others may be thinking or feeling. It is idiographic to each individual because it is affected by that person's history and capacity that leads them to
draw particular conclusions about a situation (Bateman and Fonagy, 2006). In
many ways, mentalising is the bread and butter of psychotherapy; it involves
thinking about feeling. Mental states are infused with emotion. Indeed, strong
feelings often inhibit and obstruct our ability to mentalise flexibly. Our reactions
to other people are filtered by moral judgements and attitudes which in turn are
bound up in our experience of ourselves and others.

Bogdan (2005) states that at the core of understanding others' minds is the
ascription of representational states or attitudes, which he calls "representingness"
(p. 190). We have a sense of 'representingness' regarding mental states, that is, an
implicit awareness that a mental state is always a particular version of a situation.
Acquiring this perspective of mental states is a major developmental achievement
and much of psychopathology entails losing this capacity. For example, in
depression there may be great certainty that oneself, the world and the future are
hopeless, leaving suicide as the only viable solution in extreme states of depression. Another example is those people described as 'psychopaths' are likely to
experience others as objects to manipulate and exploit rather than feeling compassion or empathy for them. Furthermore, in Post-Traumatic Stress Disorder,
trauma is continually re-experienced and relived as flashbacks, with the conviction that the original trauma is recurring.

We are mentalising all the time, making sense of the world and the way people
operate in it, including a self-perspective. Mentalising is a dynamic function that
is affected by stress, particularly in interpersonal relationships – it can easily be
lost. Paradoxically, in a therapy session when you are struggling to make sense of
your patient, you are probably mentalising well, whereas when you pat yourself
on the back for your ability to understand your patient, you have probably stopped mentalising and become overly certain of their mental state. We make inferences from what we observe and feel, undertaking this detective work implicitly
and explicitly, depending on the circumstances.

A brief history of mentalisation

The concept of mentalising is rooted in psychoanalysis although it has since
flourished in the framework of attachment theory. The use of 'mentalising' was
first recorded in 1807 (Allen et al., 2008). It was then found in the Oxford English
Dictionary in 1906, where it was defined as "to imagine or give a mental quality
to; to construct or picture in the mind; to cultivate mentally or stimulate the mind
of" (p. 3). Mentalising was first mentioned in French psychoanalytic literature in
the late 1960s, then more widely introduced towards understanding autism,
where it was conceived of as 'mind-blindness' or a neurobiological failure in
mentalising. Mentalising was notably extended by Fonagy and Target, who linked
mentalising deficits to developmental psychopathology, disturbances in early
attachment and resultant personality disorders (notably Borderline Personality
Disorder).

Mentalising describes a mental *activity,* thus Jon Allen makes the case for using the present participle verb "mentalising" to capture this action mode as opposed to seeing it as something that we do or fail to do (Bateman and Fonagy, 2006). Mentalising can be located in four domains of contemporary theory and research: evolutionary biology, neurobiology, theory of mind and attachment. We will now elaborate each of these four areas. *Evolutionary biology* or *phylogeny* shows the importance of the social brain to survival: we need to know our enemies and allies in order to stay alive. Mentalising is an essential tool in achieving this, as it enables us to know the minds (and motives) of our enemies and allies. In the area of *neurobiology*, mentalising has been evidenced by neuroimaging that shows patterns of cortical activity that allow us to map the areas of the brain involved with different aspects of mentalising. If you would like to understand more of the neurological underpinning of mentalising, there is a helpful chapter on neurobiology in *Mentalising in Clinical Practice* by Allen, Fonagy and Bateman (2008).

Theory of mind refers to the ability to surmise the mental states of others. It refers to research that identified a shift in the child's ability to attribute mental states to others in order to understand and predict social behaviour and it is usually demonstrated through the following type of experiment where two different perspectives are presented to the subject (e.g. Allen et al., 2008). A young child is shown a scenario where a little boy and girl place a ball in a cupboard. The boy leaves the room and the girl moves the ball to a new position under a cushion on the couch. The observing child is then asked where the boy will look for the ball when he returns to the room. It is a mark of development when the observing child can intuit that the boy will return to his last known position of the ball (i.e. in the cupboard), even though the child saw the ball moved to another spot. This requires the subject to put themselves in the shoes of the boy and see the world through his eyes. Theory of mind is this capacity to detect mental states and reason on the basis of those states. As you can see, this a narrower definition than mentalising and does not include affective states or the attribution of intentional states of mind.

This brings us to the domain of *attachment theory.* The availability of the caregiver to the infant empowers the infant to make adaptive choices in the face of environmental stress (Fonagy et al., 2011). Where there are limited opportunities for the infant to learn about their mind through the mind of the caregiver (to use a Winnicottian model of development), mentalising is unable to be securely established. This brings us on to another key concept, that of *epistemic trust* or *epistemic safety*, namely the individual's confidence in their caretakers as reliable sources of information and their trust in the authenticity and personal relevance of interpersonally transmitted information (Allison and Fonagy, 2016). Indeed, most of our learning takes place in the context of human relationships and interpersonal situations. Establishing epistemic trust is an evolutionary development whereby children are biologically programmed to learn about their subjective worlds only from adults whose attitudes they consider benign. Epistemic trust develops in the context of sensitive responses from our attachment figures in early childhood and leads to neural development. Thus, a secure environment and attachment context fosters robust mentalising and emotional regulation.

As psychotherapists, we need to pay particular attention to developing epistemic trust with our patients since without this, we will struggle to form a therapeutic alliance and our interventions will lack credibility. Epistemic trust results in greater resilience by triggering an 'epistemic superhighway', an evolutionary protected mechanism that signals readiness to acquire knowledge (Fonagy and Allison, 2014). Mentalising in therapy is a generic way of establishing epistemic trust; and establishing epistemic trust is essential to effective treatment. The centrality of the therapeutic alliance to psychotherapy of all modalities is probably vested in this evolutionarily preserved mechanism for cultural transmission (Gergely and Unoka, 2008). Feeling understood in therapy restores trust in learning from social experience, but at the same time, regenerates a capacity for social understanding (i.e. mentalising others). Improved social understanding alongside increased epistemic trust makes life outside therapy a setting in which new information about oneself and the world can be acquired and internalised. Ultimately, it may be that therapeutic change does not result from new skills or insights gained in the consulting room, but rather the capacity of the therapeutic relationship to create a potential for learning about oneself and others in the world outside of therapy (Fonagy and Allison, 2014). This is also suggested by research findings on the efficacy and outcomes of psychodynamic psychotherapy.

In therapy, we want to attend to early negative transference and difficulties in the therapeutic relationship because this represents a source of epistemic vigilance, even hypervigilance, namely an understandable, self-protective suspicion towards potentially damaging or deceptive information coming from others. Later in this chapter, we will look at the importance of repairing breaches in the therapeutic alliance because once epistemic trust is lost, its absence creates rigidity in thinking, sending the mentalising of both patient and therapist off-line. In these scenarios, the patient becomes "hard to reach" and interpersonally inaccessible. Chronic epistemic vigilance limits the capacity to internalise available knowledge as something 'safe' to use in order to organise behaviour. This aligns with psychoanalytic concepts of defence mechanisms and transference. Repairing ruptures in interpersonal relationships of which the therapeutic relationship is one type, usually leads to greater closeness and improved sense of relatedness.

Mentalising Based Therapy (MBT) was developed for patients with a diagnosis of Borderline Personality Disorder, who present with anxious attachment, mentalising deficits and resultant emotional dysregulation. As mentioned previously, mentalising techniques are used judiciously in Dynamic Interpersonal Therapy where mentalising is adversely affected by symptoms of depression and anxiety. In fact, mentalising deficits have been observed in a number of mental health problems. Thus, poor mentalising can be thought of as a trans-diagnostic sign of mental health problems, regardless of the specific symptoms (Fonagy et al., 2011).

How do we develop the capacity to mentalise?

In Chapter 2, we gave a brief outline of how the capacity to mentalise develops in infancy in the context of significant attachment relationships. It is worth expanding our discussion here, drawing more on the neurological as well as psychological aspects of developing the capacity to mentalise.

Researchers like Daniel Stern, Allan Schore and Colwyn Trevarthen have shown that the infant is primed from birth to particular movements and stimuli that allow the baby to differentiate the self from others in their environment and to foster bodily agency in the world. Newborn babies are pre-wired to attend to faces and face-like stimuli, probably because faces provide rich sources of social information that allow them to make social inferences (Frank et al., 2009). The human brain is primed for engagement and relationships. At around three months, the baby is drawn to stimuli that are slightly different to the self. This shift in attention to the response of others towards the baby's actions bring the baby more into the social world. Gergely and Watson (1996) conclude that emotional mirroring (also termed 'social biofeedback') fosters mentalising ability in infants and that infants learn about their emotions from 'the outside in'. The emotionally attuned responses from others link with the infant's lived experience, including their internal states, and this in turn makes emotional states meaningful and allows for them to be represented. To return to Winnicott, the infant finds their mind in the mind of their primary caregiver. The caregiver forms a mental representation of the inferred mental states of the baby and then provides that representation back to the infant in such a way that the infant feels it is both congruous and separate from their experience. For example, when the baby cries, mother responds with exaggerated facial, vocal and gestural affective displays (such as narrowed eyes, downturned mouth, rubbing their eyes, pretend crying "waah, waah" and using sing-song 'motherese') as well as verbalising the baby's possible internal states, saying something like, "Poor baby, you really are miserable today!" Gergely and Watson (1996) refer to this as *marked* and *contingent mirroring*. The baby's mental state is *marked* as separate from the caregiver by this exaggerated quality that allows the baby to see it as belonging to themselves in a symbolic way. It is *contingent* in that the caregiver's response mirrors the baby's subjective internal state in an appropriately matched and emotionally attuned way. Marked and contingent mirroring facilitates the infant's ability to form a developing sense of their own psychological self and to modulate their affective states These ideas can also be linked to Bion's ideas of containment and thinking.

This emotional mirroring between the infant and caregiver is powerfully observed in the so-called Still-Face experiments (Tronick et al., 1979) where the difference can be observed in the infant's reaction to attuned versus misattuned mirroring. You can see this demonstrated very powerfully in a YouTube clip by Tronick (see Box 7.3). During the Still Face experiment, the mother interrupts her usual interaction with her infant and stops responding to the infant's social cues, adopting a frozen face devoid of expression or emotion. The baby protests, points, screeches and eventually loses postural control in a state of despair and overload. If the mother returns to responding to the baby as usual, the interruption is usually seen as a blip and the baby is resilient enough to overcome this. However, where this happens frequently in sustained ways and in the absence of any other type of benign interaction, the effects on the baby are far more pernicious and can be translated into ongoing difficulties with emotional regulation and impaired capacity to mentalise. The infant becomes unable to internalise self-states without appropriate marked and contingent mirroring; instead they are vulnerable to impaired mentalising, with mental states being "'enacted' rather than experienced" (Fonagy et al., 2011, p. 100). Social interactions become distorted and disrupted as a result. Thus, we can see that neglect often has more damaging consequences than attachment trauma incurred by intrusive or aggressive interactions.

The impact of the parent's attachment style is critical in determining the way the baby responds. One of the best predictors of a parent's attachment style is that of their own parents (e.g. Kim et al., 2014). Thus, generational layers of transmission of difficulties can be seen. This is why early intervention is so critical in order to create benign cycles of interaction and prevent psychopathology from developing in adult life. Awareness of our patient's attachment style can also give us an idea of when and how their mentalising is likely to go off-line.

Recognising impaired mentalising

In patients with histories of childhood trauma as well as those with diagnoses of personality disorder, somatic presentations, depression and anxiety, there are likely to be deficits in their capacity to mentalise for the reasons set out above. As therapists, it is crucial that we recognise these deficits so that we can work with our patients to restore their capacity to mentalise more flexibly and robustly. Otherwise, we may find our interventions do not reach our patients because they are not in a position to receive what we are saying. Our interpretations will fall on deaf ears if we fail to account for limitations in their mentalising capacity. In Box 7.1, we list some common signs of poor mentalising.

Box 7.1 Signs of poor mentalising

- Excessive detail, over-elaborating and overanalysing
- Focus on external social factors, e.g. government, council, community, etc.
- Focus on physical or structural labels
- Preoccupation with rules and responsibilities
- Denial of your involvement in a problem
- Blaming or fault-finding
- Expressions of certainty about thoughts of or feelings towards others
- Speaking in clichés and canned language
- Intolerance of the views of others – includes prejudice like racism, sexism etc.
- Disconnection from any feelings
- Excess of feelings without much thinking
- Limited capacity to play with or explore thoughts and feelings
- Valuing only physical demonstrations of intent

It is helpful to think about three different styles of poor mentalising to assist us in recognising this in our patients. This has been outlined by Bateman and Fonagy (2006) as well as Allen et al. (2008). Although it is helpful to distinguish these different types, in practice, these are theoretical constructs to aid the therapist in identifying poor mentalising.

The first type is *psychic equivalence*. This can be considered similar to Hanna Segal's (1957) notion of symbolic equations where the patient loses the capacity for "as if" thinking, in a failure in symbolisation. In psychic equivalence, there is no difference between internal and external realities: if I feel something, it is real. Most children go through a period of thinking like this that is developmentally appropriate. This is the age at which children may become afraid of the boogie monster that lives under the bed, where the power of imagination is as great as external reality. We also see this type of concrete thinking in adults with depression and anxiety. In these cases, thinking is so restricted that we stop feeling "as if" and experience things as fixed reality. Studies show that depression is characterised by impaired mentalisation (Fischer-Kern et al., 2008). Severely depressed patients are certain that they are worthless failures and that there is no hope for them – they *are* a failure, rather than feel *as if* they are. In its acute state, this can lead to suicidal behaviour. To use a metaphor, the depressed person does not see a light at the end of the tunnel as redemption but rather as the train coming towards them! In acute anxiety states, there is a similar experience of feared risks and anticipated outcomes becoming certainties and of the person losing touch with reality, relying on the past to predict the future with great inevitability. A good example of this is Post Traumatic Stress Disorder where a war veteran will respond to fireworks as if they are reliving the battlefields of Afghanistan. Their psychic reality equates with their external reality in the moment of the flashback. In psychic equivalence mode, mentalising is fixed and cannot easily be shifted. Our countertransference as therapists is often one of exasperation and frustration in these moments. Therapists can easily get into arguments or stand offs with their patients if we try to challenge their beliefs head on when they are in this mode of mentalising.

The second type is *pretend mode* or *hypermentalising*, also described as "excrementalising" by Jon Allen's daughter, Yvonne (Allen et al., 2008, p. 39) for reasons that will become apparent. In this type of distorted mentalising, there is over-thinking that has become decoupled from feeling. The patient appears to be saying things that sound as if they are in the service of self-reflection and therapy and that suggest they are being thoughtful about their experiences. However, when this mode of mentalising is used, it is like wheels spinning in the sand without any traction or progress. Rather, experiences are recycled in a way that feels stale and creates stuckness. We can understand this as a defensive retreat away from examining painful experiences and remaining in a pseudo-intellectualised state where emotions are too threatening. It can be considered a form of depersonalisation and derealisation. Too often, longer-term psychotherapies flounder in this state of affairs. We hear about people who go over and over the same ground year after year, without any shifts to their internal or external experiences. In our countertransference, one of the best indicators of pretend mode is that we may become bored and disengaged as therapists. These are the moments when you feel your thoughts moving outside the consulting room, perhaps thinking about your shopping list or what you plan on doing after the session. This is usually a sign that the patient has also disengaged from the work of therapy. It can be tempting to let things drift in this mode but if we go along with our patient's pretend mode, we are doing them a disservice.

The third type of inhibited mentalising is *teleological mode*. This comes from the Greek words 'telos' (meaning 'end', 'goal', 'purpose') and 'logos' (meaning 'reason' or 'explanation'). It refers to an action-oriented mode of operating where the purpose is determined through the end goal. In therapy, we see this when our patients are preoccupied with actions rather than understanding. There is often pressure on others to prove their intentions to the patient through their actions. The GP has to prescribe pills to show they are taking the patient's illness seriously. The patient's partner has to text them regularly to show that they care. Some patients may self-harm to demonstrate to themselves and others that they are in great distress. These are the patients who want us to write a letter to their work place or local authority, for example, to assist them with a particular issue. These are the patients who rely on the actions of those in their support networks to indicate that they feel loved or held in mind. The converse applies so that when a loved one is absent or forgets to text them, for example, they are plunged into a state of despair, feeling abandoned and rejected. There is little capacity in this teleological state of mind to consider alternatives or hold on to an abiding sense of security in relationships. These are also patients who feel that they have to resort to actions to show other people how they are feeling. In desperate states of mind, such patients may feel they have to take drastic steps, like resign from a job or cut themselves to demonstrate to themselves and the outside world that they are in a difficult situation. These patients want external proof of their internal state of affairs in order to be taken seriously. As therapists, we can feel under considerable pressure with these patients to become rescuers and act in various ways to help our patients. For instance, we may find ourselves emailing patients like this or taking additional calls between sessions or during breaks.

Restoring good mentalising

Although we don't specifically need to recognise what form of poor mentalising our patients have at particular times, it is helpful to be aware of these different forms as well as our own countertransference to them. The way of responding to restore mentalising is similar across all types of inhibited mentalising. In the first instance, we want to recognise that mentalising is offline in order to intervene when we become aware that our patients are no longer mentalising well. When you notice that you are working very hard in a session to make sense of what your patient is saying to you, when you are trying to fill in the blanks and make connections with material that feels shrouded in mystery and is vague, then it is likely that your patient is no longer doing much mentalising and that you are shouldering too great a burden. One of the liberating aspects of assuming a mentalising stance, is that you are relieved of the burden of knowing. When we feel we know what is happening with our patients and we have great certainty, it is likely that we are in our own state of psychic equivalence. One thing we do know is that non-mentalising begets non-mentalising; in other words, poor mentalising is highly contagious. It is essential to catch it quickly.

What is critical to facilitating mentalising is a collaborative and cooperative alliance that includes a focus on episodic memory of moment-to-moment exchanges in self–other understanding, including the therapeutic relationship, where appropriate. The therapist elicits detailed, blow-by-blow interpersonal exchanges and then elaborates and clarifies these exchanges by making them increasingly explicit and conscious, eventually probing for likely feelings and motivations around those exchanges (Fonagy et al., 2011). We can see the corollary with marked, contingent mirroring. This experience allows the patient to develop increasingly nuanced views of themselves and others, to mentalise with greater flexibility by stepping out of rigid, two-dimensional and dysfunctional interpersonal patterns and to develop more flexible and rounded internal working models of self and other. In service of this aim, we ask open-ended questions and remain curious about the patient's experience of self and others. It is important to avoid making assumptions about what a patient is feeling or thinking. The therapist is encouraged to summarise and continually check out their understanding of those experiences, creating a shared narrative and encouraging greater symbolic representation of internal and interpersonal experiences. Alongside this, we can begin to introduce alternate perspectives on experiences, including attending to any ruptures in the therapeutic relationship. Empathy is an important mechanism for providing a safe therapeutic environment and building epistemic trust: therapists need to provide contingent and marked mirroring of their patients' emotional states.

The therapeutic stance that encourages our patients to think flexibly and mentalise more freely is a not-knowing, curious and empathic stance. We want to model for our patients that other people's minds are opaque to us: we are unable to read minds, as are our patients. We can eschew the need to be omniscient and know what is going on. We are curious about our patients' different experiences and the conclusions they are drawing, inviting them to help us understand why they came to see things that way. This involves active questioning to elaborate these nuances of understanding. This departs from the more reserved analytic stance that is more typical in psychoanalytically informed therapy, where there are fewer questions in favour of a more interpretative approach. In mentalising, the therapist is actively encouraged to ask questions and explore what things mean and how our patients arrived at these conclusions. In Box 7.2, we have included some hypothetical questions that therapists may ask to stimulate mentalising in patients.

Box 7.2 The sorts of questions that stimulate mentalising

- You seem to be very sure about how x will respond. I wonder why that is?
- What do you think made x say that to you?
- What did you have in mind when you asked x?
- How do you understand what happened/why x responded like that?
- Have you responded like that in the past?
- How do your friends see the situation? Your partner?
- Do you ever respond differently than the way you feel with x?

In asking questions, be mindful of asking 'what' questions that are less taxing than 'why' questions which place too great a strain on the patient's already stretched mentalising capacity. 'Why' questions may also be perceived as judgemental – "Why did you say that?" can imply a judgement, compared to "What prompted you to say that?" When our patients are not mentalising well, we need to keep interventions short and to the point. The more complex our language and the meaning of what we are trying to convey, the less chance we will be understood and the more we risk overwhelming our patients' minds.

Part of the therapeutic stance involves being empathic. We want to try and really understand how our patients are experiencing the world, to step into their proverbial shoes. This involves trying to validate our patients. If you can get a good sense of what it is like for your patient and to empathise with their existential experience of the world, you are likely to bring down their emotional arousal and improve their capacity to mentalise. Of course, this needs to be authentic empathy rather than paying lip service to the patient's experience. Otherwise, patients may feel manipulated and fobbed off, rather than genuinely understood. If we cannot put ourselves in our patients' position and feel some form of compassion and identification, then it is best to say something along the lines of, "I am puzzled about how you felt about that" or "What prompted you to respond like that – can you help me understand it better?"

Part of mentalising – indeed, an alternate definition of mentalising – is "understanding misunderstanding" (Allen et al., 2008, p. 3). When communication goes wrong – as it inevitably will do – we are presented with an important opportunity to stop and understand what went awry. We want to avoid spending too long in the dark, confused and pretending we are following what is being said. This does mean being a little more active at certain points in therapy than you might otherwise be. Again, this is an adaption of psychodynamic techniques that is tailored to particular patient groups, approaches or particular moments in treatment.

We can also encourage mentalising by taking up a contrary position to the patient. When a patient is overly emotional, it is helpful to take a more cognitive and rational perspective; and vice versa. When a patient jumps to conclusions and relies too heavily on intuition, we may encourage them to be more explicit about what they are seeing and thinking. However, if someone over-thinks everything, we may encourage them to trust their intuition more and be more spontaneous.

When it comes to how inferences are derived, some people only look at external factors like body language or actions that represent entirely another person's motivations and with these patients, we would bring their attention to the internal world of the other person and what might be going on for them; and vice versa. Lastly, if someone focuses on themselves all the time, we would ask questions to bring their focus around to the perspective of others; and vice versa. Taking up an opposing pole of mentalising usually has the effect of stimulating more flexible and rounded mentalising. To mentalise flexibly, we need to be able to use each pole of mentalising and to flex our mentalising muscle by using a full range of movement. We have to be able to think both fast and slow, to rely on internal and external attributions, to balance cognition and affect, and to keep both self and other in focus.

Another useful technique is to "stop and rewind", that is, to go back to the point in the session when you were following (i.e. mentalising) the patient and to slowly unfold events so that you can get a better understanding of what went on from multiple perspectives. This may feel counterintuitive to you, even rude. However, it is better to interrupt the patient in order to gain a better understanding of what is going on than let the patient continue to speak yet without much being achieved. You may want to say something along the lines of,

> "I am sorry but I don't understand what you were saying earlier. Can we just go back?"; or
>
> "Hold on – before you move off, can we just go back and see if I understand what you are saying happened?"; or even
>
> "Bear with me, I am just not getting it. Can you help me understand why you were left feeling like x?"

If you are able to convey that you are pausing the patient's narrative in the service of improving your comprehension of what they are communicating, in our experience this is often tolerated. Indeed, patients who are not mentalising well can flood the therapist with too much emotion and content; they often jump from one scenario to another without filling in the gaps, assuming the therapist understands things as they do. In these instances, slowing things down to allow the patient to play out what was evolving, scene by scene is beneficial to both the patient and the therapist.

Sometimes this "stop and rewind" technique can be conveyed by body language – raising your hand may be enough to signal to the patient that you want to hit pause. Allen et al. (2008) refer to this as the "mentalising hand" (pp. 199–200), the way the therapist can use a slightly raised hand with the palm extended out in the same manner the police use to de-escalate a tense situation. In one instance, a therapist helpfully employed the gesture of waving her hand slowly up and down to get her anxious patient to slow down, in a neutral way. It also served to heighten the patient's awareness about the impact her speeded-up talk was having on the therapist and facilitated the patient's capacity to self-regulate.

We may want to stop and focus on a particular aspect of an interpersonal narrative that strikes us as noteworthy or unusual. Perhaps the patient was able to respond in a different way to their usual way of reacting. Perhaps the patient jumped to a conclusion prematurely. It is helpful to mark these differences and consider what made it possible for the patient to respond in this way and to recognise the patient's progress, including taking small, baby steps towards a different reaction. It is helpful to use the mentalising stance of being curious and 'not knowing' in order to generate alternate perspectives. It can also be helpful to lay down a "transference tracer" (Allen et al., 2008, p. 189) when a link can be made from external relationships to something that may also occur in the transference relationship. By doing this, we are alerting the patient to the way that we are also valuing the therapeutic relationship as an important source of information.

At times, you may need to maintain a steady resolve in the face of pressure to agree with your patient who is mentalising rigidly and who doesn't want to allow for a different perspective. In these instances, you may want to say something like:

> "I can see how you really want me to see it like you do, but I don't think it would be right to just agree without thinking it through with you".

On occasion, this may mean challenging the patient's version of events, particularly where you feel that something is being avoided or where the way the patient is responding to a situation is unconsciously inviting others to respond in a predictably unhelpful way to them (e.g. when the patient is stand-offish to others yet complains of being rebuffed). In these instances, it can be helpful to mark your own reaction as different to the patient's, by saying something like:

> "I am not sure if you will agree with what I am about to say, but it occurs to me there's another way of thinking about the situation you've just described. Actually, there may be many other explanations".

Or you may try something like:

> "Although you say you accept the situation and don't need their help, sometimes the way you speak about it, makes me think there's more going on".

In these examples, we don't want to meet certainty with our own certainty. The mentalising stance is of 'not knowing', encouraging curiosity and questioning. If the patient remains very black-and-white in the face of your attempts to introduce shades of grey, then it is important to empathise with their certainty and validate the reasons they have for this position. We often return to the idea of empathy to restore the therapeutic alliance and epistemic trust we are co-creating with the patient. This can be conceptualised as a stepped approach. Most of the time will be spent in empathy and validation. We then move to questioning and elaborating, in the process hopefully introducing some doubts of cognition to offset the patient's certainty of affect. As we gain a better understanding of what happened and how the interpersonal event unfolded, so we can start to make links with what we have come to understand as the patient's repeated interpersonal patterns of relating. In Dynamic Interpersonal Therapy, we would be making links to the Interpersonal Affective Focus formulation at this point (see Chapter 11).

Once the patient is mentalising well, we can then make links to the way these patterns play out in the transference relationship. We are aware that we run the risk of increasing the patient's attachment anxiety and therefore bringing their mentalising off-line, so these moves to exploring the transference need to occur judiciously. At times, we may choose to increase the emotional heat of the therapeutic situation, particularly where a patient seems rather disconnected from their affect in 'pretend mode'.

Managing ruptures in the therapeutic relationship

We want to pay particular attention to difficult affects that arise in the consulting room because this is when the patient's mentalising is most likely to go 'off-line'. Any breakdown in the therapeutic relationship needs to be attended to as soon as possible. Rather than interpret the transference at this point, the mentalising approach is to acknowledge the 'elephant in the room' and take responsibility for your part in the breakdown of communication. There is a fine balance to be struck here – we are not suggesting that you beat yourself up for your clinical insensitivity neither that you avoid acknowledging culpability and suggest it is all in the patient's mind. Rather, we would acknowledge that something we have said or done has caused offence to the patient for which we are truly sorry. We may be aware of this difficulty first by our countertransference, where we find ourselves feeling very uncomfortable, perhaps choosing our words in an overly careful way – 'walking on egg shells'. The first step is to validate the patient's experience and empathise with how they are feeling, in the hope that this will bring down their levels of arousal and allow both of us think about what has happened. We remain curious about their experience of us and the more open we can be to hearing the patient's version of events, the more possible it is to hear what has gone on in the patient's mind. We don't want to introduce any alternative versions to the patient's perception of events at this stage. We may want to say something that acknowledges that there is a shared emotional experience, such as, "I am suddenly aware of feeling I have to choose my words carefully because I don't want to offend you, and I wonder if you might be feeling that you are not free to speak your mind either".

It is helpful to mark our own state of mind (as separate from the patient). We may say, "What occurs to me now is …" or "That makes me think about the time you …" We want to keep checking our understanding of what the patient is saying, for example, by saying things like "If I have understood what you've said, then …" Sometimes, therapists will say in supervision that they thought of making a particular intervention with a patient but they knew the patient would feel criticised, so they chose not to say anything to protect the relationship. We would argue that from a mentalising perspective, saying nothing will not protect the relationship and in fact, runs the risk of damaging it. Rather it is useful to openly acknowledge these anticipated reactions by saying something like, "I realise that what I am about to say might irritate you or leave you feeling criticised but this is what I have been thinking …" It is easier to acknowledge where you may have gone wrong and to validate the patient's experience of you, for example, "I can see how you may have concluded that I was bored with you when you saw me look at the clock towards the end of the session". It can be easier to begin by attributing the difficulties to the wider therapeutic situation than personalising it to yourself or the patient. Once you have ascertained and described what has happened between the two of you, then it may be possible to generalise this to similar instances that occur in other relationships in the patient's life or to allow for an alternate perspective (for example, that the therapist was keeping an eye on the clock as a way of taking care that we finish on time).

Monitoring our own mentalising capacities as therapists

It takes two people to mentalise well and the therapeutic couple is no exception to this. Part of our meta-awareness includes monitoring our own countertransference and this refers to our capacity to mentalise ourselves as therapists. We have described how easy it is for our patients' mentalising to be affected by their attachment history and emotionally distressing and arousing events. The same holds for therapists. This is partly why it is an essential part of most psychotherapy trainings that prospective therapists undergo their own psychotherapy, with the general rule holding that you would see patients for the same intensity as you have personally experienced in psychotherapy. Thus, someone who has had one or twice weekly psychotherapy would not be equipped to see patients for deeper, more frequent work. If you have had your own difficult attachment history – and many therapists are drawn to this work for this very reason – then it is even more reason to have your own psychotherapy, where you have a chance to form a trusting attachment and make sense of your own difficulties and have ways of taking care of those areas of vulnerability in your own life.

We also are vulnerable to having our mentalising go 'off-line' when we are with patients who are not mentalising easily or well. We will elaborate on these ideas further in Chapter 9 when discussing the countertransference, and although these concepts are not routinely or explicitly linked to notions of mentalising, we feel it is helpful to draw out these comparisons here. What are the signs that you as a therapist have stopped mentalising? When you start to feel great certainty that you know exactly what is going on for your patient, or when you feel completely lost and unable to think clearly, you have probably stopped mentalising. Mentalising well often involves grappling with confusion and not-knowing. We need to monitor our own reactions to our patients so that we are always stepping back and observing our own experience in the room and reflecting on it. There are times when this is more likely to be challenging. You may feel highly identified with what a patient is bringing. Perhaps it has resonance with your own life or someone close to you. You may be subject to attack and criticism by a suspicious, traumatised or angry patient or your patient may make you uncomfortable in other ways by talking about subjects that unsettle you, for example, or when your patient responds to you in a sexualised way. Sometimes we react to these points of discomfort by distancing ourselves from our emotions and becoming experts and scientists.

We run the risk in those moments of no longer relating to our patients as emotional beings but rather objectifying them. We should not be using our patients to fulfil our own needs for reassurance, closeness, admiration and so on. Earlier in this chapter, we described the risks that patients run when they objectify their relationships and as therapists, we are not immune to the same risks. Being an effective therapist involves the capacity to be subjectively affected by your patient while still being able to step back and have an objective perspective. Supervision is a helpful insurance policy against these risks although this requires honesty at sharing your difficulties openly, something that can feel difficult to do when you are also being evaluated by your supervisor. Your personal therapy is another helpful place in which to bring personal difficulties stirred up by your experiences as a therapist.

We hope that this chapter has shown that mentalising is the foundation of psychotherapeutic treatment where we are trying "to apprehend our own and others' minds as minds" (Fonagy et al., 2011, p. 102). Mentalising bridges different therapist orientations and treatment approaches: "Psychotherapists across modalities necessarily use this capacity, whether or not they conceptualize this explicitly in their theories, and good outcomes may be conceptualized in terms of improvements in mentalizing ability." (Fonagy et al., 2011, p. 102). There isn't just one way to improve mentalising capacities and the methods suggested in this chapter are not exhaustive by any means. Indeed, psychodynamic psychotherapy can be seen to facilitate better mentalising by focusing on the patient's subjective affective experiences, creating alternate perspectives by responding in flexible, marked and contingent ways to the patient, and attending to interpersonal relationships, including the therapist in the service of creating epistemic trust and safety. Mentalising techniques come into their own with severe mental disorders, such as Borderline Personality Disorder, Obsessive Compulsive Disorder, psychosomatic presentations and eating disorders. They also form part of the therapeutic repertoire employed in brief, Dynamic Interpersonal Therapy when patients are mentalising rigidly in heightened states of depression and anxiety. We hope that this chapter allows you to recognise when to employ these mentalising techniques so as to return to the typical psychodynamic interventions described in this book in order to maximise the value and effectiveness of those interventions.

Box 7.3 Useful resources

Readings

There is a very helpful chapter on Mentalising Techniques in Allen, Fonagy and Bateman's (2008) book, *Mentalising in Clinical Practice*. This book, together with Bateman and Fonagy's (2006) *Mentalisation-Based Treatment for Borderline Personality Disorder: A Practical Guide* contain practical ways of applying mentalising to clinical practice.

There are two important early papers written in 1996 by Peter Fonagy and Mary Target that detail the way mentalising develops in children:

Fonagy, P. and Target, M. (1996). Playing with reality: I. Theory of mind and the normal development of psychic reality. *International Journal of Psychoanalysis, 77*, 217–233.

Target, M. and Fonagy, P. (1996). Playing with reality: II. The development of psychic reality from a theoretical perspective. *International Journal of Psycho-Analysis, 77*, 459–479.

Online resources

The following YouTube clip (https://youtu.be/apzXGEbZht0) of the Still Face experiment, illustrates the impact of a mother denying her baby attention for a short period of time. Tronick narrates how prolonged lack of attention can move an infant from good socialisation to periods of bad but repairable socialisation, or at their worst, to 'ugly' situations, in which the child has no opportunity to return to an experience of the good object, and becomes stuck or damaged irreparably.

The Pixar Movie, Inside Out, offers a Disney explanation of mentalising. The trailer to the movie can be found on YouTube and is worth watching: https://youtu.be/yRUAzGQ3nSY.

There are some excellent talks and demonstrations of mentalising on YouTube by Anthony Bateman, Peter Fonagy and Jon Allen that are worth watching. We recommend the following:

* https://youtu.be/IzBHDSnR2jk (Anthony Bateman demonstrating the stance of empathic validation);
* https://youtu.be/BZl4OtQvDDg Anthony Bateman demonstrating the "not knowing" mentalising stance;
* https://youtu.be/oeboLKNV3PQ (clip of Anthony Bateman demonstrating how to work with an emotionally aroused patient, particularly using the stop and rewind technique),
* https://youtu.be/OHw2QumRPrQ and https://youtu.be/ugyScp3IxDl (Peter Fonagy introducing mentalising);

- https://youtu.be/sSvaXw92W7U (Peter Fonagy talking about mentalising, Borderline Personality Disorder and epistemic trust);
- https://youtu.be/vYg92Zps1Dw (a longer clip with Peter Fonagy talking about the links between psychoanalysis and attachment theory);
- https://youtu.be/KcCYLUn_uG8 and https://youtu.be/NLT7ieO3hTk (Jon Allen's introduction to mentalising);
- https://youtu.be/QB6oa4Mjplw (Mary Target describing the role for mentalising and attachment within clinical analysis);
- https://youtu.be/TXjUE7CLsO4 (Mary Target discussing affect regulation);
- https://youtu.be/ZBeEOkwLToM and https://youtu.be/mCqrgQSe2MY (Dickon Bevington describing the importance of mentalising and epistemic trust).

8   Unconscious communications

The focus on the unconscious mind is the defining aspect of psychoanalytic and psychodynamic therapies, as compared to other approaches. For the psychodynamic therapist, the required core competence is the ability to work with unconscious communication. According to the competence framework, this involves being able to facilitate the exploration of various unconscious dynamics and influences on relationships, as well as helping the patient become aware of unexpressed or unconscious aspects of their behaviour and experiences. Alongside this is the ability to work with the patient's internal and external reality since internal realities are informed by unconscious fantasy and include unconscious internal structures of the mind. In this chapter, we discuss the need to discern different types of unconscious communication when listening to our patient's verbal and non-verbal communication, including slips, dreams and embodied experiences. We also discuss how a therapist can interpret this layer of unconscious communication. This builds on the earlier discussion of interpreting anxieties and defences in Chapter 6.

Listening for unconscious communication

Psychodynamic psychotherapy is a talking therapy, where words are the currency of communication between patient and therapist. However, alongside the patient's verbalisations and narratives, it is important for the therapist to listen for what is being unconsciously communicated. The image of an iceberg is often used to represent the way what is conscious and manifest is often only a small part of the communication, the tip of the iceberg so to speak. Freud (1900) distinguished between *manifest* and *latent* content of communication. Manifest content refers to the communication that is immediately obvious and noticeable, such as the story the patient is telling the therapist: what happened, when and how. The latent content refers to what may lie beneath what is being explicitly expressed, including what is implied or omitted. Thus, when the therapist listens to the patient, the therapist is not only listening to their narratives but also attends to all the possible meanings. This includes what is implied or concealed from plain sight, the manner in which something is being conveyed and our own response or countertransference to the material. The therapist is interested in both what is being consciously expressed as well as what is not being expressed. We are not talking here about lying, but rather omissions about which the patient is not consciously aware. We are all familiar with instances where someone in distress tells us they are 'fine', yet we have a sense that they are anything but fine, that they are probably grief-stricken, shocked and afraid.

This brings us back to repression, one of the key defence mechanisms an individual utilises to protect themselves from psychic pain. You will recall from our discussion in previous chapters that Freud formulated a dynamic topography of the mind in which memories and thoughts that are too painful for the individual to tolerate in conscious awareness are then actively repressed into the unconscious. While repression represents an attempt to forget, it does not equate with the actual elimination of a memory or thought. Thus, Freud alerted us to the need to listen out for "the return of the repressed" (Freud, 1896, p. 169). The aim of therapy is to work through troubling repressed memories by bringing them into conscious awareness so that they can begin to be tolerated. This in turn gives the patient access to a fuller range of their personality and they can live in a more unencumbered way.

Freud (1923a) spoke about the need to practice "evenly suspended attention" when we are with the patient, in order to ensure we are receptive to the latent and manifest content of the patient's communications. Bion (1970), in turn, urged the therapist when entering each session to "let go of memory, desire and understanding" (p. 315). The therapist is required to have no pre-set agenda for the session by, for example, listening with pre-conceived ideas or holding on to the memory of previous sessions. You may be thinking that this is impossible: of course, we can't enter a session with a blank mind, devoid of previously acquired knowledge or knowledge of the patient, nor without any sense of what can be achieved in therapy. Notwithstanding this, Freud and Bion are emphasising the capacity for the therapist to be constantly open and receptive to the potential of something new being communicated. The basic assumption is that the therapist's unconscious understands the patient's unconscious (Heimann, 1950).

This way of listening is not easy. It requires the therapist to attend to several registers at the same time, as succinctly described by Heimann (1950):

> He [the analyst] has to perceive the manifest and the latent meaning of his patient's words, the allusions and implications, the hints to former sessions, the references to childhood situations behind the description of current relationships, etc. By listening in this manner the analyst avoids the danger of becoming preoccupied with any one theme and remains receptive for the significance of changes in themes and of the sequences and gaps in the patient's associations." (p. 82)

In the midst of a patient conveying a detailed story, it would be unhelpful for the therapist to listen out for only unconscious communication at the expense of responding to the patient's conscious account of their difficulties. The therapist needs to listen empathically to what is troubling the patient; after all, this allows the patient to feel heard and acknowledged. However, for the patient to be understood at a deeper level, the therapist also needs to be able to move back and attend to the unconscious layers of expression. The therapist may struggle to do this at all during the session, or the therapist may be receptive to various forms of communication but not know how to make sense of it, let alone interpret it in the session. Writing process notes following the session and reflecting on our experience in supervision provide invaluable spaces in which to gain a better sense of the dynamics of the patient, the session and the transference. Trainee and newly qualified therapists are likely to feel anxiety around making sense of the patient's material, including a pressure to know what is going on. However, part of maintaining an analytic attitude entails the therapist's ability to tolerate periods of not knowing without acting in by interpreting prematurely. It may take time for something to be properly understood, with careful attention to various forms of unconscious communication over an extended period of time. As we know with primary process thinking and the unconscious, there is an endless number of meanings that can be assigned. Material can be revisited from different angles as we continue to make sense of these complex dynamics. Thoughtful listening to unconscious communication is an acquired skill that takes practice: bear in mind Winnicott's metaphor of the cellist needing to become an accomplished musician which we made reference to at the end of Chapter 1.

Types of unconscious communication

So how do we attend to unconscious communication? While the unconscious can reveal itself in a multitude of ways, we are going to consider here four key avenues of unconscious communication in the therapy setting:

1   The therapist attends to the *sequence* of the patient's verbal communications, that is the free associations and links the patient makes between the material that they bring, including manifest and latent content. This includes slips or parapraxes;
2   The therapist attends to the *patterns* of the patient's verbal and non-verbal communication, that is the forms of language used as well as non-verbal behaviour;
3   The therapist explores the patient's *dreams* and the associations to dream content;
4   The therapist attends to their *countertransference*.

Let's consider each of these in more detail.

Free association, manifest and latent content

One of the fundamental rules of Freud's talking cure is the facilitation of free association (Freud, 1910). The patient is encouraged to speak whatever is on their mind, without censor or any agenda. Although the instruction is to be free of censure, Freud believed that what the patient says in sessions will be unconsciously determined and will reveal both those conflicts as well as be influenced by their resistance and other defences. What is said is not meaningless or random but can be seen to have relevance, despite this not always being understood at first.

Usually, the patient starts the session by bringing something that is consciously on their mind, such as a current worry or event of the week. From there, the patient is encouraged to continue exploring whatever comes to mind, usually by expanding on associations to earlier material. During the process of engaging with this process of freely associating, thoughts, images or memories that were outside their conscious awareness may start to surface. Free association is not an easy thing to do because it goes against the usual rules of holding a conversation. Patients may expect to be asked questions that they can then answer, or they may want more explicit turn-taking, rather than having space to explore their associations. Patients may also be unsure of what to say, even dismissing some things that come to mind as unimportant to talk about, as the following example illustrates:

> *I began the session by telling my patient, Lee, about an unexpected break in treatment when I had to cancel a session at short notice. Although I didn't give a reason for the cancellation, I sensed that Lee may become concerned about my reasons for this. Lee appeared to take it in her stride by starting to speak about the events of the week. However, she then broke off and shared an image that had come into her mind, observing aloud that this seemed rather random and insignificant, but she decided to share it nonetheless. She had found herself thinking of how the lid of her small child's drinking cup had come off unexpectedly, spilling liquid all over her. She pointed out that this was a cup that was meant to be leakproof. This free association conveyed Lee's unconscious sense that something in my private life had spilled into her session, leaving her with leaked out feelings that we then went on to explore productively.*

Patients may need some encouragement and explanation about the nature of psychotherapy. We discussed some of this in relation to the analytic setting as well as the initial consultation process. It may take the form of explaining the process of therapy, for example, by saying:

> Therapy won't involve me asking you a lot of questions; rather I am inviting you to talk about whatever is on your mind, even if it feels unimportant or difficult to verbalise.

Patients usually do have something to start speaking about at the beginning of the session, and may need prompting to facilitate free associations later in the session. For example, the therapist may say, "I wonder what else comes to mind?", "I wonder if that reminds you of anything?" or "Do you have any further thoughts?" There are times when patients say from the outset of the session, "I can't think of anything I want to talk about today". Despite the pressure you may feel to rescue the patient by setting an agenda or asking a here-and-now question, often responding along the lines, "Maybe something will come to mind" is enough to encourage some free association. Sitting with silence is another facet of tolerating uncertainty and holding a neutral, non-gratifying position. Some patient struggle to free associate, and may benefit from mentalising techniques to develop a greater reflective capacity that in turn facilitates their ability to symbolise and free associate. You may have to help your patients develop the ability to free associate by inviting them to describe the events of their day in detail, in the knowledge that unconscious processes will be operating in terms of how events are described and sequenced (Bollas, 2009).

We are always listening to the manifest story (the conscious account of what happened) and the latent content. To facilitate this, it is useful to ask yourself why the patient is telling *this* story, at *this* time, and in *this* way? It is important to think about the sequence of what is being narrated because this conveys unconscious preoccupations. What preceded the narrative in the session, including what happened in a previous session or even a throwaway comment on entering the consulting room, may relate to the current narrative and what ensues. We can consider the material that precedes and follows a dream as belonging to the patient's free associations to that dream and can think about their relevance at an unconscious level. Sometimes, we may point out what is missing from the narrative. One patient filled the session with a plethora of characters and events, but it became apparent that they seldom described how they felt about any of these events. In this instance, the therapist pointed this out by empathically observing, "You tell me what's happened, but you don't say how that left you feeling; that seems more difficult to share". The therapist may be puzzled about why the patient said something seemingly randomly at a particular moment in the session. It can be helpful to say, "I wonder what brought that to mind?" It may be that the patient changes the subject to distance themselves from a painful topic and the therapist can then point this out: "It seems we have moved away from something difficult".

The timing of what the patient says in a session is also meaningful. A good example is the doorknob moment, where the patient says something important or impactful right at the end of the session as they are about to leave the room. The unconscious (or possibly even conscious) motivation may be to avoid the ending, or put pressure on the therapist to respond in a certain way. The patient may want to say this in such a compressed way there is no opportunity to explore it, thereby expressing their unconscious resistance. It is important to bring this into awareness by saying, for example, "You said something important, but you brought it right at the end of the session, preventing us from exploring this further. Perhaps we can return to it next time?"

Freud (1901a) found parapraxes or slips of particular interest as manifestations of unconscious communication. A word may mistakenly pop up in the middle of a sentence, seemingly irrelevant and out of place and although the patient may quickly correct it, often the word has resonance with the patient. There are many examples of slips in popular culture. One such famous example is from a televised speech given by USA vice-president George H. W. Bush in 1988, reporting on the agricultural policy successes he and President Ronald Reagan had at the time, saying "We've had triumphs. Made some mistakes. We've had some sex … uh … setbacks". While there are many such humorous examples, parapraxis in therapy sessions may seem funny, but very often are meaningful and can be full of resonance.

> *Olivia began talking about her family life as the child of a messy divorce. She spoke about her "atomic family", then quickly corrected herself, saying "nuclear family". We were able to explore this slip that contained all manner of compressed and condensed meanings, as is typical of unconscious communication. The atomic family suggested something had been violently exploded, which tallied with her experience growing up torn between warring parents. There were resonances with the nuclear threat of the cold war and how her adolescence was spent in great tension, afraid of upsetting a very fragile balance between her parents. We could also think about the nucleus as the centre while the atom represented the singular, yet we also knew that the atom was made up of several different parts, the nucleus and the electrons that circled around it. These were competing internal models of her experience in her family of origin, where she felt both helpless in orbit of her parents as well as harbouring powerful fantasies about splitting up her parents.*

A useful way to allow space and encourage the patient to free associate, is for the therapist to remain relatively silent in order to allow new thoughts to emerge in the patient's mind. If the therapist rushes in to respond to every utterance of the patient, it breaks the patient's stream of thought and becomes more of a back-and-forth, structured exchange, thereby losing the emergent quality of psychodynamic psychotherapy. Opportunities for reflection are important. However, in a talking therapy, prolonged silences on the part of the patient often become a source of anxiety and shame for both patient and therapist. Silences may be challenging, and can be seen as a form of defence or resistance (Freud, 1912), or as a form of communication, where a feeling or experience is wordlessly shared (Coltart, 1991). As we have said before, we can't manualise psychodynamic psychotherapy and so it is up to the therapist to reflect on the quality of the silence in considering how to make sense of it. This requires the therapist to put aside their anxiety about saying something, and instead pay attention to their countertransference in order to attend to what the silence may be communicating.

Patterns of verbal and non-verbal communication

Some of the latent content that is communicated by the patient is conveyed through the form of *how* the patient talks or behaves in a session. We pay particular interest to the form of language the patient uses. When we narrate a story, the way we language it will convey the content of what happened, as well as the emotional and unconscious meaning of those experiences. We select certain words over others when we describe events and people. We use particular phrases or figures of speech or metaphor. The following example illustrates the power of language:

A prospective patient described how he "loved his partner to death". This was a particular expression that conveyed to me how desperate he was about being in an unsatisfying relationship to which he felt committed at any cost. Unconsciously, I was alerted to suicidal fantasies that I could then explore more explicitly with him as part of the assessment process.

Words are symbols and signifiers of meaning, and thus any utterance may have symbolic, unconscious meaning. Those patients with cognitive disabilities or in transient states of psychic equivalence or with psychotic levels of functioning, will have a more concrete style of communication, where there is little symbolisation in their narratives. We would need to be more cautious in interpreting this level of unconscious communication in the presence of these deficits.

We should also pay attention to the way the patient refers to themselves. For example, it may be that at the point the patient begins talking about an uncomfortable interpersonal conflict, there is a switch from using the pronoun 'I' to 'you', by saying, "When somebody laughs when you make a mistake, you feel ashamed", or "When someone does that, you can't help but feel angry". The introduction of the second person pronoun allows the patient to have some distance from the emotional aspects of what they are saying. It may even allow them to deflect taking responsibility for their actions. Other patients may over-use the pronoun 'I', possibly suggesting that they find it difficult to consider the perspectives of others.

Some patients keep repeating certain words or phrases, indicating some unconscious importance around those expressions, as the following clinical example shows:

Sean had grown up with a sense of not being wanted or important to his parents and struggled to form fulfilling and enduring relationships. The therapist noticed his repeated use of the word "anyway" when his voice tailed off after talking about something painful. He seemed to be indicating that he was moving on in the narrative and implicitly inviting the therapist to turn a blind eye to the hurt he had briefly been in touch with. It was helpful to point out his repeated use of "anyway" as an unintentional attempt on his part to create distance from something significant. In this way, he was unconsciously inviting me to repeat his childhood experience of feeling dismissed and unimportant, in the very place he had come to feel understood, namely psychotherapy.

Each person has their own particular style of talking, drawing on their idiographic use of language as well as their fluency and rhythms of speech all of which can vary at different times. Some patients speak more formally while others use more slang and colloquial language including swearing. This conveys the transference they bring unconsciously to therapy. Both the language and forms of communication with the therapist may reflect something about the patient's sense of personal and professional boundaries. It is important for the therapist to recognise interactions or conversations that have a more familiar and informal tone, as if the patient is talking to their friend.

The therapist pays attention to how the patient talks about themselves, others and events in their life. Who or what gets the most air time is of interest to us as a measure of their preoccupations while at the same time we are aware that less controversial areas can be focused on defensively in order to keep their distress outside the session. A patient may also make use of clichés, metaphors and other forms of symbolic language. It is important to explore what the patient implies by what they say, rather than assume we understand the meaning of a particular word or expression. For example, some patients often describe how they became "upset" about something. While on the surface, upset appears to convey meaning, it is also rather clichéd, vague and possibly understated. Does the patient actually mean they felt angry, sad, distraught or disappointed? Did they cry, shout or sulk? Similarly, other patients may use diagnostic words to describe their experience, possibly intellectualising their emotions. They may describe feeling anxious or paranoid. Rather than assume what the patient means by these hold-all terms, it is more useful to explore the different facets of their experience. For example, did they felt worried, panicked, on edge or afraid of how others were viewing them?

Non-verbal behaviour is another valuable source of information. This includes how a patient carries themselves physically, how they enter and position themselves physically in the room, their actions, gestures and way of moving, their eye contact and facial expressions. The following example shows this non-verbal level of communication operating in the session:

> Tom came to see me because he was having problems at work and with his relationship. He arrived five minutes late for his first session and entered the consulting room with apparent assuredness, walking straight up to me and holding out his hand to shake my hand firmly. He took his time to survey the room before sitting down in the chair I indicated for him. He didn't acknowledge his lateness and immediately began talking about why he was coming to therapy and what his problems were. As he spoke, he leaned back on the chair, legs spread apart and his hands clasped behind his head, glancing around the room every now and then. He noticed a jug of water and glasses and stood up to help himself to water while he continued talking. I decided to interrupt him after having seen how he made use of the space and I explained the purpose of the initial consultation, aware at some level that I felt a need to assert my authority in the space. Tom was nonplussed by my interruption and said he was happy to provide me with whatever information I required in order to help him with these difficulties. He talked freely and elaborated his narratives with such a level of detail that I felt rather swamped by the information. Aware of the time, occasionally I moved him along, aware of being pulled into a structuring function. During the session, Tom stood up several times to help himself to more water, and to take a tissue to blow his nose from a tissue box across the room, rather than the box placed within reach next to his chair. As the consultation proceeded, I found myself feeling increasingly irritated and intruded upon.
>
> In this brief vignette, Tom's non-verbal behaviour provided me with an important source of information about his relationships and why he may be experiencing conflict in his personal and work relationships. He was talkative and shared his experiences openly, but in a manner that dominated the space and shut me out from sharing any observations. His physical behaviour also occupied much of the space. Tom seemed to behave as if he owned the room, using the space as he wished with an air of entitlement. This had the effect of

distancing me, the therapist, with my growing feelings of irritation. I began to hypothesise that Tom was not really interacting with me in any meaningful way and was struggling to relate to me as a separate person. My reaction to Tom may say something about how other people experience Tom, and why he may have relationship problems. I wondered if at some level, he felt intruded upon by having to seek help and that his shame was manifesting in this reaction formation of overt confidence, rather making use of the space to explore his difficulties.

The decision about when and how to interpret Tom's behaviour is a matter of clinical judgement as would be the choice to disclose countertransference feelings. It is probably unwise to do so in an initial consultation, although it may be possible to take this up as a cautionary tale around his fear that he will not be able to be have his needs met in therapy. The therapist holds in mind their internal reflections as initial hypotheses in order to see whether a sustained pattern of interpersonal relating will emerge. After all, it may be that Tom is highly anxious at his first encounter with a therapist and this behaviour abates with time, or it may be that this is his usual modus operandi. Once the therapist has observed the patterns over time and established a rapport, it may be possible to interpret Tom's need to set the pace of the interaction and take charge in the session and his relationships in order to protect himself yet noting that it has the effect of shutting others out, relegating them to the side-line and leaving Tom even more alone.

Dreams as unconscious communication

Our fascination with dreams goes back to ancient history when dreams have been the topic of religious, philosophical and scientific interest. We are often struck by the strangeness of our dreams or the powerful emotional reactions they evoke. We do not always remember our dreams, with some standing out more vividly than others. We may remember dreams from long ago, but can't remember what we dreamed last night. We often want to understand the meaning of our dreams, and there are long traditions as well as popular cultural ideas about the significance of dream elements. It was in Freud's ground-breaking book, *The Interpretation of Dreams* (1900) that he set out his theories around the unconscious, writing that "The interpretation of dreams is the royal road to a knowledge of the unconscious activities of the mind" (p. 608). Dreams are rich in latent meaning and primary process thinking. When we interpret our patients' dreams in psychodynamic psychotherapy, we are working with their unconscious communications and therefore need to interpret beyond the manifest content (the obvious elements of the dream narrative), to explore the dream's latent content as well as the function the dream serves. Before continuing, let's consider a dream brought by a patient:

Martina was a 26-year old single woman, the youngest of three siblings. She was currently unemployed and living at home. She described her parents as "caring", having always provided for her needs, however, both of them were prone to bouts of depression and had problems with alcohol. Martina had had a string of jobs which all ended badly when she left after experiences where she found her bosses to be "useless". She had various short, unsatisfying relationships with women, most recently with Wendy; these often ended when her partners felt unable to tolerate her bad moods. Martina sought therapy because she was depressed, with suicidal thoughts. After an initial assessment, Martina agreed to start therapy, saying she felt "happy" to be starting.

In the third session she reported this dream:

I was in a big house, with lots of rooms. I was on my own in this house, walking around trying to find something. Suddenly, zombies began to appear in one of the rooms and my mission was to escape from the house. It was like I was part of a video game or movie or something. I looked around for an escape route. Then I was in this big hall, with a glass wall on one end. On the other side were some people, and they were watching me. There was one person who had on a white coat. There was a woman, who looked a bit like Wendy, but older. It wasn't her. There was another guy with a big build, and I can't remember the others. The zombies had started to come into this big hall. There were a few of them running around. I saw a young child in the hall on their own; I think it was a boy. He looked familiar. Next thing, I had a machine gun with me, and I was starting to gun the zombies down. I was trying to get the boy and myself to safety.

Freud (1900) argued that unconscious conflicts, fears and wishes are translated into the manifest content of dreams through the process of *dream-work*. Freud (1901b) further wrote that "The task of dream interpretation is … to unravel what the dream-work has woven" (p. 686). Dreams have their peculiar qualities as a result of this dreamwork, which disguises latent meaning in the manifest aspects of the dream. Some of the processes that are utilised in dreamwork are condensation, displacement and symbolism.

Condensation involves the combination of different ideas, people or places into one compressed image or element. For example, more than one person can be compressed into a single character of a dream, leading the person to describe a character in the dream as more than one individual. In Martina's dream, someone represented both her recent girlfriend Wendy (it looked like her) and someone older (her mother, perhaps?). In the earlier example of a slip, we saw how several different and conflicting ideas could be encapsulated in the neologism of "atomic family".

Displacement is the process whereby a real conflict is displaced onto something else (see the reference to displacement as a defence mechanism in Chapter 6). For example, in Martina's dream the inclusion of a zombie game in the dream may reflect her experience growing up with depressed, intoxicated parents.

Symbolism is the process where aspects of the dream stand for or symbolise something else. Akhtar (2009a) expands this: "'symbolism' stands for representing a body part (e.g. a penis), activity (e.g. eating), feeling (e.g. hate) or idea (e.g. patriotism) by a concrete object" (p. 279). Further examples include underwater as a symbol for the unconscious, or a snake as a symbol of the penis and possible sexual danger. In Martina's dream, the person wearing the white coat may symbolise the therapist (the doctor). While the symbol is conscious and/or concrete, what it stands for is often unconscious and/or abstract. However tempting it may be, we cannot resort to a dream dictionary to decode our patients' dreams. Each symbol will be used by a patient in a particular way. Notwithstanding this, Laplanche and Pontalis (1973) remind us that "an individual may choose among the senses of a symbol but he cannot create new ones" (p. 444).

In interpreting dreams, we are interested in its latent communication along with the patient's associations to the dream. In Martina's dream, the manifest content is that of a video game and danger. This may have some relevance to external reality. Indeed, Martina did spend a lot of her free time playing video games. We may also think that she was experiencing some current anxiety (danger) in her life. However, the meaningful unconscious communication lies in the dream's latent content. We can consider the zombies as a reference to Martina's experience growing up with zombie-like parents (when depressed or drunk). The young child in the dream may represent Martina's child self (disguised as a boy) who needs rescuing. Martina made an association to another dream of hers, which she then remembered:

> *I also had a second dream where Wendy and I were both sitting on a couch. We were getting intimate, but then I could see in her eyes that she was thinking of someone else, and so I pushed her away.*

Given the timing of the dream and their sequence in the session, one possible interpretation would be that the dream is expressing Martina's intense anxiety about starting therapy and whether the therapist is someone she can trust. Here, the manifest content of the dream can be interpreted in association with the psychotherapeutic material that came before it. As Meltzer (1983) states, a dream may give the analyst "the means for discerning how the work of the previous session has been 'digested'" (p. 134). The dream itself is a free association, as it arrived two sessions following the first meeting. There is a symbolic reference to the therapist (the person with the white doctor's coat) that is suggested in the second dream by the presence of a couch along with themes of anxiety about intimacy and trust.

Thus, dreams can be understood to contain unconscious expressions of past infantile experience, and/or the external, here-and-now context in which the dream occurred (why was this dream dreamed now?). Freud (1923b) observed different ways in which the task of dream interpretation could be undertaken:

1   the therapist can ask the patient for association to all elements of the dream as they occurred in the dream. These may include associations to memories from the past, for example, or to particular words or people;
2   the therapist can ask the patient to associate to a particular element of the dream (e.g. a particularly striking part);
3   the therapist can ask the patient what recent events come to mind in association with the dream;

4   the therapist can leave the patient to make their own associations, without the therapist's instruction. In this way, we can consider the preceding and ensuing material as the patient's implicit associations to the dream.

Unconscious communication through the transference and countertransference

We will discuss the countertransference and working in the countertransference in detail in the next chapter. For now, it is relevant to note that unconscious processes are at work in the transference and countertransference. The patient often communicates unconsciously through the therapist's countertransference, leading to a reformation in the way countertransference was first seen (Heimann, 1950). This is a wordless form of communication from one unconscious to the other. We may all have had experience of working with patients who have porous boundaries with others where they can intuit things that are going on in the therapist's life or mind with uncanny accuracy. The following example illustrates the way the therapist can be informed by their countertransference reactions to unconscious aspects of the patient:

> *I was listening to my patient, Lola talking in a matter-of-fact way about her interaction with her aging mother, as if it did not hold much emotional significance. And yet, I became increasingly aware of feeling intense sadness as I listened to her. I chose to interpret this, based on careful consideration of my countertransference in order to bring Lola's repressed emotions into awareness in the session. I said, "You're telling me about what happened with your mum, as if you were unaffected by it, but I wonder if there is a great sense of sadness and loss that you are reluctant to feel right now?"*

Different patients evoke different affective reactions in the therapist at different times, reflecting the transference-countertransference dynamic. At times, the therapist may feel pulled right into the patient's emotional world, perhaps feeling tears well up in their eyes. At other times, they may feel disconnected, even bored as they listen to their patient. It is important to reflect on what belongs to the therapist and what is information communicated by the patient; what is it that makes the therapist feel over-identified or distant?

Making an interpretation

The role of an interpretation is to bring into consciousness that which is unconscious, so that it can be thought about, tolerated and reflected upon. However, the timing and purpose of the interpretation needs to be considered carefully. An interpretation can be made too soon, making it difficult for the patient to connect with what has been said. Interpretations are not about appearing clever and should not include technical language. We shouldn't interpret because we have suddenly had an insight into the patient's conflicts if we judge that the patient is not ready to contemplate hearing this. At all times, we need to weigh up when and how much to say, bearing in mind the patient's possible experience of that interpretation. This draws on the generic meta-competence of using clinical judgement when applying a theoretical model.

Tuckett (2011) provides a useful heuristic for the therapist to consider when considering interpreting unconscious material in the consulting room. In this chapter, we have outlined the different forms that unconscious communication can take, and we have suggested asking ourselves the crucial question, why did my patient express something, in that particular way, at that moment in the session? In answering this question, the therapist should bear in mind the patient's background history, the process of therapy over time as well as the particular moment in the session itself. Tuckett uses the mnemonic of the window when inviting us to consider whether the unconscious communication is taking place *outside* or *inside* the consulting room. In other words, is the patient bringing something in their external life to the session to be thought about (i.e. outside), or whether the patient's thought, memory, idea, fantasy or wish originates in the consulting room, as a result of something that has happened in the session (i.e. inside the therapeutic relationship or the transference). The patient may ostensibly be describing something that happened outside, yet material from the session brought this to mind. This is a key aspect of free association in its ability to facilitate revealing unconscious material.

Eric was in his early 50s, married with two adult step-children. His wife, a music teacher, was some years older. Eric was generally a reserved man, preferring to live a quiet home-life. However, he had become increasingly depressed and lonely since his adult step-children had moved out of home, and his wife was busy with her work and hobbies. He had no friends of his own. Eric had been attending weekly psychodynamic psychotherapy for some time, arriving reliably and regularly. At first, he had been awkward and reserved, but in recent months he had begun to open up about his loneliness and wish to connect to others. In a recent session, he relayed his difficulties starting at a new school as a young teenager after his family relocated to a different city. He felt like an outsider and was bullied and intimidated by his peer group. It was unusual, a session where Eric allowed himself to be vulnerable, and shared more than he had to anyone else.

Several sessions after this, Eric arrived wearing new glasses, dressed in a colourful shirt. He appeared younger and brighter. In this session, he spoke about visitors they had over the weekend, colleagues of his wife, and how awkward he had found it. He felt self-conscious, not knowing what to say much of the time. Yet he pushed himself to be more talkative and the visit had gone alright. Eric acknowledged that he has a better understand of his social discomfort since coming to therapy and making links with his past. This was followed by a pause, where he fell silent.

Eric then said he had a dream the other day which was "a little strange". He couldn't remember much of it, other than one small detail. In the dream, he was in bed and his father came and lay down next to him. His father lay there and said, "I have been talking a lot". He remembered feeling very uncomfortable in the dream. He added that this was all he could remember.

I asked what associations he had to the dream.

He thought for a moment. He went on to recall an incident when he was aged 9 or 10 and he had woken up at night and vomited in bed. He called out to his mother but instead, his father had come in, and calmly and gently cleaned the mess up. Eric observed that this was very unlike him, as his father was typically quite absent. He added that it was the sort of thing his mother would do, not his father. After cleaning up everything, his father had taken him to sleep in their bed.

Eric seemed embarrassed while telling me his dream and this memory, something I reflected back to him.

He said he had felt uncomfortable at the time, lying in his parent's bed between them, like he shouldn't be there.

I said that I wondered whether part of the embarrassment was that he had also liked being there. I observed how struck he was by his father's nurturing response to him. Maybe he was embarrassed by his wish to be closer to his father.

Eric agreed, recognising that he had always wanted a closer relationship with his father. He elaborated how his father was not the type of father who would play football with him in the garden, or do father-son things with him. He was always working and couldn't come to key events in Eric's life, like sports days or prize-givings.

I thought to myself about what had prompted Eric to tell me this dream and this memory at this point in time. I brought to mind his feelings of loneliness and isolation, including his lack of friendships. I also thought about his growing attachment to his sessions and to me, as well as the way he had changed his appearance recently to look younger and brighter. While Eric was at one level talking about things outside the consulting room (his social awkwardness, loneliness and past experiences), I thought Eric was also communicating something in the transference of his relationship with me inside the room. I decided to interpret this aspect of the unconscious communication and said to Eric that in a way, this wish is still relevant for him. He is looking for a father figure, a male figure, with whom he can feel closer.

"Yes", he quickly agreed, "Someone to go to the pub with".

"What about the other element of the dream?", I asked, "Your father said that he has talked a lot".

Eric tentatively said that he thought that probably referred to the therapy sessions, and how he has been coming here to talk more and more.

"I think you are also saying that these sessions are becoming increasingly meaningful to you", I said, "and perhaps there is a wish that we could be closer, even go down the pub as friends".

"Yes, maybe a little", he said. "I do find it strange not knowing anything about you. There are questions I would want to ask, but I don't, because I know it is a professional relationship".

When interpreting unconscious communication, the therapist should aim to do so from a position of neutrality (an aspect of the analytic frame). Anna Freud (1954) suggested that analytic neutrality is located in a position that is equidistant between the analyst's id, ego and superego. Tuckett (2011) extends Anna Freud's insight by providing a useful heuristic tool when thinking about how to phrase an interpretation. He discusses two triangles that depict the positions that both therapist and patient can adopt (Figure 8.1).

Therapist's position   Patient's position

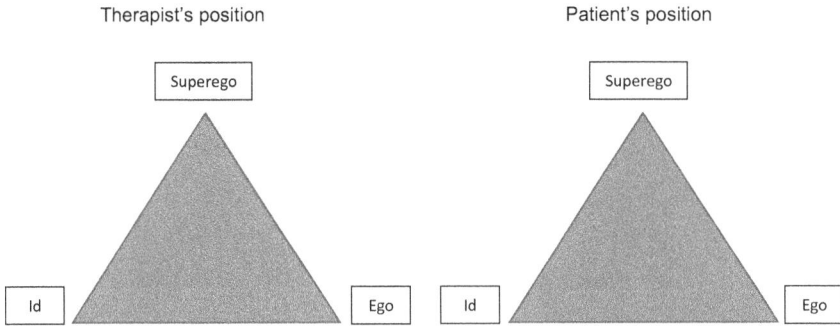

Figure 8.1 Therapist and patient position triangles
Source: Adapted from Tuckett, 2011, p. 1373

When making an interpretation, the therapist does so from any of the corners of the triangle (left hand triangle in Figure 8.1). As Tuckett states (2011, p. 1373), they may love or hate the patient (coming from an id position), judge the patient (from a superego position), or teach the patient (ego position). It is preferable to phrase an interpretation in a neutral way that is equidistant from these three positions. Returning to the earlier clinical vignette of Eric, the therapist took a stepped approach when phrasing the interpretation and chose to put things in the hypothetical ("perhaps you have this wish") in order to be as neutral as possible without being drawn into shaming or judging Eric. It could be argued that adding the clause, "even going down the pub" may have represented something of a risk because Eric may have taken this up negatively, perhaps feeling mocked.

Tuckett (2011) points out that the patient also has a triangle of different positions (right hand triangle in Figure 8.1) from which they perceive the therapist. For example, they may experience the therapist as loving or hating (id), judgemental (superego) or problem-solving (ego). The patient's perceptual position depends on the transference. The therapist, in turn, may be pulled into a particular complementary position in their countertransference without realising it (see Sandler's role responsiveness in Chapter 9). Thus, even though the therapist endeavours to make an interpretation from a neutral position, the patient may still hear the therapist as coming from the position of id, ego or superego. This creates the potential for a mutual enactment, according to Tuckett. To guard against this, the therapist needs to be able to consider not only the patient's unconscious conflict and how it is being communicated in the session, but also whether the therapist has been positioned within that conflict so as to enact something. You can see here why Casement (1985) stresses the importance of developing an internal supervisor as a tool for maintaining an analytic attitude. Tuckett reminds us that "if the analyst is unaware of the right-hand [patient's] triangle position in which the patient has placed him, he cannot possibly be experienced as speaking from the centre of the left-hand triangle, however great his efforts" (2011, p. 1375).

We have focused on this chapter on various forms of unconscious communication. The task of making interpretations bridges several different areas of psychodynamic work. We invite you to read this chapter in conjunction with the chapters on defence mechanisms (Chapter 6) and transference and countertransference (Chapter 9) where we provide other useful heuristics for making interpretations.

Box 8.1 Useful resources

Readings

We highly recommend Freud's *Interpretation of Dreams*. Although readers are often intimidated to read Freud in the original, it is an eminently readable text. After all, Freud won the Goethe prize for literature and he writes in an engaging way. You may be able to find an audio version of the book if this is an easier way to access it.

There are other books on dream analysis which are very useful:

Ella Sharpe Freeman (1978). *Dream analysis: A practical handbook for psychoanalysts*. London: Hogarth Press.

Jean-Michel Quinodoz's book, *Dreams that turn over a page: Paradoxical dreams in psychoanalysis* (2002)

Sara Flanders' (1993) edited collection of essays, entitled *The dream discourse today*, which forms part of the Routledge New Library of Psychoanalysis Series, contains a number of significant papers on this key topic.

Online resources

The Freud Museum has a helpful online resource to assist with dream interpretation www.freud.org.uk/learn/discover-psychoanalysis/the-interpretation-of-dreams/

There are several lectures available on YouTube by clinical psychologist and psychoanalyst, Professor Aleksandar Dimitrijevic for Berlin Psychoanalytic on the central concept of the Unconscious, where he reviews various conceptions of unconscious and evidence for its existence and power: https://youtu.be/Tr19yMl2WbMhttps://youtu.be/DY-BElxmGCc

In this YouTube clip, Professor Salman Akhtar revisits some of Freud's most central claims regarding the nature of the unconscious and examines their current status within and beyond psychoanalysis: https://youtu.be/gVlm 94nUmkU

This is a lecture given by Yoram Yovell, Israeli psychoanalyst, psychiatrist and neuroscientist on the unconscious and trauma as part of a presentation at the 2014 Joseph Sandler Psychoanalytic Research Conference: https://youtu.be/UEVitquDhN0

This YouTube video is of a discussion between three British psychoanalysts David Bell, Leon Kleimberg and Michael Parsons in conversation with Caterina Albano, curator of the Science Museum on the 2011 exhibition "Psychoanalysis: The Unconscious in Everyday Life" in London: https://youtu.be/MzqgKQUq92w

9 Transference and countertransference

Fostering and maintaining a good *therapeutic alliance* has been identified as a generic therapeutic competence that is common to a wide range of therapeutic modalities including behavioural, cognitive, gestalt, person-centred and psychodynamic (Hovarth and Luborsky, 1993). It has been robustly shown to be a key factor in positive outcomes for psychotherapy (see Chapter 3). The therapeutic or working alliance refers to the ability to establish a collaborative and positive relationship between the therapist and patient, so that constructive work can take place. The therapeutic alliance is developed and maintained by the therapist providing a safe therapeutic space and responding to the patient in a non-judgemental way with empathy and understanding. We want to distinguish this from the ability to work with the transference and countertransference, which represent specific psychody-namic competences alongside making dynamic interpretations and working with defences. The ability to focus on the vicissitudes of the therapeutic relationship with its primary focus on the patient's unconscious projections on to the therapist is a distinguishing feature of psychodynamic psychotherapy (Lemma et al., 2008) and is distinct from the therapeutic alliance which involves a reality-based, healthy part of the patient's ego relating to a real therapist. Zetzel (1956) argued that most patients oscillate between periods of relating dominated by the transference and other periods dominated by the working alliance, with a requirement to attend to both types of relating in psychodynamic psychotherapy.

This chapter introduces the substantive concepts of transference and coun-tertransference in psychodynamic psychotherapy. We will first examine the transference and how this has been seen over time before arriving at a working definition. We will consider how to recognise the transference in a session and explore different manifestations including positive and negative transference, the transference neurosis and the cautionary tale. We will then look at how to interpret the transference as well as working with the transference in psy-chotherapy using Malan's (2001) triangle of person. We move on to consider the countertransference, including a working definition, the interaction between transference and countertransference through Sandler's (1976) concept of role-responsiveness, how to recognise and monitor our countertransference, and particular countertransference phenomena including Winnicott's (1949) con-tribution towards hate in the countertransference, revisiting projective identification, acting out and acting in. Although we have separated out the transference from countertransference in order to examine each separately, this is a theoretical artifice because the two are in dynamic interaction with each other.

Transference

The transference is ubiquitous, by which we mean it is found everywhere. In the therapeutic situation, the transference begins before the patient has even met the therapist. The patient will have a range of thoughts, fantasies and emotional responses about the therapist, including the therapist's name, presumed age, race, religion, sexual orientation, gender, the address of the therapist's consulting room, the therapist's photograph and online presence (these days, most patients will google their therapist as a matter of course – see Chapter 14 on the role of technology in psychotherapy) and the therapist's voice and accent when they speak on the phone prior to meeting. Thus, the patient brings a range of pre-existing emotional responses and expectations to the therapist. Sometimes, these are optimistic, hopeful expectations for a positive encounter where they will feel understood while at other times, these are more negative and pessimistic predictions of an encounter filled with shame, judgement and criticism. We can consider the first scenario of an idealised version of the therapist as a defensive splitting off from more anxiety-provoking or persecutory feelings. Both extremes are concerning. However flattering and seductive an overly positive transference is for the therapist, inevitably being put on a pedestal leads to a fall from grace. We will touch on this more in Chapter 12.

The analytic setting and attitude of the therapist promotes the development of the transference. By remaining in a neutral position in relation to the patient and not responding in keeping with the patient's preconceptions on the whole, it is possible to identify and interpret the way the patient replicates their earlier patterns of relating, for example the way the patient treats the therapist as if they were a parent, sibling or other key figure (Rycroft, 1995, p. 186). The analytic setting becomes the Petri dish in which the transference can multiply. If the therapist is overly reassuring or gratifying, this will inhibit the patient's transference from developing. Of course, in brief psychotherapy there is a need for greater support and scaffolding of the patient-therapist relationship and the therapist probably adopts a more active, structuring and supportive therapeutic stance (see Chapter 11).

Rycroft (1995) states that the transference comes in all sorts of forms:

> Transference may be paternal, maternal, oedipal, pre-oedipal, passive, dependent, oral, etc., according to the object transferred and the stage of development being recapitulated; object or narcissistic … according to whether the patient conceives his analyst as an external person on whom he is dependent, whom he hates, etc. or as a part of himself; positive or negative, according to whether he conceives the analyst as a benign or malevolent figure. (p. 186)

Before continuing, let's turn to a clinical example of a very early manifestation of the transference:

> *I collected my new patient, Maggie, from the waiting room, having read the referral letter that alluded to her traumatic early childhood with an abusive mother followed by multiple foster home placements. She was late to the meeting, having already rescheduled her appointment and I found myself predicting that she wouldn't turn up today. I had given up on her before she had even arrived! Maggie was seemingly nonplussed at being late, taking her time while she gathered her possessions from the waiting area before following me to my consulting room. As she walked behind me, she complimented me on my shoes and how much she liked them. I chose to wait until we reached the consulting room before starting the consultation by inviting her to share what had brought her to seek psychotherapy today. She ignored my opening and repeated that she had complimented my shoes, but I had not thanked her.*
>
> *My countertransference included my awareness that I felt uncomfortable about the shoes I was wearing that day which were casual trainers. Her compliment did not land easily with me and it felt as if it was an invitation to sweep any difficulties around her late arrival under the proverbial carpet. It may have been that I was set up to respond like this. I had the choice of adopting a more supportive and mentalising approach but considered that since she was being considered for psychodynamic psychotherapy, part of the assessment process was to establish whether she was able to manage this way of working. I therefore said, "It seems that you are creating a diversion from your lateness by complimenting my shoes".*
>
> *Maggie became furious at this interpretation, angrily criticising my poor manners and berating my parents for the way they had brought me up so badly. I was acutely aware that she was bringing her own early experiences with her mother and projecting them on to me, so that I became the person with the inadequate upbringing who didn't know how to behave and she was relieved of her own insecurities and anxieties at the initial consultation. It would have been premature to interpret this at such an early stage, when it could have been experienced by her as a refusal to accept her projections. Instead, I observed that we had got off to a difficult start and established this as a shared problem about how we can proceed to think together about her difficulties.*

Here we have a powerful example of transference, where an experience related to a childhood figure (mother) is transferred onto the therapist. As you can see, the therapist's countertransference is also evident in this example in the anticipation that the patient is unreliable, may not turn up and feeling messed around. This may also give us some clues as to the patient's inner world and her experiences of having been messed around and let down by key figures in her life. We will return to consider countertransference later in this chapter.

What is transference?

There are different theoretical understandings of what the transference is. Freud initially saw the transference as a contaminating influence that should be avoided at all costs. He regarded the transference as the patient's past difficulties intruding into the therapy space and contaminating the relationship with the therapist, distorting their perception of the therapist. However, Freud (1914a) soon came to realise the importance of the transference as a primary route into understanding the patient's internal world. The transference provides traces of forgotten or unremembered infantile experiences with the patient's Oedipal figures (mother and father). Because of the compulsion to repeat, these infantile experiences which are inaccessible to memory are procedurally re-enacted with the therapist through the transference and come to be interpreted and known in this way. Anna Freud (1954) writes that "because these impulses (experienced by the patient in his relation with the analyst) are repetitions and not new creations they are of incomparable value as a means of information about the patient's past affective experiences" (p. 18). Unacceptable impulses towards the therapist will in turn be defended against, particularly when the patient's extreme emotions do not feel justified by the actual situation and unless interpreted, this will lead to defensiveness and *acting out*. Adhering to the transference is understood as a form of resistance, which the therapist has to help the patient break through.

Anna Freud adopted a benevolent attitude towards the defences our patients utilise. She didn't see the patient as deliberately misleading or deceiving the therapist but rather perceived the patient as being as honest as possible in giving the only form of expression to their feelings and conflicts as is possible to them at that time. She advocated tracing the stages of the transformation of the instincts and the resultant conflict in order to allow the patient to make sense of the way their ego has developed and to fill in gaps in that history, as well as taking up aspects of the transference that are ego-syntonic and that the patient does not see as repetitions of the past but rather defends against knowing about. Interpreting the transference involves taking up both the underlying id instincts as well as the ego defences and resistance to psychotherapy.

Paula Heimann's (1956) influential paper on the transference broadened our understanding beyond transference as repetition compulsion. She regarded the transference in terms of internalised object representations and unconscious phantasies, which distort all relationships, including the relationship with the therapist. Rather than being just a re-enactment, the transference externalises internalised object relational experiences and distorts object relational experiences in the here-and-now. Heimann focused on the importance of the transference as a two-way unconscious communication, requiring a receptive therapist to bring the patient's unconscious phantasies into being. She suggested that the answer to the question "Why is the patient now doing what to whom?" constitutes the transference interpretation: "It is the transference interpretation which fully re-instates the past in the present and makes it accessible to the patient's ego" (Heimann, 1956, p. 307). Kernberg (1987) describes transference as the "reactivation in the here-and-now of past internalized object relations" that include intrapsychic conflict between parts of the self. The internalised object relations are derived from actual as well as fantasised past experiences.

Betty Joseph's (1985) seminal paper on the transference broadened the transference to the "total situation", namely all aspects of the patient's responses to therapy and the therapist, shaped by past object relational experiences and past as well as current unconscious phantasies and wishes. She concludes that "everything of importance in the patient's psychic organisation based on his early and habitual way of functioning, his phantasies, impulses, defences and conflicts, will be lived out in some way in the transference" (p. 453).

Over time, the concept of transference has broadened to represent the way the patient experiences their current wishes and expectations in relation to the therapist as influenced by past object relationships. The transference is seen as a co-construction by the patient and therapist, involving present reality filtered through the lens of early experiences. These modern revisions of transference have allowed it to be seen less as resistance to progress and more as a way of allowing previously learned experiences to be continually updated and revised with each new situation (Bateman and Holmes, 1995). In brief psychotherapy, such as Dynamic Interpersonal Therapy, transference is used to explore the way an identified interpersonal and affective pattern is played out with the therapist (see Chapter 11).

To summarise, the transference can be variously defined as (Bateman and Holmes, 1995; Rycroft, 1995):

1   The process by which a patient transfers (or displaces) past experiences, expectations and feelings, both conscious and unconscious, on to figures and situations in their present-day life
2   The way the patient relates to the therapist as though they were some former object in their life (i.e. they project on to the therapist object representations acquired from early attachment relationships). This involves the activation of internalised object relationships that are externalised in relation to the therapist and in everyday relationships
3   Loosely, the patient's emotional attitude towards their therapist. This broad definition subsumes the concept of therapeutic alliance.

Understanding and interpreting the transference is an important area for insight and change in psychotherapy because it allows these early internalised relationships with significant figures in the patient's life to become accessible to conscious awareness over time so they can be understood and the patient can choose more flexible and robust ways of relating. These early internal object relationships developed at a time in the patient's life when they were in a powerless, helpless position and had to arrive at compromises to protect themselves. However, these patterns are often no longer adaptive in later life and can lead to repeated difficulties. It is largely through the transference relationship with the therapist that the patient becomes aware of these patterns of relating. Through this awareness, the patient is increasingly able to step back from implicit ways of relating to others in order to have a greater repertoire of responding that in turn elicits more constructive relationships. This is also referred to as *working through* (Freud, 1914a) where the patient's insight leads to change.

How to recognise the transference

The transference is an unconscious communication whereby internal object relationships are transferred on to the therapist. The patient's conscious response to
the therapist is also coloured by their unconscious feelings and fantasies which
leads in turn to a distorted perception of the therapist. In the clinical example of
transference with Maggie, she jumps to the assumption without any knowledge of
the therapist's background that they are poorly raised, rude and dismissive. In this
example, the transference is also communicated unconsciously by the patient's
lateness and lack of concern about the impact this may have on the therapist. We
may even wonder if it is present in Maggie's intuiting at an unconscious level that
her compliment may not feel genuine to the therapist.

To recognise the transference, the therapist needs to consider the way the
patient is behaving and responding to them. The clues are there from the very
beginning. How did the patient make contact with you? Was there something in
those early communications that alerted you to something? Was the patient
formal, casual or overly familiar, for example? Perhaps something stood out for
you in the way the patient phrased their first email or whether it was easy or
convoluted to arrange an initial appointment? Some patients get lost on their way
to the appointment, perhaps not allowing themselves enough time to find the
consulting room, only to arrive flustered, on the back foot. Others appear to
command the space, spreading their possessions across the room and driving the
communication.

The transference can be detected in the assumptions the patient holds about
the therapist. Is the patient saying things that you don't recognise as belonging to
you and your view of yourself? A paranoid patient starting out in therapy
expressed her fear that the therapist was very charismatic and would exert an
undue influence over her personality and choices. The therapist felt this had more
to do with the patient's anxiety at entering treatment than the therapist's enduring character. Is there a variance between what the patient is saying and their
body language or even tone of voice? A patient may sound polite and measured,
but their tapping leg suggests an irritation or impatience that in turn conveys a
sense of pressure to the therapist.

The patient may also be talking about something or someone else, but there
is a sense that something else is being referenced or implied, in a symbolic way.
For example, does the patient describe a situation with someone in their life or
even a TV programme that begins to sound more and more like an aspect of
their relationship with you, for instance how they feel about being in treatment
or their reaction to an upcoming break?

Another indicator of the transference is the impact it has on us, in particular
our countertransference to the patient. Are there times with patients where you
are unable to think clearly or you feel stuck, sleepy or hopeless? Do you find
yourself distracted by outside noises or events in your life while you are with a
patient? Perhaps you feel pulled into being rather cold or critical with one patient
while another patient elicits a maternal response from you. In many ways, there is

an intersubjective nature to the transference and countertransference. The relationship between patient and therapist is the Petri dish in which the cultures of earlier relationships will grow and multiply, casting light on the patient's internal and interpersonal world. We don't wish to disturb this process of projection and multiplication by revealing too much about our own identity. In order to facilitate and make use of the transference, we have to be willing to be experienced in a multiplicity of ways by our patients. One patient may experience you as patient and gentle while another may complain that you are overly cautious and walking on eggshells. Another patient may see you as powerful and opinionated while a different patient will experience you as weak and pathetic. We have to be willing to be made use of in this way, in the service of the transference and a deeper understanding of the patient's unconscious dynamics. This is where the therapist's personal therapy is important so that we can move beyond a wish to be helpful and appreciated by them, views that will hinder our capacity to be made use of by them in whatever way is required at that time. We are talking about symbolic ways of projecting on to the therapist, with the safety of the analytic frame acting as protection to both therapist and patient.

Different types of transference

Positive, erotic and negative transference

When considering the transference, it helps to classify whether it is negative or positive overall. *Positive transference* refers to the way the patient transfers onto the therapist their feelings of attachment, love, idealisation and other positive emotions that were originally experienced toward parents or other significant individuals during childhood. We can think about it as the warm, non-romantic feelings that contribute towards the establishment of a constructive therapeutic alliance.

When the positive transference takes on a romantic or sexual nature, it is termed *erotic transference*. Freud described the way this transference love is stirred up by the analytic situation, where the patient becomes more resistant and is less concerned with reality and consequences than they would ordinarily. Akhtar (2009a) described a variant of this which he termed the *malignant erotic transference*, referring to an intense seemingly erotic transference that hides marked aggression towards the therapist and is more common in female patients. It has a lot in common with negative transference and often includes the delusional belief that the therapist should or will consummate the relationship and marry the patient. We look at the clinical dilemma of how to manage erotic transference in Chapter 12.

Negative transference is where the patient transfers onto the therapist negative feelings of irritation, anger or even hostility or hatred that were originally felt toward parents or other significant objects from childhood. These negative feelings can result in a rupture to the therapeutic alliance, so it is important, particularly in once-weekly or brief psychodynamic therapy, that the therapist attends to the patient's negative transference feelings in order to avoid the therapeutic alliance breaking down. This includes getting a better understanding of the patient's experience of the therapist and acknowledging anything the therapist may be contributing towards this, knowingly or unknowingly.

When we ask someone during an initial consultation about whether they would prefer to see a male or female therapist, we are exploring which gender the patient will find it easier to form a positive transference with at the start of treatment. If a female patient describes her difficulty relating to her father and struggles to get along with male authority figures, it may be easier for her to form a trusting relationship with a female therapist. This is not to say that more complicated and ambiguous feelings will develop towards the therapist over the course of treatment, regardless of the therapist's demographics. One of the reasons we strive for neutrality in the analytic setting and therapeutic stance is to enable the transference to develop freely in whatever direction the patient takes it, without being overly impeded by external realities. The less the patient knows about the therapist's actual life, the easier it is for the therapist to become a screen on to which the patient can project their fantasies and internal world. This in turn allows the therapist to better understand the patient in the wider context of their early and current object relationships and internal psychic structures.

Both positive and negative transference can operate as forms of resistance in psychotherapy. An insistence on positive transference usually represents the patient's attempt to keep the therapist all-good, thereby idealising the therapist as someone who can do no wrong. This is an *idealising transference* which we describe further below. The negative transference represents the polar opposite in which the therapist is seen as all-bad, harmful, malicious, neglectful, obstructing and so on. The patient can then become caught up in a hostile attack on the therapist. These two positions align to Klein's concept of splitting and the patient can alternate rapidly from one to the other. We would expect that an outcome of therapy is that it promotes the patient's capacity to integrate these two distinct versions of the therapist, allowing for a shift to the depressive position, with reparative guilt replacing persecutory guilt.

Transference neurosis

While all patients will develop a range of transient transferences towards the therapist, these often settle into the *transference neurosis*. Freud (1914a) wrote that "we succeed in giving all the symptoms of the illness a new transference meaning and in replacing (the patient's) ordinary neurosis by a 'transference neurosis' of which he can be cured by the therapeutic work" (p. 154). The transference neurosis develops in the context of relative calm in other parts of the patient's life, such that their conflicts are experienced in relation to the therapist with the establishment of an intense and ongoing transference relationship. Even though the patient may experience their reactions to the therapist as genuine, they are understood to be distorted repetitions of the past. The work of therapy is to work through the transference neurosis and resolve these longstanding and implicit interpersonal and intrapsychic difficulties.

This therapy work stands in sharp contrast to the *transference cure*, that is, the illusion of positive change that occurs in the context of an idealised relationship with the therapist. The transference cure is very different to making structural changes that are reliable and enduring once therapy concludes. When there is a transference cure, there is usually an idealisation of the therapist that sustains the patient while they continue to see the therapist, but these gains quickly wear off when their contact with the therapist reduces and/or stops. This is a defensive response in therapy and in sharp contrast to the *negative therapeutic reaction* identified by Freud (1923a), whereby the patient undoes any benefit experienced from the therapist's interpretations because of an unconscious investment in remaining unwell. While the thought of making progress appeals to the patient consciously and aligns with their stated goals, we are aware that unconsciously the patient is often defended against making positive change and may want to remain in their stuck position because of the defensive function it serves. In psychology, we often talk about secondary gain, namely the positive consequences that may arise from being unwell or requiring help. Patients may fear that if they improve, the therapist will discharge them, or their families and friends will withdraw care and concern.

Self-object transferences

In Kohut's (1984) writings about disorders of the self, he described some forms of transference dynamics that can be observed with patients with a narcissistic, disturbed sense of self. Here we introduce three such variants of transference that were identified in Kohut's writing on Self Psychology.

Those patients who feel unconsciously inferior as a result of damaged ambitions may develop a *mirroring transference*. In grandiose and exhibitionistic states of mind, the patient perceives and experiences the object (i.e. the therapist) as admiring of the self. The patient may also strive to be perfect in order to win over much-needed admiration, as an external means of compensating for internal, low self-esteem. Kohut suggests that initially the therapist should provide a positive mirror for the patient in order to strengthen self-esteem. Once the patient has strengthened a sense of self through this validation, and has a positive sense of trust towards the therapist, then the work can turn to exploring and working through more conflictual affects and dynamics.

Another type of transference is the *idealising transference*, where the individual vicariously boosts their low self-esteem through identifying with an idealised object. Here, it is the object rather than the self that is experienced as perfect, leading to the self being strengthened. In the transference, the therapist is idealised as perfect and 'the best'. This defensive strategy locates the goodness outside the self but leads to interpersonal vulnerability, whereby any difficulty in the relationship is experienced as a narcissistic blow, leading to a loss of internal goodness and a depletion in positive introjects.

A third type of self-object transference is the *twinship transference*. This occurs with those patients who feel insecure about themselves, their value and abilities and this leads them to seek an object that can be used as a type of alter-ego. The other functions as an externalised twin that represents a more secure and compensatory resource. Here, the object is perceived as an extension of the patient rather than having their own subjectivity. In these cases, differences cannot be easily tolerated. This is an early state of ego functioning whereby the self feels merged with the object. It is similar to the way the parent functions as an auxiliary ego for the baby and small child.

The cautionary tale

Ogden (1992) highlights the importance of recognising and taking up the patient's cautionary tale when they enter into therapy. This serves as an early interpretation or tracer of potential negative transference and is intended to strengthen the emerging therapeutic alliance. Ogden (1992) writes:

> The patient unconsciously holds a fierce conviction (which he has no way of articulating) that his infantile and childhood experience has taught him about the specific ways in which each of his object relationships will inevitably become painful, disappointing, annihilating, lonely, unreliable, suffocating, overly sexualized and so on. There is no reason to believe that the transference relationship in to which he is about to enter will be any different. In this belief the patient is both correct and incorrect. He is correct in the sense that, transferentially, his internal object world will inevitably become a living intersubjective drama on the analytic stage. He is incorrect to the extent that the analytic context will not be identical to the original psychological-interpersonal context within which his internal object world was created i.e., the context of infantile and childhood fantasy and object relations. (p. 235)

As we discussed previously in relation to assessment, it is important to explore the patient's previous experiences of psychotherapy and receiving help prior to seeing you. These often hold clues about the patient's relationship to help and what they are worried about being repeated in starting therapy now. It is important to attend to the stories they tell you about the previous therapist who was so unresponsive, they felt very alone and unimportant, for example, or the bored therapist who dozed off or the therapist who was so controlling about what could and couldn't take place in sessions, that the patient felt dismissed and frustrated. Each scenario will reveal a different anxiety about the process of entering into treatment. It is helpful to interpret these signposts as understandable fears the patient is letting you know about and that you can both look out for to avoid this being repeated yet again. The cautionary tale may also link to a patient's likely response to their feared reactions at entering therapy, like dropping out of treatment prematurely, having a breakdown of some sort, becoming very depressed and needy or lodging a complaint with the therapist's governing body. We might say something like "I can hear that you can often end up feeling criticised and then feel you have no choice but to walk away; we will need to watch out that this doesn't happen here and that you can come back to talk about it with me if you feel like that".

In longer-term psychotherapy, these anxieties are facilitated by the analytic stance the psychotherapist takes which is less supportive and more boundaried, allowing the transference to develop more clearly and quickly. Again, this is an approach that will vary depending on the theoretical stance of the therapist, personality factors and the particular relationship of patient and therapist.

Working in the transference

What does this mean? It refers to those times in the session when you consider and then go on to explore what is happening in the therapeutic relationship. This could relate to an actual event, perhaps the way the patient felt you reacted to their lateness with irritability, or an anticipated reaction that led the patient to respond defensively about their lateness, already expecting you to be on the attack. These moments in which earlier relationship patterns are activated in the immediacy of the therapeutic relationship are often the most affect-laden and powerful way of working in psychotherapy. Psychodynamic psychotherapy is fundamentally a relational therapy and therapeutic change results from working on these long-standing, entrenched interpersonal patterns as they manifest in the transference. There is an immediacy of exchange because it is happening inside the consulting room, rather than outside over there. It is also powerful because it is happening in the 'here-and-now', rather than the 'there-and-then' of the past. This means that because it is so powerful, it is also the most anxiety-provoking area in which to engage with the patient. It arouses the patient's attachment to the therapist and can easily destabilise the patient, leading to an inhibition in the capacity to mentalise. We need to be mindful at all times about the impact our interventions have on our patients.

We can use the following diagram (Figure 9.1) developed by Menninger (1958) and then Malan (2001) which is called the Triangle of Person or, alternatively,

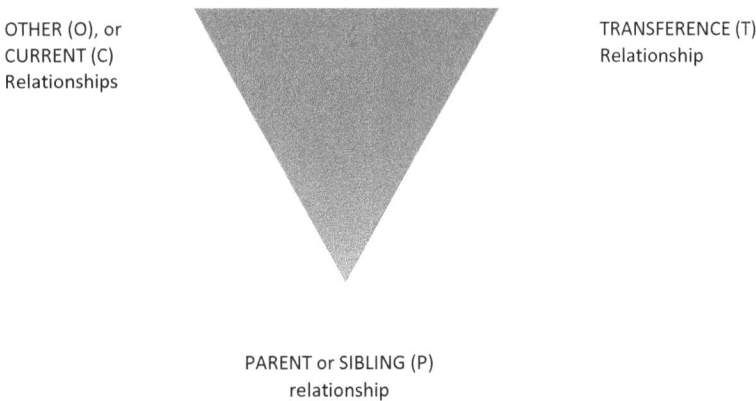

OTHER (O), or CURRENT (C) Relationships

TRANSFERENCE (T) Relationship

PARENT or SIBLING (P) relationship

Figure 9.1 Adapted from the Triangle of Person or Insight
Source: Malan, 2001, p. 90

The Triangle of Insight and which relates to the Triangle of Conflict that we introduced in Chapter 6. Malan makes the point that the two triangles of conflict and insight cover almost every intervention a therapist will make: "Much of a therapist's skill consists of knowing which parts of the triangle to include in his interpretation at any given moment" (2001, p. 91).

Again, the triangle is placed on its apex to indicate that there is an underlying element to the other two sides of the triangle. In this case, past relationships with the primary attachment figures in the family of origin underpin later relationships and in psychodynamic psychotherapy, we are ultimately trying to make these links to earlier relationships as a part of the repetition compulsion. The triangle allows us to see that three different types of links can be made (Malan, 2001, p. 90):

O/P links – feelings directed towards others in the patient's life (e.g. boss, friends, partner) derive from early relationships with parents and siblings; this relates to the current and recent past. Sometimes this is denoted as 'C' for current relationships.

O/T links – similar feelings exist between other figures in the patient's life and the therapist; this is usually about the here-and-now present.

P/T links – feelings that derive from parental and sibling relationships are transferred on to the therapist; this tends to relate to the distant past.

Making transference interpretations

This refers to any intervention that is aimed at drawing the patient's attention to the transference basis of the patient's attitude, feeling, fantasy or behaviour. Some theoretical approaches to psychotherapy place great importance on transference interpretations as the site of change.

How much importance you place on the transference will depend on several factors. Your theoretical orientation within the field of psychoanalysis will influence this. Typically, Kleinian therapists view transference interpretations as the most mutative interpretations of all. As Heimann (1956) puts it, "Whether the patient talks about a dream or a current incident or a childhood episode, the analyst's task is to perceive the dynamic line which links this with the patient's actual motives, preconscious or unconscious, towards the analyst" (p. 309). Hanna Segal (1990) went further when she writes, "In the phantasy world of the analysand, the most important figure is the person of the analyst ... all communications contain something relevant to the transference situation" (p. 8). Perhaps we have to consider whether once weekly psychodynamic work requires an adaptation in relation to how much we take up the transference with our patients.

Your level of experience and confidence as a psychotherapist will play a part too in your ability to make transference interpretations. You may feel it is presumptuous to assume the patient has strong feelings towards you as their therapist. Taking up the patient's transference towards you requires some degree of confidence in yourself as an important figure in your patient's internal world. Listening to transferential links requires listening beyond the content of the material to think about it as if your patient is describing a drama: you need to discern which role has been ascribed to you in that drama. We don't mean to imply that the patient is being overly dramatic or manipulative, rather that approaching it in this way is a useful technique to help you identify repeated patterns in relationships. For example, if a patient brings lots of stories about feeling annoyed with people in their lives who let them down and are a disappointment just as there is an approaching break in therapy, it is likely that they are also unconsciously addressing their feelings about how they feel you will be letting them down during that break.

Strachey (1934) identified truly *mutative interpretations* as those which had a sense of immediacy and credibility by virtue of taking up the transference relationship. However, this has led to an over-valuing of transference interpretations by some therapists. Greenson (1978) cautions against this, arguing that by "focusing constantly on the patient's transference distortions and ignoring the reality elements, we undermine his self-esteem and make him feel he is always wrong sick or crazy" (p. 434). He goes on to say that this leads patients "to live in the outside world as though all of life were lived on a gigantic psychoanalytic couch and people at large were either patients or psychoanalysts" (p. 434). He further warns that this type of approach will inevitably restrict the development of the transference along the therapists' theoretical biases.

Greenson (1978) helpfully distinguishes between the distortions of the transference relationship and the real relationship with the therapist, which incorporates the therapeutic alliance. Separating out these two is a useful theoretical construct but difficult to do in practice. However, he emphasises that a patient will have a range of different transference reactions to the therapist over the course of treatment that may range from more primitive to sophisticated responses, from loving to hating, aggressive responses. Alongside this, "the patient will also experience realistic and genuine reactions toward the analyst and form a real relationship.… Intelligence, sensitivity, humour, empathy, education, temperament, and taste all play a part in shaping the transference and nontransference reactions" (p. 439) for both patient and therapist. He cautions against limiting the changes in therapy to any one factor.

The classical way of proceeding with interpreting the transference is to allow the transference to develop, then interpreting from the surface to the depth, by taking up the resistance to the transference first and by addressing the ego aspects before the id (Greenson, 1978). This links with Malan's triangle of insight, discussed earlier. We start by interpreting the patient's feelings that are closest to awareness, then moving to explore the patient's defences and resistance before interpreting the more unconscious, id aspects of the underlying, hidden affect at the base of the triangle. Greenson (1978) argues that we need to work with the patient's observing ego with whom we have the working alliance: "A transference reaction, to be effectively interpreted, has to be demonstrable to the patient, he must feel that it is plausible, and he must be able to cope with the emotional repercussions of his new insight" (p. 525). This staged approach is intended to give the patient the best possible chance of hearing the interpretation openly, without too much resistance and in the service of the therapy.

How and when you interpret the transference can make the difference between your pushing something back at a patient or allowing the patient to brush away what you are saying as inconsequential, particularly if this involves taking up the negative transference. Posing transference interpretations as questions can allow patients to dismiss them more easily. Obviously, we are not suggesting you interpret with huge certainty because this will inevitably mean you are not mentalising flexibly. However, the way you say something can suggest this is what is occurring to you and this is how you are making sense of what is happening at the moment with the patient. You can say things like, "It seems to me", "I am wondering" and "I can't help but notice that …" By presenting your point of view, the patient is invited to consider this perspective and be curious about what is happening between the two of you in the room. This stimulates mentalising about the therapeutic relationship. Often patients will find this a difficult concept to understand and may want to put the therapeutic relationship into a completely different category to the rest of their other relationships. The patient may reply, "But this is a professional relationship and of course, you will behave with confidentiality and respect so I am not concerned about what might happen in this situation". It is helpful for patients to feel they can form the start of a trusting relationship with us – after all, this facilitates the collaborative work of psychotherapy. However, as we have pointed out, too much idealisation of the therapeutic relationship is problematic.

Countertransference

One of the important competences for psychodynamic psychotherapy is the therapist's capacity to be self-reflective and consider the meaning and relevance of their emotional reactions to the patient. Countertransference is made up of our responses to the patient's material, including feelings, thoughts and behaviour in relation to the patient. Our countertransference gives us clues about the patient's inner world and interpersonal experiences. At the same time, we are aware that there are unconscious forces operating in both therapist and patient, particularly given that there is a level of communication from unconscious to unconscious. It is important to monitor our emotional reactions to our patients and identify our part in any enactments, blind spots or collusions, whether indulgent or depriving. We need to weigh up how much of this has to do with our own personal material (e.g. our transferences) and how much of this has to do with the patient's projections and our being pulled into responding to the patient in particular, complementary ways.

At first, Freud (1910) saw countertransference as an indication that the therapist needed further therapy, a sign of unresolved areas of personal development and resistance to engaging with areas of shared difficulty with the patient. However, Paula Heimann brought an important new understanding of countertransference, moving away from a negative understanding of countertransference as interference, to regarding countertransference as an important source of information about the patient's psychic life: "the analyst's counter-transference is not only part and parcel of the analytic relationship, but it is the patient's *creation*, it is a part of the patient's personality" (Heimann, 1950, p. 83). This opened up the possibility of drawing on our own responses to the patient as a source of information as to what may be happening for the patient. From becoming problematic, countertransference now is seen as an opportunity. In Heimann's words, "the analyst's counter-transference is an instrument of research into the patient's unconscious" (1950, p. 81).

At around the same time, Heinrich Racker was developing similar ideas in Argentina, without any knowledge of Heimann's writings in England. Racker (1953) classified countertransference into direct and indirect types, with direct countertransference representing the therapist's emotional response to the patient while indirect countertransference referred to the therapist's emotional response to someone significant to the patient. He further divided the direct countertransference of the therapist into concordant and complementary countertransference. Where the therapist felt a concordant counter-transference, there was an empathic symmetry between the experiences of therapist and patient whereby the therapist feels identified with the projected parts of the patient. In complementary countertransference, the therapist becomes unconsciously identified with an unconscious or unwanted, projected part of the patient. Racker (1957) writes that "the complementary identifications are closely connected with the destiny of the concordant identifications: it seems that to the degree to which the analyst fails in the concordant identifications and rejects them, certain complementary identifications become intensified" (p. 312). Where the therapist feels unable to accept a part of themselves, such as their anger or envy, this in turn leads to a rejection of the patient's anger and envy. This touches on the role of projective identification in countertransference and the need for therapists to be willing to be 'made use of' in this way by patients.

A warning is required at this stage, particularly for those therapists who are at the early stages of their career. We do need to carefully monitor our counter-transference responses to the patient at all times to ensure we are not embarking on wild speculation that has no basis in the material the patient brings. It is essential that we remain reflective practitioners at all times, and part of our own reflective practice is the careful monitoring and attending to our counter-transference. When we are with patients who evoke intense reactions in us, it is important that we can step back from those feelings and consider the impact of them, including being under pressure to act on those feelings. Often these are patients who require a teleological response to their distress – we have to do something to show the patient that we care. The danger is that if we don't process these responses, we can end up being unseated analytically and run the risk of being pulled into enactments with patient.

Betty Joseph (1985) wrote about the importance of the transference and counter-transference as encapsulating all of the patient's struggles and as such, representing the 'total situation':

everything that the analyst is or says is likely to be responded to according to the patient's own psychic make-up, rather than the analyst's intentions and the meaning he gives to his interpretations. The way in which our patients communicate their problems to us is frequently beyond their individual associations and beyond their words, and can often only be gauged by means of the countertransference. (p. 453)

Role responsiveness and countertransference

The therapist has to maintain free-floating attention which as we have already suggested, is not about clearing the mind of all memories or thoughts but rather the capacity to allow all sorts of thoughts, daydreams and associations to enter the therapist's consciousness while at the same time, listening to and observing the patient. Alongside this, Sandler (1976) says the analyst also has *free floating responsiveness*. Sandler links this to the way we can be pulled unconsciously in our countertransference to enacting a particular relationship with the patient. An interaction develops between the patient and therapist whereby the patient casts concordant or complementary roles for themselves and therapist. Sandler gives the example of a patient to whom he kept passing the box of tissues every time she cried. After two years, there was an occasion where for no apparent reason, he did not respond in this manner when the patient cried. This led to the patient shouting at him for this failure, accusing him of being callous and uncaring. He replied that he didn't know why he hadn't passed the tissues at that point, but encouraged her to carry on talking so they may understand it more. In doing so, a deeper understanding of the patient's presenting difficulties became apparent that had not emerged prior to this point. The patient's earlier experiences around wetting or soiling herself were now understood as an anger that there was no adult around to clean her up. She had been unconsciously repeating an experience of wetting herself through her tears and inviting the analyst to clean her up symbolically through offering the box of tissues.

Sandler understood that the patient's transference represents an attempt to impose an interaction or interrelationship between patient and therapist. Something in the therapist's internal world corresponds to the patient's internal world, akin to Racker's concordant countertransference. The resultant feelings or behaviours generated in the therapist, either consciously or unconsciously, are not elicited by the present, real situation as much as they relate to the patient's internal world. The therapist has to be able to go along with these identifications, at times without any awareness of it.

We can link these ideas of role responsiveness to our discussion on mentalising. We know that poor mentalising begets poor mentalising. As patients become excessively concrete in their thinking, so we can feel pulled into similar ways of responding. There are different countertransference responses to poor mentalising states of mind that are useful signals to our patient's mentalising being compromised.

When the patient is in a state of *psychic equivalence*, we are likely to have a complementary response of wanting to argue with the patient and impose our view of reality on their rigidly held view of events. The patient's certainty and black-and-white thinking often leads to rigidity and certainty of our own. We may find ourselves insisting on our version of events, perhaps repeating interpretations that are not resonating emotionally with the patient. We may feel very frustrated with these patients who are convinced of their worthlessness, for example, or feel certain that they are being badly treated by others when we are struck by a different impression. We may also find ourselves holding great confusion, puzzlement in the face of the patient's certainty and feel consigned to the role of a nodding dog therapist, having to agree with everything the patient is saying.

When patients are pseudo-mentalising or in *pretend mode*, we can find ourselves similarly disconnecting from what the patient is saying. At these times, the patient is emotionally removed from what they are talking about. On the face of it, their conversation may sound very meaningful but often the clue is in our countertransference where we feel bored, even sleepy, or our mind wanders onto other matters, and we in turn may be tempted to say something equally trivial in response to the patient. If your mind has decoupled from the session and you feel emotionally distant from your patient, it is likely that the patient is also feeling disconnected in some way. Rather than sit back and let the patient continue to speak in this manner, you should intervene to re-establish contact and to draw the patient's attention to what is being avoided.

When patients are in *teleological mode*, there is a wish for action rather than contemplation and the intentions of others are measured in those actions. In such states of mind, there is often a strong wish for the therapist to do something and respond in a particular way. This may be to provide advice, medication or coping strategies, write a letter or engage in siding with the patient against a significant figure in their life. In erotic transference, there is a wish to engage sexually or romantically with the therapist. The patient may also want to co-opt the therapist as a critical or obstructive figure in the patient's life. In our countertransference, we can often feel anxious and manipulated, taken over with a focus on what needs to be done and losing sight of the patient's mental states. We notice this response particularly when a patient is suicidal and we are liable to get caught up in a teleological response, unable to be reflective at the very time we need it the most.

How to recognise and monitor your countertransference

Part of the role of a psychodynamic psychotherapist is to take up a 'third position' (Britton, 2004) where you can step back from the immediacy and heat of the therapist-patient dyad and reflect on what is happening at a meta-psychological level. This triangular space is one of the main reasons we have clinical supervision, which gives us the opportunity to think with another experienced person, our supervisor, about the third – in this case, the patient. This experience both in supervision and clinically as an internal supervisory space (Casement, 1985) allows us to retain a more objective perspective while at the same time allowing ourselves to be immersed in the subjective experience of being with the patient. This is a continuous dynamic that the therapist has to manage in the room. If we are too analytical and detached, then we do not allow the patient to make use of us; conversely, if we are too enmeshed with the patient's emotional experience, we are unable to step back from moments of role responsiveness, projective identification and acting in to recognise and then interpret this. We need to be willing to accept (momentarily at least) the patient's uncomfortable projections into us, whether these are overly negative or idealised, however ego dystonic they may be for us. We have to be open to being experienced by the patient in ways that we may not recognise as part of our self-perception. If we insist on being seen as benevolent, kind and thoughtful all the time, we will inhibit the ability of the patient to feel angry when they inevitably will experience us as critical, withholding, inconsiderate and rejecting. This is a paradox of psychodynamic psychotherapy: the therapist draws on their experience, knowledge, deliberateness and strategy (Levy, 1987) on the one hand, yet is also involved in a spontaneous and undetermined relationship with the patient that goes beyond memory or desire (Bion 1970) and that allows for moments of spontaneity, play, creativity, even mess and error.

While you are in the session, it is helpful to be both immersed in the session while also attending to the particular feelings, thoughts, associations and fantasies evoked in you as you attend to the patient. We remind you again of Winnicott's cellist analogy from the opening chapter and the way this 'therapeutic multitasking' becomes more implicit and assured with practice. This may be aided by ongoing reflective questioning about your own responses (see Box 9.1) in order to listen beyond the manifest content of the patient's messages and tune into the patient's unconscious communications. As we know, the patient communicates with us on all kinds of levels, conscious and unconscious, verbal and non-verbal. Being attuned to our countertransference is a powerful clinical instrument. We may find ourselves feeling enraged as we listen to our patient relating a seemingly innocuous story about their week. We may find ourselves feeling all kinds of bodily sensations from sleepiness to nausea to itching skin and this can be understood as a communication of powerful embodied emotional states. Alessandra Lemma has written evocatively about this in her book, *Minding the Body* (2015). When you are working remotely with patients, it is very difficult to have the same bodily countertransference you would have if the patient is in the room with you and this form of work can remove an important source of information from the therapist (Lemma, 2017, see also Chapter 14).

Box 9.1 Reflecting on your countertransference

Useful prompts to think about your countertransference:

- What are you feeling as you listen and watch your patient's verbal and non-verbal behaviour?
- Do you feel under pressure to act in particular ways?
- Does any part of your response belong to you, and not the patient?
- Is this a new feeling, thought or body sensation that you have when working with this patient?
- Have you thought or felt this way in previous sessions?

- Does the patient's story remind you of a person/situation in your own life?
- Are any of your thoughts or feelings similar to those your patient needs to express, but has not yet done so?

When your feelings belong to you (your own transference to the patient and therapy situation):

Identify your feelings and bodily reactions:

- Right now, I feel/experience/think …
- This particular patient's story reminds me of …
- Today I am affected by this patient because …

Consider your current life situation:

- What's going on for you?
- What self-care do you need and how can you take care of yourself?
- Is there a personal situation playing a significant role in your life right now?
- Who can help you with this in your network of friends, colleagues and family?

What learning points can you take away from this situation?

- My blind spots are …
- I didn't know that …
- I realise that …
- What I need is …

Let us return to the heuristic about maintaining analytic neutrality discussed in Chapter 8, whereby the therapist aims to interpret from a position that is equidistant between the ego, id and superego (Tuckett, 2011, see Figure 8.1). Anna Freud (1954) points out that if we are overly drawn to any one clinical endeavour, this results in a distorted or incomplete picture of the patient's personality and is a travesty of reality. When we are monitoring our countertransference, we need to be aware of whether we are being pulled towards one of the corners in response to our patient. For example, have we become overly punitive by assigning fault or blame, thus being pulled into a superego position? Have we become overly focused on planning real world solutions and thus overly aligned with the patient's ego, at the neglect of other, unconscious communications? Are we pulled towards feeling warm towards a very special patient, or the opposite, in identification with our id impulses? By becoming aware of our countertransference, we can recover a neutral position before interpreting and thus reduce the risk of acting this out in the session.

Maintaining neutrality involves being able to remain circumspect about the actuality of what happened in the past or present of the patient's life. We should be alarmed when we hear versions of people's lives that are very two-dimensional, where certain characters are depicted as all-good or all-bad. Our countertransference is a useful early warning system. Notice when we start to feel indignant or enraged with someone in the patient's life, perhaps even co-opted into this role by the patient or holding feelings that have been disowned by the patient and given to us to experience (i.e. projective identification). It is useful to consider everything that is described as possibly containing elements of projection. Analytic neutrality includes avoiding siding with one or other person in the patient's world, as well as avoiding siding with one or other aspect of the patient's personality. For example, we can be drawn into a punitive, disapproving, even sadistic position in response to a patient's masochistic wish to be punished.

If you are in your own psychotherapy, this can be a useful place to explore what may be stirred up for you in your own clinical work so that you can better understand your countertransference to your patient's material and separate it from your personal responses and your own issues that may be resonating with the patient.

Particular types of transference-countertransference dynamics

Hate in the countertransference

Winnicott (1949) writes that the main task of the analyst of any patient is to maintain objectivity in regard to all that the patient brings, and he points out that a special case of this is the analyst's need to be able to hate the patient objectively. He says that one of the key ways the therapist expresses hate is by the existence of the end of the 'hour'.

> However much he (the analyst) loves his patients he cannot avoid hating them, and fearing them, and the better he knows this the less will hate and fear be the motive determining what he does to his patients. (p. 69)

and

> If the analyst is going to have crude feelings imputed to him he is best forewarned and so forearmed, for he must tolerate being placed in that position. Above all he must not deny hate that really exists in himself. (p. 70)

These ideas are often difficult for budding therapists to acknowledge and accept. It is useful to think about the way opposing feelings are usually held simultaneously and that we need to be willing to think about both. In psychic terms, the opposite of love isn't hate, after all: it is indifference (a quote attributed to Eli Wiesel but originally found in Austrian psychologist Wilhelm Stekel's book, *The Beloved Ego*, 1921). Winnicott describes the ways hate can be found in the primary relationship between mother and baby, a relationship that is also characterised by profound love. Like the mother of an infant, the therapist must be willing

> to bear strain without expecting the patient to know anything about what he is doing, perhaps over a long period of time. To do this he must be easily

aware of his own fear and hate.… Eventually, he ought to be able to tell his patient what he has been through on the patient's behalf, but an analysis may never get as far as this. There may be too little good experience in the patient's past to work on. What if there be no satisfactory relationship of early infancy for the analyst to exploit in the transference? (1949, p. 72)

Winnicott distinguishes between those patients who have had 'good enough' parenting and that allows for those experiences to be discovered in the transference, as opposed to those patients with such adverse childhood experiences that the therapist is the first experience of a benign object for the patient. In the case of such patients, he describes the process of the patient requiring objective hate of the therapist before being able to accept objective love. He writes that "I suggest that the mother hates the baby before the baby hates the mother, and before the baby can know his mother hates him" (p. 73). What does he mean by the mother hating her baby? Winnicott provides a list of many reasons, which includes the baby being a danger to the mother's own body in pregnancy and childbirth, the baby being an interference to her own personal life, the baby being relentless in his needs and demands, and many more. This is an ordinary, garden variety of hate we are talking about here, not the sort that will result in Social Services knocking on the door!

Winnicott likens this early relationship of mother and baby to psychoanalysis with regressed patients who relate to the analyst like an infant to a mother, without being able to see her as separate (Think about the similarity with the Kohutian twinship transference). Winnicott reminds us about the need to know about your hate in the countertransference in order to contain it. He goes on to say,

> The most remarkable thing about a mother is her ability to be hurt so much by her baby and to hate so much without paying the child out, and her ability to wait for rewards that may or may not come at a later date. (p. 74)

This is an essential aspect of the analytic stance; the absence of the talion reaction (of an eye-for-an-eye). Winnicott draws our attention to the analytic stance of abstinence and the importance of monitoring our countertransference so we do not get caught up in wanting acknowledgement from our patients who may not yet be able to see the therapist as a separate person.

Projective identification and countertransference

Projective identification is linked to countertransference, in both its pathological and benign forms, (i.e. as containment and a form of primitive communication). We can sometimes become aware of our response towards a patient that feels alien or unusual to us, something that we would not usually feel in those situations. We may find ourselves feeling very critical for example, or overly admiring and affectionate. This is different to projection, where a patient may attribute something to us that feels separate, even foreign. You will remember that in projective identification something is projected *into* the other. For the therapist, there is a sense in which

something of the patient's experience belongs to you (the clue is in the word identification) and that you come to recognise with time that it has much more to do
with the patient than you, after all. This is a very primitive form of communication.
In its earliest forms, it is the means a baby has to communicate with parents before
language has been acquired. The infant can convey very primitive emotional states
in this way with the ultimate aim being their survival. In therapy, we can consider
projective identification as the patient's attempt to convey something to us that
cannot as yet be put into words or communicated more consciously. Projective
identification can sometimes manifest at a somatic level in the therapist, bypassing
symbolic expression through words. The therapist may feel overcome by feelings of
nausea or pain, as in the following example:

> *Kiran had a very disturbed childhood history of abuse and neglect. As she related these*
> *painful stories to me in a session, in a matter of fact way, I found myself developing painful*
> *earache that made me want to stop the session. I became concerned that I was ill but after*
> *the session ended and my earache subsided, I realised that this was most likely a projective*
> *identification in which I became someone who was unable to hear what she had to say. In*
> *this scenario, it is also possible that I felt overloaded by such disturbed material that my*
> *ears shut down, in which case this would relate to my own defensive system.*

As you can see, this is not an exact science and we do need to take responsibility
for our own contribution to the countertransference experience. Was Kiran projecting her unbearable pain into the therapist? Perhaps she could put into words
what had happened to her, but she could not feel it. Alternatively, was the
therapist, for their own reasons (the therapist's transference), unwilling to hear
Kiran's story that assaulted their ears?

Pathological forms of projective identification are not commonplace and are often
very disturbing to receive. It is a particular version of Sandler's role responsiveness:
the way the therapist is drawn into responding to the patient in a particular way that
is unique to that patient and yet is not typical for the therapist. You would not expect
patients who are seen in psychodynamic psychotherapy to regularly employ this
means of communication. It is usually a sign that a different form of treatment
should be considered, either a more intensive treatment that allows the therapist to
work at a deeper level and with greater regularity and containment, or a more
structured and/or supportive treatment approach like counselling, trauma work or
CBT. This is a decision you may have to make as the therapy unfolds and it can
result in you titrating your clinical work and interventions with your patient if there
are no alternatives and ending treatment is not possible.

Although Freud used metaphors of therapist neutrality by depicting the clinician as a blank screen, mirror or detached surgeon, the reality is that we are not
neutral. Part of being aware of our countertransference and reflecting on our
reactions to different patient material is to be aware of our own prejudices, strongly
held beliefs and blind spots. You may have a negative transference of your own to a
particular patient or presenting difficulty and it is important to avoid the omnipotent
position of believing you can help anyone and everyone. We know of highly

experienced therapists who willingly engage with disturbed and perverse patients yet state that they would find working with anorexic patients too challenging, and vice versa. There will be some presenting difficulties that may feel too difficult or provocative for you to work with – this is idiographic and personal to each therapist and it is important for you to acknowledge your limitations.

Acting out and acting in

The term *acting out* was first used by Freud in relation to his patient, Dora, who "acted out an essential part of her recollection and phantasies instead of reproducing it in the treatment" (Freud, 1905b, p. 119). Acting out was seen as a form of resistance as well as a way of remembering through behaviour rather than by verbal recollections of the past. Although it was originally applied in the restricted sense of the analytic setting and the transference, the term has since been used more widely to refer to the way patients act in impulsive, socially or morally unacceptable ways outside the therapy setting, including addictions, eating disorders, perversions, alcoholism and drug addictions (Akhtar, 2009a). This gave rise to the term 'acting in' (Zeligs, 1957) to distinguish this specific form of transference resistance by direct actions of the patient during the psychotherapy session, including body movements and postural changes that may reveal unconscious conflicts. For example, a patient thrashed about on the couch in a way that revealed the exciting and uncomfortable transference relationship that was less evident in the verbal material they brought. Acting in can also refer to more complex exchanges with the therapist which disclose repressed memories or desires that find expression in the transference. This has been referred to as enactments, the way the patient induces the therapist to join with the transference fantasy and is akin to both the concepts of projective identification as well as role responsiveness (Akhtar, 2009a, p. 94). With both forms of acting in or out, "something is put into action instead of words. Repeating has replaced remembering in these instances." (Akhtar, 2009a, p. 2). Again, this can be seen as a form of resistance as well as communication of mental states that perhaps have no other way of being represented or mentalised. As such, it can be understood as an interim step between acting out and free association (Zeligs, 1960). We need to be aware of our own countertransference in response to the patient so that we are better able to interpret their acting in.

The role of therapy can be seen to facilitate the patient's capacity to represent emotional states verbally and symbolically with increased capacity to reflect on these states (i.e. to mentalise), rather than through discharge in actions and deeds. Van Waning (1991) describes how this shift from direct action into expression in thoughts and words is possible:

> only in a relationship in which the analysand feels understood (in empathy and interpretation), in which anxiety and unpleasure can be tolerated and contained; a relationship which can survive the hurt and rage and in which the optimum frustration whereby the analyst can be truly 'used' is possible. (p. 550)

Box 9.2 Useful resources

Readings

These are some of the seminal papers on transference and countertransference:

Heimann, P. (1950) On counter-transference. *International Journal of Psychoanalysis, 31*, 81–84.

Heimann, P. (1956). Dynamics of transference interpretations. *International Journal of Psychoanalysis, 37*, 303–310.

Joseph, B. (1985). Transference: The total situation. *International Journal of Psycho-analysis, 66*, 447–454.

Sandler, J. (1976). Countertransference and role-responsiveness. *International Review of Psycho-analysis, 3*, 43–47.

Strachey, J. (1934). The nature of the therapeutic action of psycho-analysis. *International Journal of Psycho-Analysis, 15*, 127–159.

Winnicott, D. W. (1949). Hate in the counter-transference. *International Journal of Psycho-Analysis, 30*, 69–74.

Online resources

The School of Life have a short film on transference that includes a useful illustration of how this operates in our everyday relationships: https://youtu.be/TPMrWGUfkl8 and https://youtu.be/QX_cp1K514E

Patricia Coughlin talks about the phenomenon of countertransference in this brief clip and in the second clip, she addresses the concept of transference resistance with a useful clinical example of her working with a patient around these issues: https://youtu.be/ZJgWWDLdLtE https://youtu.be/prg_U7a4lA4

There is a dramatisation of erotic transference in the TV series *In Treatment* with the first patient in Series 1, Laura. As the work continues, so you get to see more of the therapist's counter-transference: https://youtu.be/15B7vCpSoz8

This is another video from Berlin Psychoanalytic by Professor Aleksandar Dimitrijevic, psychoanalyst and clinical psychologist in which he addresses what transference is, how definitions have changed, and how to address it in treatment: https://youtu.be/vQIxTzRyrRQ

We can recommend this lecture by Don Carveth on countertransference and projective identification, with reference to Klein and Bion. He is Emeritus Professor of Sociology and Social and Political Thought and a past Director of the Toronto Institute of Psychoanalysis https://youtu.be/048FdwaHuLc

Here is another lecture by him on transference: https://youtu.be/Ku3AWc9adGo

10 Endings

In today's speeded up world where we are impatient as data loads on our computer or phone, where road – and even pavement – rage is becoming an increasing phenomenon of modern life and we can have most goods delivered to our home the same or next day, the notion that psychotherapy takes time is an alien and difficult concept to grasp. Notwithstanding this, there has been a trend for psychodynamic psychotherapy to become longer and longer in duration. We are typically focused on keeping patients engaged in therapy, aware of the depth of difficulties and extent of work in this joint undertaking. Most psychotherapy trainings concentrate on retaining training patients in treatment, with planned endings a neglected part of the preparation for working as a psychotherapist. Alongside this, some therapy settings inevitably place endings centre stage, such as a university counselling service where students pass through and inevitably graduate, or the NHS where the constraints of public health funding require limits to be placed on treatment, or a hospice where terminal illness brings its own reality of finality and ending. In this chapter, we will explore issues around ending psychotherapy, including how to evaluate when it is appropriate to end treatment, particularly when this is not agreed from the start or determined by external factors like a pending move, financial constraints or arrival of a baby. The ability to manage an ending is a generic competence for all therapists and it presents an opportunity to work through other losses and separations in the patient's life. The therapist's role is to help the patient understand both the conscious and unconscious meanings of the ending, to review therapy and say goodbye, and to articulate feelings around this ending in order to reduce the possibility of a premature ending or other enactments (Lemma et al., 2008). Although we are primarily considering the finality of psychotherapy in this chapter, there are other, smaller endings to which we can apply this line of thinking, like the ending of each session, breaks between sessions, missed appointments, unplanned breaks and holidays.

Termination vs ending

In the literature on endings, psychotherapists tend to refer to this as "termination", a word that conveys a sense of finality at ending: it is after all often used for abortions and removing someone from their job. So why have psychotherapists adopted this terminology? Schlesinger (2014) explains that endings and termination are not synonymous:

> I reserve the term termination for the process of bringing the treatment to an end electively and with the agreement of both parties that the maximum expectable benefits have been obtained. Its distinctive features are that it is planned, and it gives full consideration both to a review of the treatment and its accomplishments and disappointments and to the problems associated with ending, especially those associated with separating from the therapist and in particular freeing the patient's gains from the fantasy that they depend on remaining a patient. (p. x)

By contrast, Pedder (1988) suggests that the term termination should be used for psychotherapy that has been brought to an end prematurely and objects to termination being an odd and unsatisfactory term for "what should be a healthy developmental process" (p. 485). It is interesting to reflect on how we have absorbed this brutal term into the terminology of psychotherapy, as if recognising that there is an unconscious resistance to the finality of the ending that needs to be confronted. Every act of ending can be seen as a micro-aggression, whether this is calling the end of time on the session or taking a holiday break. It can be difficult to get hold of the feelings aroused by these endings because patients often resist owning them, for example by saying that of course they knew there was an agreed endpoint or holiday break. Some patients will respond by taking control of these smaller endings, for example, by looking at their watch as the session progresses or ending the session themselves before the therapist can call time.

In working with the end of a session, we want to understand and interpret the abrupt feeling of disconnection and loss that is triggered, recognising how difficult it can be for some patients to hold on to a continuous sense of the therapist between sessions. The patient's reaction to these lesser endings and breaks is important information for the therapist about the way they are likely to experience termination of treatment. This assessment starts when we meet a prospective patient and informs our thinking about the best type and frequency of treatment to offer the patient. Those patients with insecure attachment histories who quickly form a close bond to the therapist are likely to find endings very painful. Once we are aware of the dangers posed by breaks and endings to our patients, we are in a better position to anticipate this and open up a line of communication with the patient. After all, what we want to avoid most of all is acting out around the ending. This can take the form of patients ending with us before we can discuss ending with them or taking a flight into health, presenting as if everything is now sorted. Unplanned endings are very difficult for both patients and therapists to process because so much is left unsaid. It can be likened to sudden deaths where we are left unable to process unresolved aspects of the relationship.

Developmental perspectives on endings

Developmentally, endings are part of the life cycle and there are particular times in life when we have to face separations and endings as part of life's developmental challenge. These tend to fall at the beginning and end of the life span. As infants and toddlers, we experience separation anxiety when our primary caregiver leaves our line of sight and this has to be managed in a variety of ways in order to develop a sense of autonomy and identity. The caregiver functions in many ways as an auxiliary ego to the baby and small child. Through a series of gradual frustrations, and with the help of transitional objects (Winnicott, 1953), the small child develops the capacity to manage more independently. This can be affected by constitutional differences, with some babies being far more sensitive to separation and loss than others.

If the process of leaving is too much (abrupt and overly long separations, for example) or too little (such as enmeshed relationships where separateness cannot be tolerated), then difficulties can arise. As we go through life, we have to move away from our family of origin into our peer group and then we may leave to study or work away from the family, eventually going on to form bonds with our own partner and perhaps forming a family of our own. There are further losses heralded by the developmental chain of events, including empty nests as children leave home, retirement as we say goodbye to our work identity and the sense of purpose this has provided, the limitations posed by aging and health difficulties, and then death. Of course, death can present earlier in our lives. This may be the untimely death of a parent, sibling or child as well as other possibilities that are killed off through events like infertility, miscarriage, abortion, serious illness, disability or injury, missed opportunities, divorce and so on.

In all of these endings, we have to face a process of mourning the implicit and explicit losses. Much has been written about mourning and the stages of grief we go through. Elisabeth Kübler-Ross (2009) is best known for her descriptions of the five phases of grief: denial, anger, bargaining, depression and acceptance. Although these are described sequentially, it is commonly accepted that the stages are not linear and not everyone will experience all five of them. We have included them here because they may be helpful in recognising some of the experiences your patient may have as the ending approaches.

Freud described the process of loss in his seminal paper, *Mourning and Melancholia* (1917a), where he differentiated between the process of mourning the lost object or experience that allows the patient to reach acceptance on the one hand, and melancholia, a more malignant process in which the person is stuck in the experience of loss. Freud (1917a) writes that in melancholia, "the shadow of the object fell upon the ego" (p. 249). This metaphor suggests that the individual has identified so closely with the lost person, that their own identity has become tied up with that person. The loss of the other is therefore felt to be a loss of part of the self, including a loss of the capacity to love. Freud goes on to describe how the hostility released from this painful experience can then be turned back on the self:

the ego can kill itself only if … it can treat itself as an object – if it is able to direct against itself the hostility which relates to an object and which represents the ego's original reaction to objects in the external world. (pp. 251–252)

The sense of hopelessness that loss brings leads the patient to a passive state of waiting to die or a more active, self-directed anger of suicidality. Ignês Sodré (2005) likens the loss to the longing for the mother whom the patient feels has disappeared forever: "a feeling that it is the dark shadow of the object's absence which takes over the ego" (p. 125). There are both murderous and despairing states of mind, which inhabit the melancholic person separately and absolutely.

We see this most commonly in patients with narcissistic features where the loss of the object is experienced as a narcissistic wound that depletes their ego resources. There can be no working through of the loss and it results in an unresolved depression where the attachment to the lost object cannot be relinquished: "on the contrary, there is in fact a tremendously possessive, intense relationship with the object taking place unconsciously in the internal world" (Sodré, 2005, p. 127). Rather than a slow acceptance of the loss of the other (as seen in mourning), there is an unconscious refusal to give up the object. Freud referred to this state as melancholia; today, we would describe it as clinical depression.

How does this relate to the process of ending psychotherapy? It is important to recognise whether the patient is going through the stages of gradual acceptance of the ending of treatment and relinquishing ties to the therapist (mourning) or whether there is a more malignant process of melancholia taking place. The ending of therapy is likely to trigger associations to other endings that are recapitulated. Where those endings have been complicated, there is more likelihood that the patient will struggle to manage terminating therapy. Does the patient allow the therapist to have their own, separate state of mind? If you feel under pressure to see things exactly as your patient does and where any difference between the two of you is vehemently denied by your patient or causes them distress, then your patient is probably having a melancholic reaction to ending treatment.

Difficulties around addressing the ending should alert you to the presence of hate for the lost, loved object, something that may be openly expressed by your patient or may be more obscured from direct view. The patient may feel there is something wrong with them and that this is the reason why you are ending treatment. Part of working through the ending is getting to understand and bring into awareness these (often unconscious) fantasies. Patients will have their own ideas about why the ending is taking place and their fantasies will resonate with their particular histories and personalities. Lemma (2016) has described some of the different types of unconscious fantasies around ending, delineating these into psychotic and neurotic fantasies around ending. Psychotic fantasies about termination include manic flights to health or disavowal of the ending altogether, while neurotic fantasies may include Oedipal rivalries at feeling displaced by the new 'baby' patient taking up their place.

When to end?

Ending therapy raises the question of the appropriate length of treatment. In general, we would say that the earlier the patient's disturbances and the more severe the impact of those disturbances on their level of functioning, the longer the length of treatment. This is important in relation to managing patient expectations at the time of assessment. Again, the pressures of today's take-away culture can lead people to want a quick fix. Perhaps it is human nature that we would all want to take the easy way out if we could (something Freud touched on in his formulation of the pleasure principle). However, for lasting change (as opposed to a transference cure) and for therapy to be meaningful and helpful rather than ineffective, or at its worst iatrogenic, we do need to make a recommendation as to who would do better with brief versus longer term treatment. Part of this initial discussion forms the basis of the framework for termination. We have touched on these issues in Chapter 5 on assessment and formulation, and will return to them in Chapter 11 on brief psychotherapy. The clues as to how a patient is likely to manage the ending are to be found in their early history and significant attachments. Patients on both ends of the relationship spectrum ranging from a deficit of attachments (avoidant and dismissive attachment styles) on the one hand, to those with sticky, adhesive attachments characterised by enmeshment and dependence (preoccupied attachment styles) on the other, are likely to struggle more with endings than those patients with sustained and varied relationships (secure attachment style).

If you are working in an open-ended way, what are the signs that a patient is ready to end? The ending can be generated by external events as well as by signs of internal progress. The decision to end therapy will often be related to the experience of perceived progress in therapy. When reviewing the work of therapy, it is important that the progress is seen by your patient as something they participated in with you and not attributed solely to the therapist's skill and experience. It is important to acknowledge that the impetus to stop treatment may be mutually agreed and arrived at, or it may be decided by one party. If we don't acknowledge our own part in the decision to end treatment, we run the risk of presenting ourselves as the omnipresent, bountiful breast-therapist who will continue to see the patient until they feel they have had a sufficient 'feed'. Perhaps we are most likely to be caught up in this dynamic with those patients with awful histories of deprivation and neglect. We run the risk of falling into a saviour complex by wanting to ameliorate those difficulties by being the patient's good object. We may have narcissistic fantasies that we can do a much better job than their key attachment figures and previous psychotherapists.

There are other occasions when you may feel that the patient is caught up in an unhealthy dependency, and where you have a sense of prevailing stagnation and stuck-ness. How long you choose to persist with this will vary from therapist to therapist. There can be times when a patient remains quiet for long periods of time and the particular quality of that silence qualifies the experience: is it a space for reverie and reflection or does it feel deadened and deadening? There are those situations where we may consider the patient is using the therapist in a sadistic way and our repeated attempts to interpret this are ineffective in changing this dynamic. It is up to the therapist, together with the input of regular supervision, to decide how long to continue therapy under conditions of stasis and conflict. There are no clear guidelines as to when to do this because it is idiosyncratic to each patient-therapist pairing. Indeed, it will also differ according to the theoretical orientation and clinical experience of therapists and supervisors. We emphasise the importance of supervision in making these assessments and in keeping ourselves in check from acting out with patients around these important decisions. We can collude with our patients in avoiding an ending; we can be drawn into enactments around agreeing premature endings and we can also have generative endings. Supervision allows us an important space for reflection and assists us with making these complex decisions around ending treatment, among other benefits. The ability to make use of supervision is an important generic therapeutic competence.

Deciding when to end

How do we evaluate when a patient is ready to end? We are drawing on our own countertransference: our observation of what our patient is bringing to sessions and what it feels like to be in the room with them. Where patients represent people in their lives in two-dimensional ways as witches, ogres or saints and angels, we remain sceptical as to the patient's capacity for change. So, as we consider whether a patient is ready to terminate therapy, we would expect them to be able to hold greater complexity in the way they present both their objects and themselves. If we link this to Kleinian theory, we would expect the patient to be functioning more from the depressive position, where there is a capacity for ambivalence and nuanced ways of relating. As we listen to our patients talk about their lives outside the consulting room, we would expect to hear fewer examples of major dramas and conflicts in their relationships and that they are better able to resolve any conflicts they are experiencing in a more satisfactory manner. If we connect this now to Freud's structural model of the mind, we would expect the patient to be functioning increasingly from their ego, and that their ego is strengthened and is less at the mercy of the demands of the id or an overly harsh superego. The patient's superego should have been modified by the process of psychotherapy including their identification with the psychotherapist, with whom they will have experienced a different type of object relationship.

We may also think about ending when the patient appears to have *decathected* the therapy, by which we mean that the patient has withdrawn their libidinal energy in the therapy. The patient may appear to have lost momentum or to be less engaged in treatment. For example, the patient may arrive a little late, miss the odd session or even book holidays that cut into term-time. The clinical material they bring may feel less emotionally alive. As you can see, this can be understood as either a sign of progress and readiness to end or as resistance to further work. It is up to the therapist to make sense of which way to interpret this.

In arriving at a decision about when to end therapy, we consider how our patient manages the breaks between sessions and over holidays. Are they able to hold on to a sense of us as a helpful object and what is it like resuming therapy after periods of extended absence? We would also consider how our patients are coping with other endings and transitions in their lives, since this is another indicator for their readiness to manage an ending. We would reflect on the ways our patients have managed recent setbacks in their lives. If they have been able to regain their equilibrium and capacity to mentalise flexibly without regressing or reverting to earlier, maladaptive coping strategies and fixed ways of mentalising, then this is another indicator of reliable progress. In this sense, change can be recognised not only by what is present but also by what is now absent in the patient's life. We may notice that the patient no longer brings repeated scenarios of being embattled with work colleagues, family, friends and other relationships. Perhaps the patient now desists from escapist and self-defeating responses to adversities (such as alcohol, drugs, promiscuity, pornography or isolation) and is more able to consider and tolerate their emotional states.

We would expect to see signs of progress in important areas of our patients' lives. Those patients who entered treatment unable to form lasting relationships or progress their work lives may now be increasingly able to trust others and break old defensive patterns of breaking off relationships when their own abandonment fears are triggered. They may now be able to gain employment, support themselves and realise their potential. We would expect to see a reduction in defensive strategies. Patients who self-sabotage and undermine any progress they make, may now be more able to accept their successes. Erikson (1963, pp. 264–265) purported that Freud said the important tasks of adulthood are "to love and to work". This apocryphal quote of Freud's has no basis in his writings but is borne out by other observations, such as the account of Richard Sterba (1982), a Viennese psychoanalyst:

> When once the discussion in a meeting turned to the question of what means we have at our disposal to motivate a patient to undergo analysis, Freud pointed out that we promise him relief from his symptoms, an increase in his working capacity, and an improvement of his personal and social relationships. (Sterba, quoted in Winter, 1999, p. 121)

Although this sounds simple on the face of it, we are striving to balance an ability to have a productive and satisfying work life with the capacity to have mature loving relationships. This offers another way of evaluating if someone is ready to end therapy. If we return to Freud's aim for treatment to transform "hysterical misery into common unhappiness" (Breuer and Freud, 1895, p. 305), this is yet another consideration of when to end therapy, namely when the patient's difficulties feel more manageable. This suggests a more realistic view of terminating psychodynamic psychotherapy as opposed to a wish for happiness and a 'total cure'.

We do need to consider external factors that may play a part in putting ending on the agenda. For patients with financial difficulties, this practicality is likely to make continuing treatment difficult. Sometimes, the patient will suggest ending treatment rather than exploring a reduced fee structure for a period of time, perhaps in anticipation of feared rejection by the therapist at such a proposal. However, where patients are strapped for resources – be those financial, emotional, or practical (like time constraints or the demands of other relationships and work) – we do need to give weight to these external realities. Patients may get married, move location, take on new jobs or undertake studies, have babies, need to care for elderly relatives or any other myriad of life events that may require them revisit their decision to undertake psychotherapy.

It is important to distinguish between these external reasons and resistance in the course of the therapy. Has the proposed ending coincided with a period of work where you are starting to get in touch with painful or highly defended areas of the patient's life? If that is the case, then ending may represent a manic flight away from areas of disturbance. Is the patient using thoughts of an ending to test how much the work and the therapeutic relationship really means: will you fight for them to remain in treatment with you or will you be pleased to see the back of them? Other patients may want to deflect their own need for therapy on to the therapist such that it is you who needs them, rather than the other way around. Of course, there can be an element of truth to this, particularly when you are training as a psychotherapist and keeping patients in treatment for particular lengths of time is a requirement of the training.

Generative endings

The process of ending psychotherapy is an important stage of the work in which we have several tasks to undertake. We are reviewing the progress the patient has made with us over the course of therapy and considering both the areas in which the patient has made improvements as well as areas that have remained stuck or undeveloped. In this way, we are trying to get a balanced view of the patient's life and personality. There may be a tendency in the ending for patients to either idealise or denigrate the therapist. We would want to encourage a balanced approach in which gratitude can be expressed alongside regret for opportunities missed, work unfinished and goals unmet.

Just as we facilitate our patients bringing together conflicting feelings towards the same objects, so we want to encourage patients to review and reflect on their feelings towards us, and the work we have done together. Alongside Winnicott's concept of the good-enough mother, we would include the 'good-enough' psychotherapist and psychotherapy. An ending will always be imperfect. There is inevitably more work that could be done, and in this way, endings and beginnings dovetail into each other. In many ways, it is like gardening: you can dig, water, fertilise and sow the plants that grow, flower and bear fruit yet the work of gardening is ongoing. Every season brings new tasks and there is always something that needs tending. The cycle of nature is like the cycle of life and whenever we choose to stop therapy, there will be a relentless and ongoing series of events, that continue to present themselves. It is up to the therapist and patient to judge whether they feel suitably equipped to cope with those future challenges once therapy has concluded.

Schlesinger (2014, p. 16) lists four factors that affect the way patients will end (and begin) treatment:

1   What transferences have developed towards the therapist and have these been sufficiently analysed?
2   What expectations did the patient bring into treatment?
3   Was there a degree of regression in treatment? The more severe the regression, the more difficulty in ending treatment.
4   What was the strength of attachment formed to the therapist? He cautions that this is not necessarily linked to the length of time in therapy because some patients form very strong attachments very quickly.

Schlesinger concludes that "the major determinants of difficulty around ending are characterological, reflecting the developmental level reached by the patient, and the degree to which he is object related and can make and sustain attachments" (p. 16).

Endings, recapitulated losses and resistance

As patients approach the end of treatment, so earlier losses are often activated and brought into focus. The death of a beloved grandparent can sometimes come to the fore in the work, despite never having been focused on prior to this, for example. There is a chance to revisit previous losses, that are then recapitulated and reworked. The patient can 'relapse' into earlier symptomatology because the ending can trigger regression to primitive states of mind. There is a reactivation of attachment anxiety as the ending approaches and as this is worked with, so it can abate and be understood. Endings can be painful for some patients.

As the ending approached, Grace made her feelings very clear. She accepted we had to end but did not want to talk about ending with me. She said in no uncertain terms that she was not willing to share how she felt about stopping therapy yet at the same time, she conveyed a sense that she could very easily replace me. She described a new gadget she had bought that allowed her to monitor her body functions, like her pulse and body rhythms. She earnestly conveyed how this process of biofeedback would allow her to self-regulate her feelings and physical reactions. It seemed to me a very powerful metaphor for an always available therapist, and a denial of the pending separation. Yet, the act of talking about ending felt humiliating to Grace, and she was resistant to exploring her feelings around this. On reflection, it seemed to me that she was unable to mourn the loss of this or any relationship. I was reminded of how she told me she would bin clothes she no longer liked or wanted. I felt myself to be a cruel therapist who was prematurely weaning her and indeed, this was a shorter piece of work than ideally indicated given Grace's troubled childhood and challenging relationship history. I was able to share my thoughts with her about how the material she was bringing related to our ending by marking these as different to hers, and pointing out how she may not want to hear my thoughts about our ending. This allowed me to hold on to my separate mind and process the end of therapy in the face of her omnipotent and manic defences. I was left with great concern about Grace as we concluded our work together and I wondered about her capacity to hold on to the understanding we had achieved together. Although there was clearly more work to do, I was cognisant of her youth and her wish to get on with her life. She had an experience of feeling understood by me and of us working together to make sense of her troubled life. Despite it being imperfect, I trusted that Grace would be able to find her way back to help in the future.

Mourning is a process that takes time and similarly, endings require time to be processed. As this is not an easy part of the work, it is understandable that both patients and therapists often avoid facing this task, perhaps continuing work as usual, not taking up material in relation to fantasies around ending or leaving the final date of termination vague. The actual ending then takes the patient by surprise. We are aware that this can happen even when you are diligently preparing a patient for ending. Defences are powerful indeed, and if a patient at an unconscious level does not wish to acknowledge the ending, it will drop out of their mind.

Some patients revert to previous coping strategies in the face of the ending and there is a propensity for acting out at this point in treatment. This can take a myriad of forms. Some patients may become caught up in a new relationship and defensively escape into the excitement of a fresh beginning, presenting this as the solution to all their difficulties. Other patients may already have a replacement therapist lined up in the wings. In these ways, the feelings of aggression towards you for ending treatment are deflected. We have known patients to cancel sessions as the ending approaches, hoping to stretch out the period of ending. Indeed, some patients may now ask to be seen fortnightly or monthly. On the whole, we would recommend against moving to intermittent sessions as you approach an ending. Part of the work of psychotherapy entails engaging in regular weekly sessions interspersed with planned breaks. Attending fortnightly or less frequently than that, dilutes the therapeutic relationship and the intensity of the process. In many ways, it avoids facing up to the pain of ending, as if you could gradually part. We know that when a small child is anxious at a parent's pending separation, the more ambivalent the parent is and the more they linger in the child's presence, the harder the separation is for the child to bear.

As with all of these scenarios, there is no formula that can be applied. It is important that this is spoken about in the therapy room and that you understand and acknowledge the particular meaning endings have for your patient. The more something can be symbolised through words, the less likelihood there is for acting out.

Endings from the therapist's perspective

Endings affect both parties involved in the work. For therapists, the process of ending also marks a time of reflecting back on the work done, and changes achieved. Therapists working in a public mental health setting like the NHS, may be required to complete an 'End of Treatment' report for their service, or to write a discharge letter to the referrer, giving them some feedback about how the patient engaged in psychotherapy and the progress they made. We have included an example report structure in Appendix 3, for those readers who are interested.

Therapists also have to process their feelings of loss at bringing psychotherapy to a close. Unlike other partings, this is unusual because typically there is no further contact between therapist and patient. Some patients may ask to stay in touch with you after the work concludes. You may want to think about what that will mean. If your patient wants to add you to their Christmas card mailing list, will you send them a card in return? It can be tantalising to step back from someone's life after you have been an integral witness to their struggles and do not know how things will turn out for them. In some ways, it can feel like someone has torn the last chapter out of the book you are reading, and you will never know how the story concludes. Perhaps this is an inevitable consequence of the analytic setting. Just as we frustrate our patients' curiosity in the therapist's external life in order to explore their unconscious fantasies about us and what we represent for them, so too, we have to accept that we remain an outsider in our patients' lives. There is a level of discipline and restraint required to embark on this profession and in this area, you have to let go and trust that although you probably will never see each other again, you remain a key part in each other's internal worlds. Just as our patients are impacted by us, so too we are affected by these private and highly personal moments of exchange with our patients. We cannot share them easily or freely with anyone, even more so in light of increasing requirements for privacy.

Box 10.1 Useful resources

Readings

Freud's 1937 paper, *Psychoanalysis Terminable and Interminable* is a good
  starting point for further reading.

We can also recommend these two papers:

Holmes, J. (1997). "Too early, too late": Endings in psychotherapy – an
  attachment perspective. *British Journal of Psychotherapy, 14*(2), 159–171.
  This paper can also be found at: www.journal-psychoanalysis.eu/termina
  tion-in-psychoanalytic-psychotherapy-an-attachment-perspective-2/
Pedder, J. R. (1988). Termination reconsidered. *International Journal of Psychoanalysis, 69*, 495–505.

Online resources

The following YouTube video is a talk on termination of a psychoanalysis:
  some notes on theory, technique and clinical material by Italian analyst,
  Stefano Lussana https://youtu.be/i00Pk_T7xJ4

Part 3

Adaptations and practicalities

11 Brief applications of psychodynamic work

There is a parody of brief therapy on YouTube, entitled 'Stop It' that is comedy gold: the actor Bob Newhart plays a psychiatrist consulting with a patient who has a phobia of being in a confined space. It captures the change in zeitgeist in America from long-term psychoanalysis to brief cognitive-behavioural therapies. Interestingly, therapists from opposing paradigms reference this clip, each claiming it shows their approach in a favourable light. The clip highlights the nature of therapeutic change and inevitably raises the question about how long therapy should be. After all, Bob Newhart's character suggests five minutes is all that is required to cure complex difficulties!

We typically consider psychoanalysis, psychoanalytic and psychodynamic psychotherapy as intensive treatment that lasts for many months and years. This is the usual, open-ended way of working, particularly in private practice. Longer-term psychodynamic psychotherapy used to be offered more routinely in public mental health care services, like the NHS. However, such provision has been eroded as demand for more cost-effective, brief therapy has increased. Long-term treatment in the NHS often means one year of individual psychodynamic psychotherapy. Included in the psychodynamic competences is the ability to apply the psychodynamic model to the patient's needs, including identifying and implementing the most appropriate psychodynamic approach. In some settings and with some patients, this may entail providing time-limited psychodynamic therapy. The psychoanalytic theories outlined Chapter 2 remain the substantive body of work that therapists draw on in time-limited therapy. However, some important theoretical and technical considerations need to be made when working in brief psychodynamic therapy (we refer to therapy rather than psychotherapy in this instance to differentiate it from more open-ended work).

This chapter will provide an introduction to the theory and practice of brief applications of psychodynamic work. We will mostly draw on the model of Dynamic Interpersonal Therapy (DIT), a brief model of psychodynamic therapy that was developed by Alessandra Lemma, Peter Fonagy and Mary Hepworth (formerly Target) in 2010. It arose in response to the Improving Access to Psychological Therapies (IAPT) initiative in the United Kingdom, in an effort to ensure that a psychoanalytically informed model would be offered alongside CBT, as one of the non-CBT approved treatments for depression. In this chapter, we consider how brief psychodynamic therapy differs from longer term psycho-dynamic psychotherapy, and consider the necessary adaptations that are required. We will also discuss the suitability criteria that therapists should consider in deciding whether this form of treatment is appropriate for a patient.

History of brief psychotherapy

Wolberg (1980) points out that up to the beginning of the twentieth century, psychotherapy was, in fact, mostly short-term. As described in Chapter 2, Freud began working with Breuer on hysterical symptoms using a cathartic approach, often accompanied by hypnosis, whereby patients were asked to relive painful memories and feelings that had been forgotten. This work was accomplished in a small number of sessions. For example, Freud saw the composer, Gustav Mahler, for one extended session to cure his problem with impotence and he treated conductor, Bruno Walter, in six sessions for a partial paralysis of his right arm. Some of Freud's more famous cases, like the 'Rat Man' or 'Dora', were seen for eleven months and eleven weeks respectively. This early analytic work lent itself to a clear focus, namely understanding and shifting the presenting symptoms. In the beginning, transference was not emphasised and the therapist took an actively challenging, supportive and psycho-educational stance. When Freud abandoned this approach, his technique shifted to emphasise free association and that ushered in a sense of timelessness and greater passivity on the part of the therapist. This, together with the move to the couch, resulted in an open-ended treatment, something Freud (1937) referred to as 'analysis interminable'.

As psychoanalytic work became longer and longer, so time-limited work was denigrated. Ferenczi's 'active therapy' of the 1920s emphasised active and supportive therapy that extended to therapists providing physical comfort to deeply disturbed patients in order to remediate early parental deficiencies. In a letter to Ferenczi, Freud (1931) condemned his approach as "the kissing technique" (p. 423). Ferenczi, together with Rank and Adler were all concerned about the length of psychoanalytic treatment. They stressed the way early deprivations and conflicts were repeated in the therapeutic relationship, advocating a more active stance by comparison (Coren, 2010; Gustafson, 1997). However, they were condemned and ousted by the psycho-analytic community, as 'not psychoanalysis' (Mitchell, 1997).

Over the years, a range of psychodynamic brief therapy models have been developed, all with their own not-so-catchy acronyms. Indeed, Gustafson (1997) points out that each school of brief therapy seems to have at best an average shelf life of twenty years, as if the end is inherent in the beginning of these brief iterations of psychotherapy. We can trace the trajectory of these movements through the decades, resulting in a range of models of brief psychodynamic therapy, each of which emphasises different mechanisms of change. Messer and Warren (1998) classified a number of these models according to whether they draw on a drive/ structural model of psychic development or a more relational model. According to their classification, we can group the different existing models of brief psychody-namic therapy (we've also included more recent models), as follows:

1 *Drive/Structural models*, which are generally based on the classical Freudian principles, that focus on drives and the psychic structure of the id, ego and superego. These include Davanloo's Intensive Short-Term Dynamic Psychotherapy (or ISTDP), Malan's Brief Intensive Psychotherapy (BIP), which he brought into line with ISTDP, and Sifneos' Short-Term Anxiety-Provoking Psychotherapy (or S-TAPP);

2 *Relational models* which generally draw on interpersonal and relational psychoanalytic theories, including aspects of object relations, interpersonal psychoanalysis and ego psychology. These include Luborsky's Time-Limited Dynamic Supportive-Expressive Psychotherapy (or SE), Strupp's Time-Limited Dynamic Psychotherapy (or TLDP), Kernberg's Transference Focused Psychotherapy (or TFP), Hobson's Conversational Model, also known as Psychodynamic Interpersonal Therapy (or PIT), and Lemma, Fonagy and Target's Dynamic Interpersonal Therapy (or DIT);

3 *Integrative models* that combined elements of both drive and relational models. Mann's Time-Limited Psychotherapy (or TLP) is an example of this;

4 *Eclectic models* of brief therapy that combine psychodynamic and other techniques. These include Ryle's Cognitive Analytic Therapy (or CAT) and Young's Schema Focused Therapy, both of which combine psychodynamic with more cognitive therapy approaches.

There are a number of other brief models of therapy, most notably CBT. However, we are referring above to those that are psychodynamic or include psychodynamic principles. We are not going to outline each of these models, and will instead focus on the adaptations and therapeutic stance that need to be taken when working in brief psychodynamic therapy. When discussing examples of specific techniques, we will draw on DIT in particular, as this is a model that is increasingly being used in the NHS, and is gaining in popularity in other parts of the world including America, Europe, Australia and China, and also has an evidence base. DIT draws on object relations theory, interpersonal psychoanalysis, the mentalisation model, and attachment theory, all of which are outlined in Chapter 2 (see also Lemma et al., 2011).

What do we mean by brief?

In private practice, the ending is agreed jointly by the therapist and patient. However, in public health services like the NHS, limited resources mean that time limits are imposed from the outset. Usually this means a year of individual, once-weekly psychotherapy; occasionally, longer and even less infrequently twice or three times weekly treatment is offered. From the perspective of those who offer intensive psychoanalytic treatment and who see their patients four or five times weekly for years on end, this can seem to fulfil the brief of short-term psychotherapy. So, what makes therapy 'brief'? For the purposes of this chapter, we are considering brief psychodynamic therapy to be a limited number of pre-agreed sessions decided with the therapist and patient at the start of therapy. In adolescent services, a brief consultation model can be seen to be helpful and fosters independence in line with the developmental tasks of this age. In brief models like DIT, sixteen sessions are typically offered since this is felt to allow a long enough period for meaningful change to take place. The brief models outlined above range in length, depending on factors like the presenting difficulties of the patient and the experience of the therapist. At the longer end of the spectrum, ISTDP extends up to 40 sessions with more entrenched difficulties, like diagnoses of obsessive-compulsive disorder.

Malan (2001) points out that brief psychotherapy requires a conscious opposition to one or more of the factors that contribute to the lengthening of psychotherapy, including whether there is resistance on the part of the patient, whether there is a more significant and necessary focus on past issues rather than present difficulties, and various aspects of the transference dynamic. In psychotherapy, the patient's resistance inevitably means they have an unconscious investment in keeping their difficulties in place. This leads them to resist the therapist's interventions because change threatens their status quo. The therapist's belief in the over-determination of symptoms means that every symptom is seen to have its roots in several different memories and feelings, all of which then have to be uncovered in order to relieve the symptom. Alongside this, is a belief in the necessity for working through problems from different angles and depths in a reiterative process. An emphasis is placed on early childhood relationships and experiences which are seen as the source of the current difficulties and which are privileged over here-and-now difficulties. Establishing and resolving the transference neurosis is an integral part of treatment, whereby the patient addresses the strong feelings they have for their therapist that originate in earlier relationships. As the ending approaches, this often leads to a relapse associated with negative transference as patients feel angry at being abandoned. Another lengthening factor is the dependence and reliance the patient develops towards the therapist, that often leads to regression to earlier childhood patterns of relating. There is a tendency towards therapist passivity and a willingness to follow the patient's lead, as the principle of free association is adhered to, with the therapist more interested in following the patient's unconscious associations. This contributes to a sense of timelessness by focusing on the patient's primary process thinking, where time is fluid and boundless. The therapist is held to a high standard by adhering to demanding goals for stand-alone treatment without allowing for discontinuous treatment. All of these factors are highlighted by Malan (1975) as contributing factors in the ever- increasing length of psychotherapy and analytic treatments.

In comparing features of working longer-term with working in a time-limited way and building on Malan's observations, Angela Molnos (1995, p. 42, reproduced here with permission) helpfully summarises this, as follows (please note that T stands for transference and D for defence):

- [5-15 years] ONE YEAR or less
- [3-5 times a week] ONCE WEEKLY
- [couch] FACE TO FACE

- Sense of [~~timelessness~~] SPEED & PROGRESS
- Therapist is [~~less active~~] MORE ACTIVE
- Pt's [~~free associations~~] attention is FOCUS
- Focus on the [~~past~~] present, out there & HERE-&-NOW
- T. [~~interprets~~] T/D IMMEDIATELY
- [~~Transference neurosis~~] T/D IMMEDIATELY
- [~~Regression~~] STRENGTHENING THE PATIENT'S EGO
- Focus on [~~exploring the ucs~~] the problem – PATTERN
- Focus on [~~sexual impulses~~] LOSS, ABANDONMENT, RAGE & problem-solving

Brief work is an adaptation of longer-term work and requires adjustments, as the above list suggests. Although different models of brief psychodynamic therapy all have a different emphasis, it is possible to discern the factors that are common to all. Brief psychodynamic therapy is not suitable for all patients, which means that a rigorous selection process is crucial. There is some thought as to which presenting difficulties are better suited to brief psychodynamic therapy, with some models advocating that the following respond better to brief work: grief reactions; separation and loss issues; and unresolved Oedipal issues. Difficulties of an Oedipal nature to do with triangulated interpersonal relationships occur later in development and are suggestive of the patient's greater ego strength. Patients need to be able to form a positive therapeutic alliance relatively quickly with the therapist in brief therapy.

Sydney Blatt's (1974) research at the Menninger Clinic into the treatment outcomes of patients with *anaclitic depression* (namely, depression stemming from abandonment issues with others experienced as rejecting and the self as unloved) and *introjective depression* (namely, depression resulting from a punitive superego that experiences others as critical and the self as unlovable) found that patients with anaclitic depression responded better to brief psychodynamic therapy than those with introjective depression where better results were achieved with longer term psychotherapy. This is explained by the capacity of anaclitic depressed patients to form a therapeutic alliance readily whereas introjective depressed patients often feel criticised and ashamed at being patients and take longer to feel safe with the therapist. This may seem counterintuitive: after all, why would we offer brief psychodynamic therapy to patients with abandonment issues? Notwithstanding this, it does mean that issues of rejection and loss are placed squarely at the centre of the therapy, given that in brief work, the ending is there from the beginning. It also means that the ending will probably be painful. We are not suggesting that you only see patients with anaclitic depression for brief psychodynamic therapy. However, it is important to bear this in mind when assessing patients, particularly in weighing up their capacity to form a therapeutic alliance. What works for whom is not an exact science and researchers are still trying to pin down the mechanisms for change in psychotherapy.

By necessity, brief psychodynamic therapy requires a specific focus to which patient and therapist adhere. Psychoanalytic theory informs brief work, including the formulation that the therapist arrives at with the patient. It is not possible to address all the patient's difficulties in time-limited work, so priorities have to be set. The therapist then selectively attends to the agreed focus of the work, with inevitable inattention of other areas that are beyond the scope of treatment. Struggling to find a focus is usually a contraindication for brief work. A limited number of sessions is contracted from the start. The sessions are typically once weekly, with some models advocating spacing of later sessions (for example, fortnightly) as the ending approaches. The therapist has to be more active in brief psychodynamic therapy than in open-ended work, and as a result, tends to be more supportive in this way of working. Psychotherapy is demanding and this is particularly the case in brief work. Holding a supportive stance provides a counterbalance to the challenges of engaging quickly in identifying problem areas and addressing dysfunctional patterns of relating.

Selection criteria for brief psychodynamic therapy

We have already discussed the criteria for suitability for psychodynamic work in some detail in Chapter 5. Here, we are going to add further considerations when thinking about brief psychodynamic therapy, including where there are very real time constraints (e.g. the prospective patient is a student, about to go travelling or lives part of the year abroad or where the therapist has their own time constraints such as approaching retirement or health insurance funding restrictions). When assessing for brief therapy, the therapist needs to identify whether they can find a focus for the work and to weigh up the patient's capacity to work in a more circumscribed way.

The following questions may help with this:

- As you listen to the patient's material, do you feel that you can discern a relational theme emerging that would allow you to find a focus for the work?
- Do you have a clear sense of why the patient is presenting with difficulties now, or is this a more diffuse and chronic presentation that may be more entrenched and therefore require longer term therapy?
- Does the patient have sufficient ego resources to make use of brief therapy, or are they highly defended, easily offended, struggling with extensive symptoms and so on? We will elaborate on this below.
- Does the patient feel motivated to engage in therapy or have they been told to attend by their long-suffering partner, for example, or been dragged there by an anxious parent?
- Are you able to build a therapeutic alliance during the initial consultation, and when the patient does share their concerns, does this appear to bring them some relief?

When assessing for brief psychodynamic therapy in particular, we need to get a sense of the patient's early relationships and identify at least one positive significant attachment figure since this is a good prognostic indicator for establishing a working alliance. By monitoring our countertransference during the initial meeting and using it to inform our sense of the patient's presenting difficulties, we have access to another source of evidence to guide us in the assessment process.

Patients with very rigid defences are likely to find all forms of psychodynamic therapy challenging, particularly given its exploratory and emergent qualities. Patients who are mostly focused on wanting to reduce or get rid of their symptoms or those who seek advice about what they should do, tend to do better with more directive therapy approaches, such as CBT or Interpersonal Therapy (IPT). In assessing suitability for brief psychodynamic therapy, we consider the patient's ego strengths. What do they do with their week and what support systems and relationships do they have? Brief models of work usually include more supportive elements than longer-term, psychodynamic psychotherapy. In DIT, the therapist can also make use of mentalising techniques when working with patients whose reflective capacities are curtailed at times. So, it is not necessarily about the patient fitting the model of brief work but ways we can adapt the model of therapy to best meet the patient's needs. We are also interested in whether patients are motivated to make changes and conversely, their levels of resistance to change. It is always helpful to ask about previous experiences of therapy since this gives a good indication of their relationship to help in the past and can highlight likely difficulties and concerns in entering therapy now, namely the cautionary tale (Ogden, 1992).

With brief work, we would not expect the patient to have too much instability in their lives (for example, uncertain living arrangements or major financial concerns). We would want to rule out serious substance abuse or significant eating disorders, since these are best treated by a specialised service or approach. Similarly, if patients do not have a good grip on reality because they have psychosis or severe trauma with dissociative symptoms, then brief therapy may be more harmful than helpful. Although we have said that some abandonment issues lend themselves to brief work, we would evaluate the patient's attachment history carefully and rule out those patients with multiple separations and losses that indicate great complexity and severity. These difficulties tend to present themselves as characterological difficulties and are probably too entrenched to shift within brief therapy. As with all psychotherapy, we would carry out a careful assessment of risk and evaluate the patient's capacity to manage their suicidal thoughts and impulsivity. If there is evidence of self-harm and other risky behaviour, then brief work is usually contraindicated.

As Molnos (1995) puts it: "As a general rule, the earlier the psychic damage, the more likely it is that the patient might need longer rather than shorter therapy" (p. 23). Notwithstanding this, occasionally, you may want to offer brief work as a 'trial of therapy' to see if a patient can make use of a psychodynamic approach. For some patients, having time-limited work feels safer and allows them a way of engaging in therapy without feeling trapped. A proper assessment of the potential risks does need to be made. It may be easier to offer a trial of therapy when there is the possibility of a subsequent referral to longer-term work.

Therapeutic stance in brief psychodynamic therapy

In Chapter 4, we considered the analytic attitude that informs psychodynamic psychotherapy. The techniques in brief psychodynamic therapy are no different from those used in longer-term approaches, however, they are used more judiciously and explicitly. For example, the therapist has to be more active in building a therapeutic alliance and will probably be more supportive towards this end than in open-ended work.

The different models of brief psychodynamic therapy each emphasises slightly different aspects of psychodynamic work. As the name suggests, Transference Focused Psychotherapy (Yeomans et al., 2015) places an emphasis on working in the transference of the therapeutic relationship as the key area for change while ISTDP (Davanloo, 2000) tackles the patient's defences head on by challenging the ways the patient avoids facing underlying anxieties. In DIT (Lemma et al., 2011), therapists work with a particular interpersonal and affective focus (or IPAF) that is based on an internalised, early object relationship, namely the way we perceive ourselves in relation to others and the emotions that link that experience. The work of the sessions then focus on the IPAF in the patient's interpersonal narratives including attending selectively to the transference where the agreed pattern has been activated. We will elaborate this further below. DIT uses mentalising techniques judiciously to restore mentalising in patients so that 'therapy as usual' can continue. Alongside this, the therapist uses their usual repertoire of techniques including clarification, interpretation and confrontation.

Brief psychodynamic therapy places higher demands on patients, some of which emanate from the time pressure of the limited number of sessions. Unlike ISTDP, DIT does not attempt to dismantle the patient's defences but rather encourages the patient to consider the cost of employing these coping strategies that usually maintain their dysfunctional patterns of relating.

The therapist needs to believe that change is possible within the time limits of brief psychodynamic therapy and to approach therapy with goals that are realistic, hopeful and achievable. Not all therapists will find themselves suited to brief psychodynamic therapy. It is more demanding of your time, attention and energy. It results in greater patient turnover and the uncertainty that this can bring to your practice. The therapist is more active than in longer term therapy, in particular around building a therapeutic alliance by taking up any negative transference quickly and exploring this. Rather than encouraging regression and over-dependence on the therapist, in brief psychodynamic therapy, we aim to strengthen the patient's ego functioning. The circumscribed pattern forms the focus for the work and is agreed explicitly between therapist and patient. In this sense, the therapist is far more transparent in sharing their formulation of the patient's difficulties than in open-ended work.

Trajectory of brief psychodynamic therapy

In brief psychodynamic therapy, there is usually an initial phase that involves engaging the patient and building the therapeutic alliance, exploring their presenting difficulties and how this relates to their early significant relationships and attachment figures in order to develop a focus for the work. There is a middle phase where the patient's day-to-day life is usually the focus of the work and the patient brings interactions and events that can be understood in keeping with the focal pattern. The patient may have set some goals with the therapist so that there is also an emphasis on stepping out the agreed pattern by making some changes. Finally, there is an ending phase where the work is concluded, including evaluating the experience of brief psychodynamic therapy, what has been achieved and what remains to be done. Using the DIT model, we will now outline the trajectory through brief therapy with some illustrative clinical material.

Initial phase: identifying a focus

As mentioned above, the therapist and patient require a defined focus for working in brief psychodynamic therapy. In DIT, we use our understanding of the patient's interpersonal relationships and relational difficulties to arrive at the *Interpersonal and Affective Focus*, or IPAF (see Figure 11.1). This is a formulation that draws on object relations and attachment theory and captures both past and present relationship difficulties. We listen to the stories the patient brings about their experiences with other people and identify their repeated experiences across different domains and time frames. As Freud's repetition compulsion (1914a) suggests, we inevitably seek out the same types of relationships with others based on aspects of our early relationships. In brief psychodynamic therapy (as well as open ended psychotherapy), the aim is for patients to become aware of these repeating patterns so that they can make a conscious choice to respond differently. Sometimes, it is very apparent to the outside observer that this is going on but when we are personally caught up in something, we often lack the objectivity to recognise these patterns. The IPAF brings one such significant and recurring pattern to the patient's awareness. For this reason, it is important that the pattern chosen as the focus is at the heart of the difficulties that brought the patient into therapy and that it occurs in the past as well as the present and across several different relationship domains. It should have emotional significance for the patient. Let us turn our attention to the three dimensions of the IPAF.

First, there is the *Self-representation*. This is the way the patient typically feels about themselves in particular relationships. We are listening for the problematic aspects of those interactions. It is important to differentiate between the idealised version of the self and the underlying view of the self that is usually more conflicted and hidden from full view.

Then there is the *Other-representation*, the way the patient repeatedly experiences other people. When you listen to the narratives of the patient's life, you may notice that certain dynamics keep cropping up. The patient may find themselves feeling taken advantage of by others who manipulate and exploit their weakness. You may hear stories of unavailable, out-of-reach others who are distant, perhaps ambivalent, elusive, dismissive or who run hot and cold. You may discover stories of others who are untrustworthy and unreliable.

With these repeated interpersonal self-other interactions, there is an emotional fall out, namely the affective impact of this. We know that most experiences of depression and anxiety can be linked to attachment threats, real or imagined, actual or anticipated. We are interested in exploring the *affects* that anchor and connect these experiences of self and other. Is the patient left feeling despair, shame or deep sadness? Is the primary emotion one of fear, panic or unease? Are there other affects that the patient tries to keep out of awareness, like anger, humiliation or envy?

If we think back to Blatt's (1974) work on anaclitic and introjective depression, we can already see two very different and archetypal IPAFs: 1) the rejecting other and unwanted, unloved self with resulting likely feelings of despair and anger and 2) the critical other and unlovable, worthless self with corresponding feelings that may include shame and anxiety, respectively (Figure 11.1). The IPAF formulation is

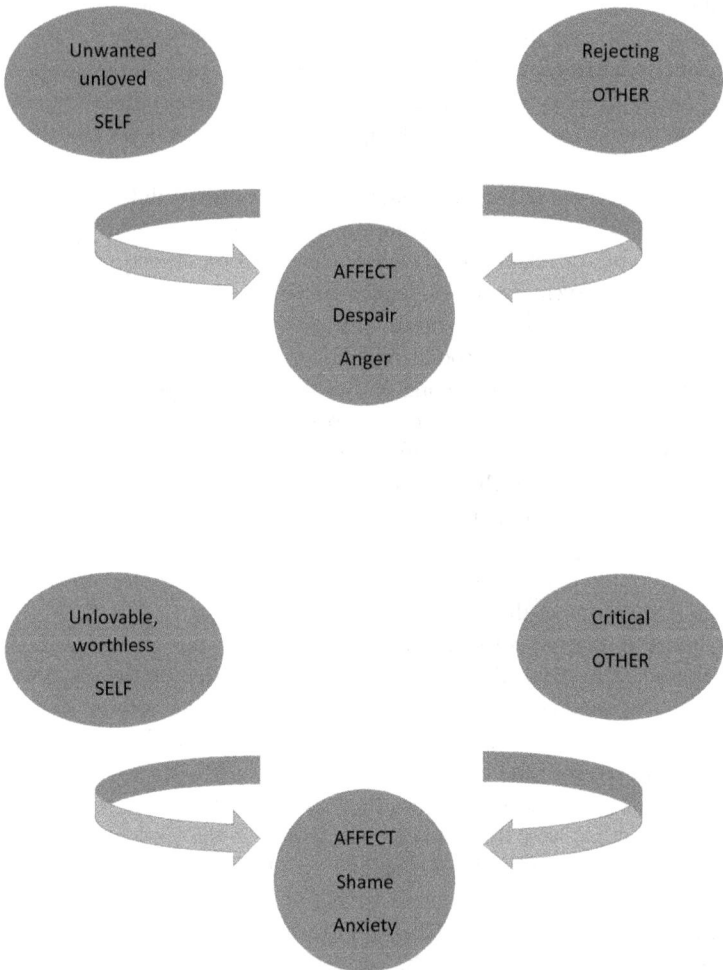

Figure 11.1 Two examples of an Interpersonal Affective Focus for DIT

most effective when it uses the patient's own words and imagery that are unique to their world and life experiences.

We develop this formulation based on our understanding of the repeated patterns evident in the patient's interpersonal relationships. These are problematic difficult interactions that stand out again and again in a range of different relationship domains and over time, for example in family relationships, friendships and with work colleagues. We are looking for a pattern that makes sense of why the patient has come for help now and that is powerfully connected to their difficulties. We would expect this pattern to have its origins in childhood and to make sense of current relationships with partners, children, parents, siblings, friends, work colleagues, acquaintances, even strangers. In Chapter 2, we described how attachment theory outlines the way the quality of our attachment relationships with our primary caregiver forms an internal working model for future relationships. So, what we are looking for here is a recurrent pattern of attachment, and the associated affect states that have become procedural models for ways of being in the world with others.

We gather this information during the first three sessions, which can be regarded as a prolonged assessment. In the fourth session, marking the end of the initial phase, we then share our understanding of this formulation with the patient, and agree the focus for the remaining sessions. Part of sharing of the formulation with the patient is helping them understand the defensive function of the IPAF, namely how it serves to protect them from parts of the self that are difficult to know about and are often projected into others. When identifying the affect that links the self and other representations, we are aware that the patient is more conscious of some affects and less conscious of others. In sharing the pattern, we titrate how much we feel the patient can manage to hear. In brief work, we are largely working with conscious and pre-conscious levels of awareness. However, in the course of the work, deeper layers of understanding will often emerge. In this sense, the IPAF is a starting point that we continue to refine over the course of the middle phase, much as we would polish a rough diamond.

Let's illustrate how a DIT case would proceed using the example of 'Rebecca'. This clinical material is adapted from Abrahams (2017, reproduced here with permission).

Rebecca approached me for therapy following the birth of her much-awaited daughter. She had struggled to fall pregnant and was delighted when she was able to conceive by IVF, yet six months on, she felt irritable and easily in tears. She was most concerned when she felt annoyed with her baby for waking her up several times a night and for her inconsolable crying. Rebecca compared herself to other mums in the new parent's group she attended, and felt she was the imposter. However beautifully dressed her daughter was, she felt the others could sense that she was not a good mum and didn't deserve to have a child. Rebecca was very careful about what she said to the other parents, often finding herself ruminating over these interactions and looking for signs that they were judging her and finding her inadequate. Her usual coping style was to set high standards for herself and present the best version of her in order to stave off any criticisms. However, she felt so exhausted and barely able to look after her daughter, let alone herself, her home or her relationship. Rebecca felt extremely frustrated with her partner and had pulled away from him, snapping at his questions and easily feeling attacked when he asked her about dinner or how she had spent her day. She had a difficult relationship with her own mother, often feeling she didn't measure up to her younger brother, who was the apple of her mother's eye. She was close to her father and had a more straightforward and uncomplicated relationship with him, feeling he was supportive even if he didn't always know how to show it to her. She was due to return to work from maternity leave in six months' time and because there was a clear onset to her depression and she felt she didn't want to engage in a longer piece of work at the moment, we agreed to brief psychotherapy.

In DIT, we would be interested in the onset of depression and anxiety symptoms that have their links in interpersonal triggers. We want to know 'why now' and what the prompt has been, not just for the start of depression and anxiety, but also for seeking therapy. In the case of Rebecca, the transition to being a mother was proving tricky.

In the fourth session, I shared the interpersonal and affective focus of the work, the IPAF, with Rebecca. I explained that having heard her telling me about her early and current relationships, I had the impression that she repeatedly experienced others as critical of her, belittling and sitting in judgment of her and I could link this to interpersonal narratives she had given me about her early and current relationship with her mother, her boss at work, some of her longstanding friends, her experience in the new parent's group as well as her fantasies about her baby. In the transference, this pattern was evident between us when she became noticeably anxious when I told her I would share my thoughts about the pattern and responded by saying she welcomed negative feedback as she needed to improve and knew she was failing at this therapy. All of this helped me feel I was on the right track in arriving at this pattern. I was aware in my countertransference that it was easy to feel pulled into being harsh with her as well as experiencing the converse: on occasion, I felt I was not getting it right as a therapist and was afraid of saying the wrong thing and being a disappointment to Rebecca.

After agreeing with this descriptor of others as critical – the part that resonated more powerfully for her than being judged or belittled – I moved on to share my formulation of how she experienced herself in turn as inadequate and second best. I gave her examples of how this applied to her early relationships with her mum and her brother as well as how she felt like this in her job. Rebecca suggested that she feels she is worthless and an outcast. This was a more powerful version of the IPAF self-representation than I had suggested, and it was useful to learn that we could intensify the descriptor we eventually settled on, the self as worthless outcast. I proposed that when Rebecca felt a worthless outcast and experienced others as critical, this led to feelings of fear, guilt and resentment that were uncomfortable to bear. She agreed and we were able to see how the resentment inevitably led to her feeling critical of others in turn, leading to a reverse of the IPAF.

In DIT, we are interested in the dynamic aspects of this formulation: just as the patient absorbs a particular version of themselves in relation to their key attachment figures, so there will be times when they project it on others, in an effort to rid themselves of this painful experience. It is not always possible to share the reverse IPAF with the patient when we are negotiating the IPAF. In the course of therapy, we are continually evaluating the impact of what we are saying on the patient. Does the patient become increasingly defensive and resistant? Is the patient overly compliant and agrees with everything we say? Is the patient reflective and able to elaborate on what we have said by providing another account of how this rings true for them? All of this is useful feedback and allows us to titrate the formulation and our interventions. Our aim is not to water down the formulation so that we end up with something overly palatable for the patient. Rather, we want to push the patient to think about challenging aspects of themselves in relation to others with the view to making some change in relation to this pattern. We are supportive of the reasons the patient may have arrived at this pattern and how the patient defends against the painful affects to which the pattern now gives rise. In DIT, we are respectful of the patient's needs for defences and we are not aiming to challenge these directly and break them down; rather we draw the patient's attention to their defences and the cost of keeping them in place. In the case of Rebecca, the pattern serves a defensive function by protecting her from getting close to others and knowing about her own aggressive feelings; instead she locates her aggression in others and writes others off as having nothing of value to offer her.

Middle phase: focusing on interpersonal dynamics

In the middle phase of DIT (typically sessions 5 to 12), we focus in detail on various interpersonal dynamics, using the IPAF as a focal framework. The aim is to deepen our understanding of this dynamic and work through the affective cost of these patterns. The focus of the work rests mostly in 'here-and-now' interpersonal difficulties, while keeping the childhood origins of this pattern in mind. Brief psychodynamic therapy is not about making reconstructive interpretations. We work in the domain of here-and-now relationships, with the patient's early experiences embedded in the IPAF. In this brief approach, we would not routinely make interpretations linking to past events and relationships because this is unlikely to lead to lasting change in a short space of time.

   In the middle phase of DIT, the therapist draws on the techniques and theoretical framework of psychodynamic psychotherapy which have been outlined in the previous chapters, including a mentalising stance to facilitate the patient's ability to reflect and interrogate their own and others' mental states. The DIT therapist adopts an open approach by listening to the narratives the patient brings, linking them to the stated focus of the work including where this connects to the transference. The middle sessions of DIT are most like 'therapy as usual' with the IPAF as the spine of the middle phase of the work. By repeatedly referring to the IPAF and continuing to refine it, we are more likely to remain on model. We are also able to work with our patient's unconscious processes in the middle phase. We take up the patient's defences and resistance more actively, pointing out the cost of these defences in the hope of mobilising some change while still respecting the need for them.

Returning to the case of Rebecca:

> *Through the middle phase, we explored the events of the week, tracking her levels of depression and anxiety at the start of each session by using a set of questionnaires to measure her symptoms. At first, I pointed out how Rebecca played down the severity of her scores on the symptom measures, not wanting to alarm me and trying to be a good patient by showing me she was doing well. Yet this was also a defensive manoeuvre in the face of her IPAF, and when the events of the week didn't match up with the low scores she reported at the start of the session, I was able to gently challenge this. We began to understand how she contributed to not being fully seen by others, leaving her feeling overlooked because she minimised her difficulties and distress. We also explored whether others were indeed feeling disappointed or critical of her, in instances where she perceived others in this way. For example, when her partner asked her how her day was, he may not be implicitly criticising her for not having done much or the house being a tip; instead, he may be genuinely interested in her. As the work went on, Rebecca was able to see how she was contributing to keeping the IPAF in place, particularly when she became prickly in anticipation of being criticised. Inevitably, this would put the other person on the back foot and Rebecca would then feel justified that they did hold critical and negative feelings towards her. In the work of the middle phase, there was a deepening of the IPAF that emerged that had more to do with her fear of being rejected and feeling unwanted. This provided us with a more nuanced understanding of her interpersonal difficulties.*

In the middle phase, we expect the formulation to shift as we get to know the patient better. The formulation is fine-tuned with ever emerging information, both in the relationships and experiences the patient reports as well as the unfolding therapeutic relationship.

Ending phase: reviewing and thinking ahead

In brief work, the ending is there from the beginning and we work actively with it throughout the course of therapy. In DIT, the ending involves the therapist writing a draft goodbye letter to the patient, which is then worked on together over the remaining sessions as a reminder of the work that has been done. This has been adapted from Cognitive Analytic Therapy (Ryle, 1990), where a letter is given to patients during the ending phase. The letter acts as a transitional object, assisting the patient with the process of leaving therapy and it also serves to help patients with future difficulties.

Sharing the goodbye letter is often an evocative and charged experience. The letter does several things: it is a summary of the patient's background and referral that informed the IPAF; it sets out the IPAF, namely the pattern the therapist and patient worked on throughout the therapy, as well as detailing the various coping strategies the patient employs; and it points out what happened over the course of therapy, the changes the patient was able to achieve, as well as remaining unfinished business. The letter also addresses the impact of this pattern on the therapeutic relationship. The letter is presented as a draft so that the therapist and patient can continue to collaborate around its content as the therapy is concluded. It is important that patients feel they can contribute towards the farewell letter so that it functions as an accurate record of their experience to consolidate that work and assist with relapse prevention.

When we get to session twelve, we prepare our patients for the letter that the therapist shares in the thirteenth session. Patients have a range of fantasies about the meaning of both the letter and the ending. We work very actively with those fantasies and try to put words around the particular sense our patients make of the ending. How does the ending tie in with their childhood experiences? Do they feel replaced by another, more worthy patient? Do they feel we have grown bored of them and are discharging them? In the previous chapter, we discussed aspects of working with endings in more detail that are relevant here.

Below is an example goodbye letter, related to the work with Rebecca:

Dear Rebecca

As our sessions together are coming to an end, I thought it would be useful to write down some of my thoughts about the work we have done. This letter is for you to take away as a reminder of that work and the changes you have made, as well as an acknowledgement of some issues you continue to struggle with and work on.

You came to see me when you realised you were feeling increasingly hopeless and irritable after the birth of your daughter. We agreed to meet for sixteen sessions of DIT to address your concerns about repeating your own challenging relationship with your mother with your daughter.

We understood that you felt unable to stand up to your mother throughout your childhood and put your needs aside in order to try keep her happy. You felt you were a deep disappointment to her and tried your best to be the type of daughter you felt she wanted by becoming a gymnast even though it wasn't what you enjoyed. You explained how this pattern of demanding mothers and disappointing daughters goes back several generations and that your mother had a distant relationship with your grandmother. This made you even more guilty that you were repeating this pattern with your daughter when you felt disappointed at her inability to sleep through the night.

We identified a recurring pattern as the focus for our work together, the way in which you experience others as critical and rejecting and then experience yourself as the worthless outcast. This pattern evokes strong feelings of fear, indignation and guilt. We also saw how there were times when the pattern was reversed: you would become critical, thereby giving others (most often your mother) your unbearable experience of feeling useless.

One of the ways you guard against your fear of being criticised is to be perfectionistic and focus on gaining others' approval. However, this inevitably leads to you feeling depleted and ignored, which reactivates the pattern. You also observed how you skew things by focussing excessively on all the 'bad' things you get wrong, discounting your worthy qualities, and evidence to the contrary. We also saw how your preferred relationship style is to be more self-sufficient and manage without relying on others because you fear being hurt by them. Yet this comes at a great cost of isolating yourself and reducing any sources of support. Indeed, having a baby has forced you to question this strategy and review it.

Over the course of therapy, you have been able to see your relationship with your daughter in a different light, for example, recognising the ways she is connected to you and how you were the best person to comfort her when she was ill recently. We have also focused on your relationship with your mum whose comments about your mothering felt undermining and angered you. Rather than pull away and sulk like you used to do when you were a teenager, you tried explaining to her how hurtful her comments felt to you and this allowed for a different type of exchange to take place between the two of you. Although you are aware this is early days, you are hopeful at getting into a more benign pattern with her. With your partner, you have been able to show him your doubts and insecurities in a different way so that he has been able to offer you the support you crave but which you had been denying yourself by being so inaccessible to him.

We saw how this pattern played out between the two of us, particularly at those times when you would put yourself down in the sessions, mocking your efforts in a sarcastic way by anticipating that I was going to 'put the boot in' and then getting in first. We also saw that when I invited you to think about things from your mother's viewpoint, you experienced me as pressuring you to placate her and see things only from her viewpoint. We were able to explore this misunderstanding between us and over time, you have become increasingly able to feel a boundary between your own experience and your mother's, without accepting all the responsibility and taking on the role of the 'bad daughter'.

You are continuing to work on these relationship patterns and you have made good progress in the goals you set yourself, including being easier on yourself, worrying less about mistakes and gaining perspective on your relationships by exploring what they mean by something that strikes you as critical. You have been less 'spiky' as a result. We saw how your relationship questionnaire shows this change, with a little more anxiety about being hurt by others replacing the self-sufficiency you had adopted to protect your vulnerabilities. New developments in the future, like your daughter starting to crawl and becoming more independent and your anticipated return to work, will bring forthcoming challenges in creating loving relationships in which you feel close without becoming enmeshed or distant. I hope this letter is useful in highlighting the insights you have made and that you can use it to help you continue with the valuable work we have started.

With best wishes

Why offer brief psychodynamic therapy?

It is not always the case that more is better when it comes to psychotherapy and there is a place for brief psychodynamic therapy alongside longer term psychotherapy. Some patients specifically request brief work and it is important to work out whether this is part of a wish to speed things up in order to find shorthand outcomes; there may also be a wish to stay away from difficult areas and not 'go too deep'. This resistance would need to be explored when assessing the best way forward.

There may be external circumstances in the patient's life that lend themselves to brief psychodynamic therapy, like pregnancy, limits on student visas or a period of time before travelling or taking up a new job. Patients may want to focus on a particular difficulty rather than embarking on open-ended exploration. There are sometimes external circumstances in the therapist's life that make brief psychodynamic therapy the best way forward, such as pending retirement and a wish to cut back on open-ended work, or where you live between two locations. There can be financial and time constraints that make brief psychodynamic therapy a more viable option. Where patients have medical insurance, they are usually funded for a limited number of sessions per year and offering brief therapy can be an affordable and effective option. When offered in a public health context like the NHS, there are clearly budgetary constraints that mean DIT can be offered to a wider remit of patients.

Brief psychodynamic therapy is informed by psychoanalytic and psychodynamic principles but the structure and support it provides means it is more accessible to a wider population. Although there are economic arguments for offering something for most people, brief psychodynamic therapy is often a very effective and meaningful intervention in its own right. Howard et al. (1986) explored how many sessions were required to produce clinically significant change and found that the measurable rate of change is fastest in the earlier stages of therapy, with diminishing returns the longer therapy goes on for. A significant proportion of patients improved the most in the first few sessions of therapy. There have been outcome studies of the various brief psychodynamic therapy models that demonstrate their effectiveness against non-analytic treatment (e.g. Fonagy et al., 2019). In Chapter 3 we reviewed some of this research, indicating the effectiveness of brief (and long-term) psychodynamic therapy. Our experience has been that in 16 sessions, considerable work can be done with an immediacy and focus that longer-term work may not always have.

Box 11.1 Useful resources

Readings

The following book provides a detailed manual for working in the DIT model:

Lemma, A., Target, M., & Fonagy, P. (2011). *Brief dynamic interpersonal therapy: A clinician's guide*. Oxford University Press.

The clinical material used in this chapter is taken from this article: Abrahams, D. (2017). Dynamic Interpersonal Therapy: Working with perceptions of the self and other. *BACP Healthcare Counselling and Psychotherapy Journal, 7*(3), 8–13. The article is available online here: www.bacp.co.uk/bacp-journals/healthcare-counselling-and-psychotherapy-journal/july-2017/dynamic-interpersonal-therapy/

The following book provides a useful, comprehensive overview of brief psychodynamic therapy: Coren, A. (2010). *Short-term psychotherapy: A psychodynamic approach* (2nd edition). Palgrave Macmillan Limited.

Patricia Coughlin (2016) has written a helpful book, *Maximising Effectiveness in Dynamic Psychotherapy* that includes lots of clinical examples derived from Davanloo's model of ISTDP.

The following journal paper clearly explains seven models of brief psychotherapy:

Demos, V. C. and Prout, M. F. (1993). A comparison of seven approaches to brief psychotherapy. *International Journal of Short-term Psychotherapy 8*, 3–22.

Online resources

While the resources around DIT are limited to those who have completed the training, you can find some useful information on YouTube about ISTDP, with Patricia Coughlin. The following clip shows how to work with the patient to find a focus https://youtu.be/DDKEGwXiNsY while this clip looks at working with Malan's triangle of insight https://youtu.be/eVOgXhq49ek

There are some resources about Time Limited Dynamic Psychotherapy with Hanna Levenson on YouTube at https://youtu.be/yTHM2o3dvao. She has written a book called *Brief Dynamic Therapy* (2010) which is published by the American Psychological Association and has an accompanying teaching DVD about the Strupp-Binder model of Time Limited Dynamic Psychotherapy.

You can watch Stanley Messer speaking about Brief Psychodynamic Therapy on YouTube https://youtu.be/1dui1PmjKDo. He is the co-author of *Models of Brief Psychodynamic Therapy: A Comparative Approach* with C. S. Warren which appears in the reference list.

The Bob Newhart clip referred to in the introduction to this chapter can be found on YouTube at https://youtu.be/4BjKS1-vjPs

12 Challenging situations and clinical dilemmas

Harry Stack Sullivan is known to have said "beware smoothly going therapy" (quoted in Akhtar, 2009b, p. 99). In thinking about difficult and challenging situations that can arise in psychotherapy and how we might deal with them, we run the risk of being overly prescriptive. So, the scenarios that follow and the ways we might tackle them from a psychodynamic perspective should always be thought about in relation to a specific patient and their particular circumstances in order to avoid a 'paint by numbers' approach. Having said that, it is helpful to consider these scenarios in advance so that you can feel more prepared to deal with them as and when they arise. Dealing with difficulties and dilemmas requires the capacity to make clinical judgements in the course of a therapy, a meta-competence for any therapy work. For the psychodynamic therapist, this involves the basic competence of being able to respond to difficulties in the therapeutic relationship. One such difficulty is working with resistance in psychotherapy, which we covered in Chapter 6. In this chapter, we will consider further challenges and dilemmas in relation to the analytic frame and with reference to the therapeutic alliance and relationship. We will also consider ways of managing risks in the clinical setting (which also forms part of the psychotherapy assessment).

Challenges to the analytic frame

As already discussed previously, an important component of psychodynamic psychotherapy is maintaining a consistent setting and analytic frame. This is not always an easy task, and the therapist may face some challenges to this, some of which we touched on already. Here we expand on a few specific difficulties that therapists will probably come across at some point.

Lateness

The analytic frame is intended to provide a structure for the work of psychotherapy such that any deviations can be considered in light of the patient's dynamics. It is not uncommon for patients to have difficulties with aspects of the frame, like punctuality. Kegerreis's (2013) paper helpfully explores how we can make sense of repeated lateness in psychotherapy. She sees this as an enactment around the analytic frame that is worthy of consideration. Perhaps it represents a defensive manoeuvre to deny vulnerability and dependency in the face of a regular psychotherapy appointment? Some patients will allow sufficient time for possible transport delays while others may not want to be in the position of a needy patient, waiting in the waiting room, preferring the pressure of rushing to their appointment.

Denial of the reality of time or omnipotent attempts to master time can be seen as a refusal of this most fundamental element of our human existence. Hartocollis (1983) writes about how being late for appointments or failing to meet deadlines serves to protect compulsive individuals from the anxiety-provoking idea of time and its equivalent, death. Accepting the reality of the finiteness of time can for many patients mean acquiescing in a relationship to reality that is unbearable, leading to considerable effort being expended in order to omnipotently deny this. A variant can be seen in patients who use magical thinking to express their defiance of reality. Some patients are habitually late, not centrally because of the immediate transference dynamics but rather because it is intolerable for them to accept limitations on their omnipotent fantasies: it is difficult to accept how much time is actually needed to get from A to B.

Kegerreis (2013) states that "time acts both as a currency in our relationships with others and as a most fundamental element in our relationship with ourselves" (p. 451). She goes on to say that there is a powerful sense that if the patient could come on time in a relatively straightforward way, a considerable proportion of the therapeutic task would have been achieved. The demands of time correlate with other demands the patient encounters in their external world as well as in their early life with authority figures, dating back to their father. Kegerreis also points out that the converse, namely punctuality driven by a punitive superego with an accompanying state of heightened anxiety, is also problematic and needs to be part of the work of therapy.

Absences – extended, planned and unforeseen

Winnicott (1949) described that the end of an analytic session can be seen as an expression of the therapist's hate for the patient, as can other breaks in therapy. The patient may react to this with retaliatory lateness and absences. It is not uncommon for patients who have disturbed early attachment histories to react to breaks in the work by taking their own breaks, either before or after the therapist's dates. This defensive attempt to make the break more manageable has the paradoxical effect of extending their absence from therapy.

In Chapter 4, we discussed issues of breaks, holidays and cancellations mainly from the perspective of the therapist setting up a clear therapeutic contract. We suggested that therapists give their patients advance notice of annual leave, on the understanding that our patients take their holidays at the same time, thereby avoiding disruption to the therapeutic work. Where the patient takes an absence from therapy or advises they cannot attend a session, it raises the question of whether to replace and/or charge for missed sessions. It is important that you explain your policies clearly when you contract with your patients at the start of the work. It is unfair to change the goal posts without having given forewarning. However, if you have explained to your patient that once the time is in your diary, it belongs to them and that they are responsible for paying for it, then it is a reasonable assumption that you will invoice for that time. It can be helpful to distinguish between the patient's reasons for missing a session. Where a patient has advance notice of a work commitment or an important hospital appointment that conflicts with their session time, then you may want to consider offering an alternate time, assuming you have options available in your diary. However, if the patient is cancelling their sessions to go on a holiday or because they have scheduled something discretionary, this is more likely to be an expression of resistance or hostility and should be interpreted accordingly. Patients may be testing to see what it means to their therapist that they have cancelled their session, particularly when they reassure the therapist that they will pay for the missed appointment. Often this conveys their conviction that the therapist is only in it for the money and doesn't really care whether the patient attends or not. It may even extend to a fantasy that the therapist is happier not having to see the patient at all. So, as therapists, it is a balancing act between conveying the importance of the commitment both parties are making in undertaking this work together while not becoming overly punitive and judgemental.

Silences vs over-talking

In some ways, these two extremes represent similar challenges to the therapist, albeit in different directions. Those patients who retreat into long silences as well as those patients who fill all the space with their words serve to keep the therapist at a distance. This is probably because they are frightened by the thought of joined-up thinking or emotional contact. The quality of a patient's extended silence will create different countertransferences that can help differentiate between helpful and stuck quietness. Some space to reflect and get in touch with thoughts and feelings is part of the valuable, emergent aspect of psychodynamic psychotherapy for patient and therapist alike. These spaces can be productive and calming, allowing new associations to emerge, for affects to be felt and for experiences to be consolidated. By contrast, other silences feel more like psychic retreats (Steiner, 1993) where the patient disappears into a cut off, disconnected bubble that serves a protective function in that moment, rendering the patient inaccessible to the therapist. Sometimes, this retreat communicates to the therapist the way the patient experienced their depressed parent, for example.

Freud (1912) regarded silence as a form of defence and resistance to the transference. Later theorists, however, consider silence as a form of communication (Khan, 1963; Coltart, 1991). Khan (1963) understood silence in his work with a particular patient as a transference communication of unconscious memories that were related to a disturbed early relationship with their mother. This can be illustrated with the case of Aishwarya:

Aishwarya was the youngest of two girls. She had been depressed for much of her adult life, feeling that she was unloved by her mother who had wanted a son. During the course of therapy, it emerged that when Aishwarya was just under three years old, her mother had a still-born son, and fell into a deep depression. Aishwarya came to therapy for her difficulties in establishing and maintaining an intimate relationship, resulting in her feeling very lonely and depressed. She made good use of the first year of therapy and fruitfully explored her past, but the recent ending of a brief yet hopeful relationship had left her very low. She was also experiencing some work stress and feared for her job. In recent sessions, she had fallen quiet, saying there was little point talking because it wouldn't change anything. She felt hopeless that therapy could help her.

I said, "Your experience in your family and with other people, is that it is difficult to reach out to one another when you need someone. Here too, you feel you do not want to bother me with your sadness and worries, convinced that I won't care". She disagreed with me, then fell silent again. I found myself wondering if she was angrily shutting me out and felt a heavy sadness in the room. Several sessions followed where she was mostly quiet, with four sessions of near total silence. I felt frustrated and unsure how best to respond. If I prompted her or interpreted her uncommunication, she could experience this as an impingement. If, on the other hand, I too remained silent, she could experience me as disinterested. I became worried that she would end therapy, and struggled with feeling useless and ineffectual.

During one extended period of silence, I prompted her by asking, "Any thoughts?" to which she responded "Nothing", and a further silence ensued. During the stillness, I noticed myself growing sleepy and drifting in and out with my thoughts, in a state of reverie. At one point, my thoughts turned to her brother, and then I caught myself with the realisation that she did not have a brother – it had been a still birth. I started thinking about her answer, "Nothing", and how my tiredness felt deadening. The time went by slowly, but there was a different quality to it. It no longer felt unbearable and I felt less irritated with her. It seemed to me that it was not a defiant silence, but rather a shared experience of emptiness.

It was interesting that in this session, I had a vivid thought of Aishwarya having a brother, only to recall that this was a loss grieved by her mother, who became deeply depressed. It occurred to me that her silence was a wordless communication to me of her early relationship with an initially engaged and available mother who became unable to attend to her young daughter through her grief [becoming what Green (1986) refers to as the internalised 'dead mother']. *Towards the end of the session, I noted, "Sometimes, it is difficult to put things into words, but I think you have shared with me how alone you feel and perhaps what it is like to feel that there is no one there who cares". She nodded and tears flowed down her face. In the next session, she started talking again, and we began to explore her relationship with her mother in this next stage of the work.*

The opposite of this is the talkative patient. Speaking with pressure and great detail, often recycling events and insights without much affect, can be understood as a defensive manoeuvre that patients can engage in when they feel anxious in the consulting room. The resultant knock-on effect for therapists is that there is often no space to think in the face of an ongoing bombardment of words and content. It can be helpful to observe this overwhelmed and overwhelming experience you are being given, and how this is likely to be the experience that the patient often has, as was the case with Aishwarya above. Your counter-transference is an invaluable source of information. Some therapists may choose to allow the patient to speak until the pressure gradually wears off; others will intervene to slow the patient down and ask them to return to a point when you were following what they were saying. This is a stop and rewind technique to restore mentalising, as explained in Chapter 7.

Difficulties around payment

Like time boundaries, paying for psychotherapy is another part of reality that can throw up difficulties around the therapeutic relationship and can also be the receptacle for hostile feelings towards the therapist. Coming late and not paying for sessions in a timely manner can become expressions of resentment around having to pay for help. When seeing patients in the NHS, this may not be overtly present, but you may become aware of other ways in which patients may devalue therapy.

In private practice, you will need to agree a fee that is acceptable to both you and the patient, along with arrangements for how accounts are to be paid. We refer you back to the earlier discussion of this topic in Chapter 4. Some patients' financial circumstances mean they cannot afford to pay a full fee, and you would then negotiate with your patient a reasonable fee that is also acceptable to you. Just as Winnicott spoke about the endings of sessions as expressions of hatred from the therapist towards the patient, so too we can think about the regular bills in therapy as painful reminders that patients have to pay a professional for their services.

Where bills remain unpaid after the end of a consultation or period of treatment, this often indicates that the patient feels there is unfinished business with the therapist. Depending on the particular patient's dynamics, this can be seen as an expression of dissatisfaction with what the therapist has provided on the one hand, or a wish to remain connected to them without severing the link on the other. After all, by continuing to leave a bill unpaid, the therapist remains in contact with the patient by sending them invoices to prompt them to settle their account. We have found it helpful to include an accompanying letter where you suggest the patient contacts you should they need some allowance for paying the amount.

Non-payment is uncommon but does occur. It places the therapist in a difficult position because you have to weigh up whether you had a clear enough contract with the patient to charge for a missed session, for example, as well as the potential costs to you in time, effort and possibly reputation in pursuing an unpaid invoice. After all, this is not the type of debt that can be handed over to a collector. Once a therapeutic relationship is established, there are ethical considerations about withdrawing treatment owing to non-payment. In the event that a patient's medical aid will only cover a set number of sessions, you should discuss with the patient how they intend to fund the remaining treatment once they have used up their allowance. This is preferable to having to put treatment on hold while you both wait for a response from the medical aid to a request for an extension of funding. Where therapy bills mount up, the situation needs to be understood and addressed with the patient. You may want to consider a payment plan or a temporary reduction in sessional fees or frequency of treatment. Some patients may feel uncomfortable to receive a reduction in the fee, not wishing to receive any favours and such allowances can be inhibiting in therapy, particularly if the patient is to feel free to explore all aspects of their feelings towards their therapist, good and bad. It may be that you and the patient have to assess how financially viable it is for them to continue seeing you, and this may lead to exploring alternative, reduced fee options including group therapy and treatment in the public health sector.

Difficulties with bills can arise when someone else in the patient's circle is paying for their treatment, or even where the money has been gifted through an inheritance, for example. In these cases, extra-transference factors can interfere with settling the account. The patient may find it easier to miss sessions when the financial impact is not ultimately theirs. It would be easier to find a fee that the patient can cover themselves, or suggest that they get financial assistance with expenses other than therapy bills. In our experience, difficulties also arise when patients are seen through reduced fee schemes and there is a sense of getting 'too good a deal'. Psychotherapy should be valued appropriately, in our view, and paying trainee psychotherapists low rates that are often below the minimum wage, does not help in this regard.

Patients bearing gifts

Freud (1917b) writes about the way the baby presents the gift of their faeces to the mother and how with time, "this instinctual interest derived from the anal source passes over on to objects that can be presented as gifts" (p. 100). Thus, a gift can be seen as a token of affection, a bribe, request for forgiveness or even a masked expression of hostility. Accepting those gifts in turn can be seen as acting out in the countertransference, offering reassurance to the patient and potentially avoiding uncomfortable aspects of the transference. The meaning of a gift needs to be considered on a case by case basis so that the patient's action can be understood and analysed. On the whole, and in keeping with the principles of analytic restraint and neutrality, gifts tend to be discouraged in psychodynamic psychotherapy. In describing a series of gifts his patient presented over the course of treatment, Evans (2005) illustrates the multiple developmental meanings of the magical action of gift-giving which he sees as falling between acting out and dreaming and whose symbolic meaning can be explored in rich and enlightening ways.

Gift-giving often stems from unconscious motivations and can be seen as "a form of acting out of transference reactions" that should be analysed where possible so that the vicissitudes of the transference can be understood and put into words (Kritzberg, 1980, p. 100). On the face of it, a gift is "an expression of benevolent feelings, appreciation and gratitude to the helping therapist" (p. 101) while at other times the patient may not be conscious of their motivations for giving a present at that particular time. The gift itself may hold symbolic meaning for the patient. For example, Kritzberg (1980) describes receiving a wooden gadget from her patient that was a spirit level, compass and bottle opener in one, and how she was able to glean the meaning of these various functions in relation to the therapy. In this way, the gift was a condensation of several meanings, functioning in a similar way to a dream.

There are ethical issues in accepting gifts, particularly if you are working in a public health setting. There, the guiding principle is often that the gift should not be of a high monetary value and where possible, should be shared among the team rather than kept by the clinician. It would be over-simplistic to declare that all gifts are wrong and should be refused, however, we would ask you to reflect on the various layers of meaning that a gift may hold for the patient so that these can be fully explored.

Marion arrived at her session and proudly placed an enormous green apple on the table between us. She proclaimed that these were the same apples she ate when growing up and she wanted me to have one, too. I found myself in a dilemma, aware of Marion's history of emotional deprivation and repeated experiences of her mother's greed that left Marion feeling short-changed while at the same time, I registered Marion's excitement at finding this new resource that she wanted to show and share with me. This was a Marion who would be feeding me rather than being the hungry, needy patient she struggled to be. I thought about the trope of bringing an apple for the teacher as well as the expression of being the apple of someone's eye and I wondered about the way this apple was an attempt to keep me sweet as well as expressing her wish to be my special patient. While this was an inexpensive gift, it felt rich with meaning. After some thought and discussion with Marion as to her thoughts and fantasies that lay behind this action, I elected to return the apple to her, feeling that it was better to be the mother-therapist who could allow her to have her own internal resources without enviously divesting her of these. This gift could be seen as a pull for the therapist to become a depriving figure while also representing Marion's wish to share an aspect of her life that she valued.

Language and working with interpreters

We will consider issues of working with diversity and differences in the next chapter, but here we want to introduce the related topic of working with patients who speak a different language, and may require an interpreter. Such issues do not typically arise in private practice, although the ability to communicate clearly with each other in a language familiar to both therapist and patient is something that needs to be assessed and considered. It may be that the best action to take is a referral to a colleague who speaks the patient's language fluently.

For those working in public health settings, there is a greater possibility of working with interpreters. It could be argued that this creates a difficult barrier to therapeutic communication, being properly understood and in tune with unconscious communication in the session. There are delays in the work that takes twice as long to conduct. It also introduces a triangular dynamic between therapist, patient and interpreter, with possibility for splitting or rivalries to occur.

On the other hand, where patients have limited or no access to psychotherapy in their home language, it would be unethical to turn someone away because the therapeutic setting would not be ideal. We are typically talking about assessments and time-limited psychotherapy because working with an interpreter in long-term psychotherapy may pose too great a challenge and strain on resources. We have both had experiences of working with interpreters in our clinical work in South Africa as well as in the UK and when teaching in China. Swartz and Rohleder (2017), in writing about conducting research interviews with interpreters, outline some useful suggestions that are relevant for clinical work. They stress the importance of proper preparation. The researcher (in this case, therapist) should meet with the interpreter to discuss and agree how the process of interpretation will work during a session, with the therapist and interpreter having a clear understanding of each other's roles, including that everything is to be translated, with no utterances omitted, rephrased or summarised. Interpretation works best when the conversation is structured such that the interpreter works with small chunks of spoken words, rather than allowing for lengthy statements that they then try to interpret. It is also important to agree the terms and process of the interpretation with the patient, including clear discussions around the limits to confidentiality and anonymity. After the session, it is useful for the interpreter and therapist to debrief by reflecting on the experience of the session, including the emotional reactions of the interpreter (as potential countertransference material). The interpreter can also give some indication of nuances in language or culture that are not easily communicated in the moment, for example, where the patient used an odd turn of phrase or a metaphor that is familiar to the interpreter, but not the therapist. Working with an interpreter slows the process down and can offer useful pauses where the therapist and patient can digest what is being said.

Challenges in the therapeutic relationship

Ruptures in the therapeutic alliance

Ruptures are an inevitable consequence of being human and working with sensitive and challenging areas in psychotherapy. Indeed, although we try our hardest to avoid such rifts, the research suggests that the process of repairing significant challenges to and deterioration in the therapeutic alliance can be seen as therapeutic in its own right (e.g. Safran and Muran, 2006; Safran et al., 2014). However well-intentioned and attuned a therapist is towards their patient, the chances are that they will say something that feels harsh, too blunt or sharp, hurtful and insensitive to the patient at some point in therapy. Some patients will let us know immediately that this is what has happened and although it can feel challenging to the therapist, it is also very useful information that allows us to investigate the rupture, once we have validated their experience. Other patients will conceal their immediate reaction and over the course of time, we intuit that they have been affected by something we said. Perhaps they fall silent or begin to speak in an apathetic, cut off way. They may change the topic and move to speak about a peripheral area of their lives in order to recover their equilibrium. Other patients will respond with a narrative that conveys a cautionary tale for the therapist about their anticipated response.

It is useful to go back and understand what has gone wrong so that this can be incorporated into a deeper understanding of the patient's dynamics. Monitoring our countertransference is an important part of picking up on these misattunements: we may feel uncomfortable, as if we are walking on egg shells with the patient; we may feel sleepy and disconnected, often a sign that aggression is being defended against; we may feel pushed into responding in a particular way with the patient, whether this is by acting, judging, caring and so on.

Elizabeth returned to her session after a work trip in New Zealand and was confused about the time of her session. She buzzed and buzzed at the door while I was seeing another patient and eventually, I went to answer. She backed down when she realised she had the wrong time and easily agreed to return at the designated hour. However, on her return, she quickly expressed her anger at being turned away abruptly by me, particularly as she had been having a difficult time and really wanted to come to her session that day. Indeed, we may think that unconsciously she arrived half an hour earlier precisely because she wanted to be seen so much. She felt hurt by my curtness and was highly critical of me. It was difficult to resist pushing back as she pointed out how wrong I was. After all, it wasn't my mistake! However, I knew that saying this would exacerbate the situation, and so I acknowledged how awful it was for her to arrive thinking she was on time for her session and find me unable to see her because I was with another patient. I agreed that I may have been rather short with her and apologised for this. I went on to explain that I felt caught in a difficult situation because there was another patient who was in the middle of their session and I was aware of the interruption this was causing them. I did not respond as sensitively as I might have to the Elizabeth's earlier arrival and I could see that this was painful. By acknowledging her feelings and validating them, the patient's emotional arousal reduced and she was able to see the situation from both her and my perspective as well as the perspective of the other patient. We were able to go on to explore her trip and how challenging her life was at the present time. We had been working together for some time and our working alliance was better established by then. This allowed therapy to endure the rupture and for that alliance to deepen.

With patients who have a pattern of disengagement and avoidance, it can be helpful to highlight this when exploring the possibility of working together in order to pre-empt how you would deal with a rupture should it arise.

Chantal wanted me to promise her that I would never say or do anything offensive to her in therapy so that the space could feel safe for her. This was not a promise I could undertake and I responded that while it would not be my intention to be offensive or uncaring towards her, it may be that I occasionally say something that causes her offence, albeit unintentionally, and it would be my hope that she could return to discuss it with me. I added that it would be a real pity if these difficulties that she has sought help for, result in a repetition of the same patterns that she wished to address here in therapy.

Erotic transference and countertransference

As discussed in Chapter 9, some patients may develop sexual feelings for the therapist that feel very powerful and real to them. Therapeutic boundaries can be challenged by patients' flirtatiousness and attempts to subvert the therapeutic relationship into a romantic encounter. This can represent a wish to have a different type of relationship and to get away from the experience of being dependent on the therapist for their care, help and thoughtfulness.

Instead, the therapy situation is altered in the patient's fantasy to a mutually rewarding relationship in which the power differentials and differences between patient and therapist are denied. The patient recasts themselves as a lover who can provide for the therapist, thereby denying any maternal transference of dependence and need. How far these fantasies go will vary from patient to patient and may determine whether they put the future of therapy at risk. Some patients will not be able to explore transferential feelings of attraction towards the therapist without becoming confused about the realities of the psychotherapy frame. The challenge facing therapists is continuing to explore these transferences without becoming overly gratifying and seductive on the one hand, or censorious by shutting it down on the other. Working through these sexualised feelings can allow patients to work through their inevitable losses, perhaps revisiting the loss of the first love object, the mother who is unattainable as an erotic object. Maroda states that "the patient who loves and desires her analyst has an opportunity in the present to grieve all that has been lost in the past, and all that can never be" (quoted in Barrett, 2003, pp. 168–169).

Sexualising the therapeutic relationship can be an act of aggression in an attempt to unsettle the therapist and deny their professional identity. Rather than being a patient, therapy is turned into a potential conquest where there is pressure on the therapist to demonstrate to the patient that they love and approve of them in this particular way. The patient may have learned to express their love in sexual forms and may wish to return the love they feel for the therapist in action, rather than symbolically. The therapeutic relationship is unusual in its intensity within the particular analytic boundaries, and patients may have confusing and powerful feelings towards the therapist.

The erotic countertransference is a subject that is not addressed often in the literature. Perhaps this countertransference response raises most urgently the need to differentiate between our own unanalysed responses (or more accurately our transference to our patients) from a response that is being elicited by the patient's psychodynamics. Shame around the former can make this area very difficult to bring to the awareness of our supervisors, let alone ourselves. If you do find yourself becoming sexually attracted to one of your patients, it is advisable to monitor your feelings carefully in your clinical supervision as well as your personal therapy. It may be a sign that you should return to personal psychotherapy if you are no longer in your own treatment. Part of the analytic stance entails paying attention to our countertransference, including the feelings, thoughts and images that enter our minds. If you find yourself feeling particularly warm towards a patient and making special allowances, this is an early warning signal. Another sign would be finding yourself making self-disclosures that are not in the service of the patient. These are advance warnings of ways in which the therapeutic boundaries are starting to become stretched.

The challenge is how to approach these reactions from a position of curiosity so that we can consider why these feelings are occurring now and whether they can be used in a constructive manner (Barrett, 2003). It is not usually advocated that the countertransference of the therapist is interpreted to the patient. Rather, the task is to accept these erotic feelings without guilt, shame or distance while managing the crucial rule of abstinence. These feelings may be particularly challenging to a therapist if they are accompanied by sexual identifications and longings that run contrary to the therapist's sexual orientation. In this way, we are forced to face our own "polymorphous perversity", the term Freud (1905a) used to describe early stages of development where our sexual longings are more fluid.

Let us return to the television series, *In Treatment,* to illustrate this. In it, the psychotherapist Paul Weston (played by Gabriel Byrne) finds himself becoming involved in a relationship with his patient during a particularly vulnerable time in his personal life. The therapist's personal vulnerabilities have clouded his clinical judgement and he starts to look towards his patient to meet his own needs for validation and love. Their roles become reversed and this clearly is harmful for the patient, whose treatment has been subverted. Indeed, the frequent representation of therapists breaking boundaries on the large and small screen suggests a preoccupation with this outlier behaviour. Stepping outside the patient-therapist relationship is always unethical and grounds to be struck off your professional register. The principle of abstinence allows fantasies to be explored in words rather than in actions. Particularly when we are working with vulnerable patients, it is incumbent on us to hold therapeutic boundaries very clearly.

Patients who ask questions and request advice

Asking lots of questions can be seen in several different ways. The patient may be trying to deflect attention from themselves or rectify the inevitable power balance in the therapy session by putting the therapist in the firing line and asking them to account for themselves. While we would consider it relevant to answer some questions and help the patient orient themselves to therapy, excessive questions may betray other anxieties that need addressing first rather than responding to the content of the questions. Remember that an analytic attitude requires abstinence on the part of the therapist. When faced with a request, it is helpful initially to explore the motivation and fantasies behind the request rather than gratify it immediately. There is often continual pressure on the therapist to act rather than think. Since we are trying to encourage a space where we can slow down this pressure to respond immediately, it is important to find ways of stepping back from the strain posed by a question to consider what may lie behind it. Repeatedly answering questions or providing reassurance won't help your patient in the long run.

> *Sally was a suspicious patient who ended many of her initial sessions by asking for reassurance that the personal information she had shared with me during the session would be kept safe. It was important to address the way her anxiety arose as the session was coming to a close, leaving her feeling unsafe and not trusting that I could keep her material safe in my mind during the intervening week. It was possible to think about her reluctance to trust the confidentiality of therapy and to link this to Sally's early experiences of feeling betrayed and let down by her parents.*

In a similar way, giving advice to patients is not part of the psychodynamic stance. It pushes us into an expert position. This may resonate with the patient's wish for an authoritative parent figure who will 'take charge'. The patient may have a punitive superego that wants to be let off the hook should things go wrong; by following your advice rather than the patient's own instincts, the therapist is seen to carry the blame should things not work out. The patient may be afraid of their own agency, tending to take a more passive position. By repeatedly asking for advice in the knowledge that this is not a part of the psychodynamic approach, the patient inevitably re-enacts an experience of the therapist-other as withholding and repeats an experience of feeling short-changed. This suggests a similar dynamic is at play in the patient's significant relationships and that its re-occurrence in the transference should be interpreted. As you can see, some type of explanation of the approach you will be adopting is an important part of orienting the patient to psychodynamic work.

An exception to this stance is dealing with risk issues. If a patient presents with suicidality, then we do need to engage with this and intervene if we feel the risk is unacceptable. This is an important consideration in assessing the patient's suitability to work psychodynamically at the frequency you have proposed. Should a patient feel very stirred up by therapy and this leads to an exacerbation in their symptomatology, including risk, then an external assessment or additional support should be considered. This may include a referral to the GP for medication, an increase in sessions or putting treatment on pause, even ending therapy. We discussed this topic in greater detail in Chapter 5 and will go on to explore ways of dealing with suicidality later in this chapter.

Patients who challenge therapeutic boundaries

Occasionally the patient asks the therapist more personal questions. It is natural for patients to be curious about the person they are seeing for therapy and some may not inhibit themselves from asking questions. These can range from questions about the therapist's background and personal information such as whether they have children, their sexual orientation, religion or theoretical orientation.

The patient may also ask the same type of questions they would pose to friends or family members, such as "Where are you going on holiday?" or "Where did you buy your shoes?" All these questions should be thought about rather than answered there and then. It is often those moments at the doorstep of the consulting room on entering or leaving the session, where the boundaries of the analytic frame are most at risk of being challenged and where we are most likely to be unseated from our analytic stance.

There are useful responses that you can give to create a space that allows you to step back from the pressure and wish to gratify the patient's question with an answer. You may say that you can see the patient is very curious about you and that you are interested in their questions, but your role isn't to answer them. You can follow that up by enquiring how the patient feels about your response. Another approach is to understand and interpret the purpose served by the questions. This will vary from person to person and you will be guided by your understanding of the patient together with your countertransference. At the more benign end of the spectrum, the patient may feel that they are opening up to you and that their questions are an attempt to rectify the imbalance and find out something about you; perhaps they even feel it is impolite to speak only about themselves without also enquiring after you. After all, this is a rather unusual situation for most people to have a therapist at their disposal who is thinking with them about their difficulties and concerns while making minimal demands for reciprocity (other than arriving on time and paying the bill). For other patients, boundary challenges may be linked to a wish to make the therapist feel uncomfortably exposed, or on the more perverse end of the spectrum, to take voyeuristic pleasure at focusing on the therapist's world or intruding into their privacy.

Some patients can express their wish for the therapist by making contact between sessions by emailing or telephoning the service and asking questions in that way. It is best to encourage the patient to discuss this with you in the session rather than get involved in contact between sessions. This is all part of holding the analytic frame and we discuss this further in relation to the challenges of electronic communication in Chapter 14.

The 'good patient' and/or the idealised therapist

Some patients may be overly compliant in therapy, wanting to please us and be the good patient. This may underlie a fear that the patient will be thrown out of therapy if they are too problematic. Again, this probably mirrors dynamics from early childhood where they had to develop a false self and suppress their authenticity in order to feel safe with their key attachment figures. While this may give the therapist an easy life, it is ultimately unhelpful to the patient who is unlikely to benefit from therapy spent in service of someone else. We are aiming to help the patient recognise the diverse range of feelings they hold towards us, not just the pleasing and acceptable ones. The patient may find it surprising to be invited to express their hostile and unacceptable feelings towards the therapist and discover that we are willing to engage with them without the talion response of retaliation.

Some patients' compliance extends to putting the therapist on a pedestal and idealising them as perfect and beyond reproach. This often occurs in patients with a narcissistic presentation, where the humiliation of seeking help is counter-balanced by viewing the therapist as wonderful and brilliant, thereby finding an acceptable way of engaging in treatment. It can be rather tempting to let this idealised transference run its course rather than disrupt it, particularly if you are new to therapy and/or have other patients with more hostile transferences. After all, who would not find solace in having a patient always saying we are extremely helpful, brilliant and insightful? However, we also know that being raised to such dizzy heights usually presages a painful fall. For this reason, we think it is important to bring this defence of splitting to the patient's attention. Again, it is likely that this will be happening in other parts of their lives. Idealisation suggests the operation of splitting and the paranoid-schizoid position. It would be a sign of progress to shift towards the depressive position where good and bad can be more integrated, including in the transference. You can recognise their need to feel they are in safe hands and as such, they want to insist on you being beyond reproach; yet we also know that there will be a wide range of emotions they could feel about you, and you are interested in knowing about all of them. An idealising response can be used to insure against any possibility of being hurt or let down by others, but it also contributes to keeping the status quo in place.

Risks in the clinical setting

Suicide and safeguarding risks

When discussing assessment of suitability for psychotherapy, we have to weigh up the level of risk presented by the patient, and whether we can manage it within our work setting. A careful assessment of risk at the outset of therapy does not mean that risk will not change at a later point. Indeed, an assessment of risk needs to be dynamic to account for continually changing circumstances and factors. How do we look out for risk in our patients, bearing in mind that people who feel seriously about suicide often don't disclose their risk to others? You may be using outcome measures with your patients if you are working in an NHS setting, with most measures including risk questions. These are important communications between you and your patient that should be taken seriously.

> *Daniel used to score 'several days' on the last question of the Personal Health Questionnaire (PHQ-9), indicating that he had thoughts of harming himself or being better off dead. When I explored what he meant by this, it became apparent that he considered smoking and binge drinking as manifestations of self-harm. In this instance, it occurred to me that he needed me to take his distress seriously, even if that meant that he inflated the level of risk on the questionnaire. In his mind, this was an act of self-damage and he was challenging me to take this seriously as an aspect of his self-destructiveness and suicidality.*

When a patient indicates that they feel deep despair, it is important to engage in as open a discussion as possible about this. If you pose a question to a patient along the lines, "You don't think about killing yourself, do you?" you are unlikely to get an honest answer. The patient will probably feel that you are unwilling to consider these violent and dangerous thoughts inside their mind as acceptable to you and may become even more likely to keep them hidden. If you are able to have an open discussion with your patient about their suicidality and bring these impulses and fantasies out into the open, then the chances of your patient acting on those wishes diminishes. Some patients are more impulsive than others and have made previous suicide attempts. It is important to get a full history of any previous suicide gestures or attempts in order to establish how serious and chronic this is. When patients write a suicide note, it usually suggests a more serious, pre-meditated state of mind. Some patients begin taking steps to put their affairs in order, like drawing up a will, buying a funeral plan, giving away clothes and personal effects, and posting comments on social media that suggest they are saying their goodbyes. However, with other patients, this is a closely guarded secret. Campbell (1995) writes about the pre-suicidal state in patients where they are in a desperate split, both expecting their body to die while at the same time imagining they would continue living in

> a conscious body-less state, otherwise unaffected by the death of their body. Although killing the body was a conscious aim, it was also a means to an end. The end was the pleasurable survival of an essential part of the self, which I will refer to as the 'surviving self', that survives in another dimension. (p. 315)

As therapists, we think it is important to signal to our patients that we are willing to speak about those areas of their inner and external lives that are often deemed too distressing to raise with family members and friends. Enquiring in an open way about whether someone has thoughts of ending their life and exploring these fantasies openly is essential. Some patients will have passive thoughts that they would be better off dead. Occasionally this can be expressed as a wish to go to sleep, to wake up and feel renewed after the suicidal fantasy. Although this is less risky than a more active plan to kill oneself, it can result in the same end and also needs close attention. If your NHS service uses outcome measures as part of its regular practice, it is incumbent upon you to attend to the risk questions and explore these answers in the session. Any questionnaire is a communication to the therapist and needs to be brought into the session. It can be seen as an indirect expression of the wish for help or the patient's aggression towards the therapist (if, for example, scores remain high and the implied criticism is that the therapist is unable to help the patient).

You may become aware of risks to others, rather than the patient. For example, a patient may talk at length about their homicidal fantasies towards their ex-husband or parent. In these instances, it is important to weigh up how much of this is fantasy or reality. Is the patient capable of acting on these thoughts? The role of substances is an important consideration for patients who easily become dysregulated and impulsive. The riskier a patient is, the more challenging it becomes to work with them in private practice. The benefits of an NHS setting include the support of the institution, or the "brick mother" of the containing mental hospital admission (Henri Rey's term, cited by Garelick, 2011).

The risks may include safeguarding risks towards young or old people that the patient cares about. If you have any questions in your mind about a safeguarding issue, it is important to flag it with your clinical supervisor and if they are not available, to raise it with the ethics committee of your professional body. It has been shown in the awful tragedies of children who died after chronic abuse (in the UK, examples such as Victoria Climbie and 'Baby P'), many different professionals noticed what was happening but didn't raise their concerns with anyone. It is always better to attend to your worries by alerting someone than to dismiss them as irrelevant. Although reporting a patient to the relevant services (in the UK, this is Social Services) is likely to damage the therapeutic alliance and may result in treatment ending, it is our duty to respond to concerns we have for vulnerable children and adults. These could be elderly people who are reliant on the patient for support and unable to speak up, or it could include people with learning disabilities who lack capacity to consent. For those who work in the NHS and mental health charities, there is usually annual safeguarding training to ensure staff are aware of the legal requirements to report these issues and to highlight the rights of the patient. In our experience, we recommend being clear with patients about your reasons for being concerned and explain that while you are not certain about what is going on, you can't rely on their reassurances that everything is fine since you have not had sight of their child, for example. Social services are able to make a home visit and assess the impact of the parent's mental health on the child as well as provide appropriate support.

When reporting risks, we need to monitor our own superegos and strike the balance between becoming overly punitive or lax. Some services that work with risky offenders are more accustomed to managing and holding certain risks. There usually needs to be corresponding support for the therapists through supervision, team work and so on to allow higher levels of risk to be tolerable to the team. We have included some comments on burn out among therapists in Chapter 4 and would like to bring your attention to this again here. This touches on the risks posed to the therapist through doing this line of work, something we invite you to keep a close eye on.

Regression in psychotherapy

When you are assessing the suitability of a patient for psychotherapy, we need to bear in mind the capacity of the patient to regress once they enter treatment. Regression can take the form of a severe depressive breakdown and may also have psychotic features. Earlier breakdowns are a good prognostic indicator of the severity of any future breakdowns. Therapists need to address this directly with patients and enquire about their existing support systems. Patients who are living away from their family or are estranged from their support networks are more at risk than those with people in their lives that care about them and to whom they feel emotionally connected.

If you are concerned about a patient's capacity to keep themselves safe, then you need to bring this to the patient's awareness as well as that of their emergency contact person. You may find you have to adjust your way of working when a patient is vulnerable and particularly when their grasp on reality is shaky. Taking up a more supportive and reality-oriented position at such times is helpful. The patient is likely to be in a state of psychic equivalence, with impaired capacity to mentalise, so you can make judicious use of the mentalising techniques from Chapter 7.

Box 12.1 Useful resources

Readings

Don Campbell's paper (1995), The role of the father in a pre-suicide state, *The International Journal of Psychoanalysis, 76*, 315–323, explores the different fantasies that underpin suicidal acts and how to attend to these to avoid them going underground and undetected.

The book, *Assessing Risk: A Relational Approach* by Blumenthal, Wood and Andrews (2018) provides a thorough exploration of the area of risk by drawing on the authors' experience in the Portman Clinic working with violence and sexual offending.

There is an interesting article online that explores various ethical and cultural facets around gift-giving in therapy between patients and therapists by Ofer Zur at www.zurinstitute.com/gifts-in-therapy/

Robert Michels' (1977) article, Treatment of the difficult patient in psychotherapy, *Canadian Psychiatric Association Journal, 22*(3), 117–121, provides a discussion of what constitutes a challenging patient as well as those factors that contribute towards difficulties in therapy that link to the therapist's experience levels as well as the states of therapy.

Online resources

There is an interesting talk by psychoanalyst and psychiatrist, Glen Gabbard on working with so-called difficult patients on YouTube, https://youtu.be/oUDuLmjTaZ4

13 Working with difference

Psychodynamic practitioners are not immune to prejudices and discomfort about diversity and difference. While we all probably view ourselves as humane, open and empathic, we are nevertheless products of social and cultural contexts where there are likely to be biased and at times problematic views and assumptions about deviations from the dominant culture. We do not have to go too far into our history to observe the cruelty and horrors inflicted on groups of people deemed by the majority population as inferior, and even irrationally perceived as dangerous. Even the so-called 'psy' professions (namely, psychiatry, psychology and psychotherapy) have colluded with discriminatory and oppressive practices. For example, psychoanalysis has had a troubled history with homosexuality (see Lewes, 2009). Even today, some psychoanalytic practitioners and other mental health practitioners are disturbed by the view that homosexuality is 'normal' and may even advocate for conversion therapies. Only fairly recently have UK professional bodies agreed to oppose any practices that seek to convert a person's homosexuality to heterosexuality. There is an ongoing fraught and polarised social examination of how transgender identities are to be understood. For those individuals who identify as gender diverse, this debate is yet another painful example of how their existence and realities are questioned and even repudiated.

As outlined in the introductory chapter, one of the basic psychodynamic competences is to pay attention to both the internal world and external realities of the patient. Another competence is the ability to grasp the patient's 'world view'. In psychodynamic practice, we are often concerned primarily with the intrapsychic aspects of our patients' lives: their interior conflicts, internalised objects, urges, motivations, defences and so forth. We can contextualise the intrapsychic mind in an interpersonal context of the key attachment relationships of childhood. We pay relatively less attention to the social, cultural, economic and political realities in which our patients – and ourselves as therapists – are located. As Juliet Mitchell (1974) reminds us, 'the personal is political and the political is personal'. We cannot think of our patient's internal world and mental health without thinking of the possibly hostile world they live in. Nor can we as therapists think of our professional identity without considering how we may be positioned in society in relation to privilege and oppression. We can extend Winnicott's notion of the 'holding environment' beyond the maternal/paternal environment to include society more broadly, and to apply not just in childhood but throughout the lifespan. Increasingly, psychotherapy has an important role to play in this arena. In the UK, psychotherapists have contributed to discussions around the influence of the #MeToo movement, Black Lives Matter, Brexit and the wider socio-economic and political context of individual mental health. This socio-economic and political context is present in the consulting room. Thus, we cannot work only with the internal world of our patients, without placing equal importance on their external world. While we can conceptualise a struggle with internalised oppression, we should not neglect attending to objective realities of social, economic and political oppression.

Some practitioners may be anxious about working with differences in their work – whether this is working with patients who are sexual or gender minorities, of another culture, or with a racialised identity. Some of this anxiety may be an unconscious (or even conscious) fear of the Other as well as anxiety about 'not knowing' and doing or saying something 'wrong'. Often diversity and difference are thought and spoken about in terms of difference residing in the other; *they* are different. This is certainly so when the subject is a member of the dominant group. In these instances, individuals from the dominant majority culture and identity tend to view the world from the perspective of their identity representing the norm, perceiving those with non-normative identities as the ones who are different. It is important to recognise that differences exist *between* people. It is not just that the patient is 'different' and the therapist is not: you both have socially constructed identities that differ from each other. Thus, we cannot consider racism in terms of the experiences of ethnic minorities without also considering whiteness as an identity. Furthermore, we may focus our attention on one aspect of perceived difference, without giving much attention to the various points of difference and sameness that exist between two people, such as age, gender, sexual orientation, class, ethnicity, political views and so on.

We have chosen to focus in this chapter on a few specific areas of diversity, namely sexual and gender minorities, racialised and classed identities, and disability, exploring assumptions and biases that are contained in the body of psychoanalytic theory as well as more broadly. We then look at how psychotherapists can practice reflectively to be able to work effectively across differences. We hope this will allow you to apply this approach to other areas of diversity that we have not been able to address in this chapter.

Sexuality and gender diversity

Freud arguably demonstrated an openness to thinking about sexuality as fluid and diverse, and in his writings, he often explicitly regarded homosexuality as a non-pathological variant of human sexuality. Freud (1905a) depicted humans as psychically bisexual and did not regard the sexual instinct as biologically matched to an opposite-sex object choice. While on the one hand, he regarded homosexuality in terms of diversity rather than 'perversity', his theory of a hierarchical psychosexual development placed male-female genital copulation at the pinnacle of maturity and he described homosexuality in some of his writing as an 'arrest in sexual development' (Freud, 1935). Subsequent classical psychoanalytic theorists took a much more anti-homosexual stance, describing it in terms of perversity, rather than diversity. For example, Fairbairn (1952) regarded 'homosexuals' as essentially 'perverse' and 'psychopathic' incapable of having mature object relations. Much of the early psychoanalytic writing on homosexuality refers to 'the homosexual' as an object of study. In the USA, psychoanalysts such as Socarides and Bergler (reviewed in Lewes, 2009) were vociferous anti-homosexuality theorists, regarding it as a pathology and advocating for conversion therapy; that is therapy that aims to 'treat' homosexuality by conversion to heterosexuality.

Times have changed, and psychoanalysis has moved on. In 2011, the British Psychoanalytic Council issued a statement declaring that homosexuality is not a pathology and opposing discrimination on the basis of sexual orientation. In 2014, most of the mental health professional bodies in the UK, including the British Psychoanalytic Council, the British Psychological Society, The British Association of Counselling and Psychotherapy and the UK Council for Psychotherapy signed a memorandum of understanding against the practice of conversion therapy for sexual orientation, condemning it as unethical and harmful (see Box 13.1 for reference). This memorandum was updated in 2017 to include opposition to conversion therapy for non-normative gender identities. In 2019, the American Psychoanalytic Association issued a public apology to the LGBTQ (lesbian, gay, bisexual, transgender, and queer) community for the part they played in labelling homosexuality as pathological and the resultant trauma and oppression experienced by those individuals.

These welcome changes do not mean that everything is fine in psychoanalytic and psychodynamic theory and practice. Much of our body of psychoanalytic theory has an explicit heteronormative bias that we still need to move beyond (Hertzmann and Newbigin, 2020). Our theories are saturated with binaried assumptions, such as male-female, masculine-feminine, heterosexual-homosexual, paternal-maternal, active-passive, and so on. These concepts are presented, discussed and taken for granted as biological truths, rather than constructs and theories. Schafer (2002) refers to them as "organising concepts" (p. 26) which arrange our thinking into a hierarchy of normal-abnormal, aligning sex, gender, gender roles and sexuality in one neat, heteronormative line. The heterosexual, active, masculine male and heterosexual, passive, feminine female are typically regarded as the norms against which diverging identities are seen as problematic.

Most of the writing in the psychoanalytic tradition has been authored by heterosexually identified theorists and psychotherapists, given that for many years anyone identifying as homosexual was barred from undertaking a professional training. The ostensible reason for this was that 'homosexuals' were understood to have a narcissistic character pathology that supposedly rendered them incapable of mature, healthy object relations. With the revised thinking over recent decades, psychoanalytic theories about homosexuality have become increasingly contested and reformulated (for example Domenici and Lesser, 1995; Lemma and Lynch, 2015; Hertzmann and Newbigin, 2020). Increasing attention is now paid to the complexity around identifications of sexuality and gender. For example, the American psychoanalytic writers Isay (1986; 2010) and Rose (2007) theorise male homosexuality and the Oedipus Complex by taking into consideration same-sex primary object choice, namely the boy's desire for his father.

Another important shift in thinking has been recognising the need to understand any psychological and interpersonal difficulties in gay men and lesbian women not as characteristics of 'homosexual pathology', but rather as the consequence of familial and social prejudice and oppression (e.g. Lynch, 2015; Rohleder, 2020). Thus, when heterosexual therapists work with gay, lesbian and bisexual patients, it is important to consider the realities of exclusion, rather than viewing them only as psychic fantasies.

Sexuality and sexual identity have always been considered in relation to gender, in particular male and female biology, gender identifications and gender roles, where biological sex is seen to determine gender, and in turn sexuality. More recently, gender has become a contested concept. Social scientists have for many years conceptualised gender as separate to sex. Sex is understood in terms of biological markers (genitalia, hormones and X/Y chromosomes) while gender is seen as a social construct that is shaped and determined by social and cultural norms. Judith Butler (1990) in her seminal work *Gender Trouble* argues that gender is not predetermined, and that one cannot easily consider gender identity as decided by biological sex. She contends that we 'accomplish' our gender identity through negotiating societal and cultural expectations about being a woman and being a man. We are not born a man or a woman; instead we learn to 'perform' as such. Butler maintains that there is a social policing of gender and sexual identity, where homosexuality is prohibited and heterosexuality is expected, and this gives rise to expectations around how men and women should behave accordingly.

In recent years, psychoanalytic conceptualisations of sex and gender have been further challenged by understandings around transgender and gender non-conforming identities. As mentioned above, concepts related to gender can be thought of as organising concepts around which ideas of normality and abnormality are defined. Wren (2020) purports that the acceptance of the male–female binary in psychoanalytic writing is the bedrock assumption for sanity. However, she goes on to state that there is little evidence that suggests that the acceptance of a cisgendered identity (namely, an individual who identifies with the sex assigned at birth) is nothing more than social conformity. In recent years, young people in particular are challenging this gender binary by identifying as gender diverse: gender fluid or gender non-binary. Others feel a sense of incongruency with their sexed bodies and gender identity, and are pursuing physical solutions for gender reassignment. In writing about transgender individuals, Lemma (2013) argues that chronic, early parental missatunement may explain the distress that some individuals feel towards their bodies which they experience as incongruent with their gender identities. Their experience of distress is eased when their gender identities are mirrored in their bodies and the responses of others.

Gender diverse identities are protected in the UK under the Equalities Act 2010, which respects the right for people to live in their preferred or perceived gender. However, this has given rise to highly charged debate and concern from various sectors of society about the increase in referrals for gender reassignment surgery, particularly in young women. In the current psychiatric nomenclature, 'gender dysphoria' is still understood as a psychopathology, giving rise to different opinions about appropriate treatment protocols. Wren (2020) describes a current "crisis of meaning" (p. 191) surrounding childhood gender, the body and identity, in particular deciding who has the authority to 'know' and make meaningful decisions. The present conflict surrounding the debate makes finding proper space for reflection and discussion near impossible. There may be a missed opportunity for careful thought that a reflective analytic approach could offer. However, this is a fast-moving field, and there is very little contemporary psychoanalytic writing about this.

Various professional bodies have published guidelines for therapists working with sexual and gender diverse patients, including the British Psychological Society (2019) and the British Association for Counselling and Psychotherapy (2019). These guidelines emphasise that sexual, gender and relationship diversity are not in themselves indicative of psychopathology, and they call for practitioners to respect diversity and support their patients' self-determination in developing their identity, relationships and practices. Emphasis is placed on understanding the social, cultural and political context of their patients, the resultant experiences of stigma, discrimination and oppression, and the impact this has on their mental health. The guidelines further stress the importance of self-reflection and receiving adequate training so that therapists are aware of their own gender, sexual and relationship identities, and the inevitable biases they bring to their clinical work.

Some therapists may be anxious and concerned that the memorandum against conversion therapy prohibits them from exploring potential issues posed by their patients' sexual or gender identity. This may be a misreading of the guidelines which do not discourage the exploration of what things mean for the patient. There is a difference between exploring and understanding the patient's experience and perspective, and driving that exploration along moralistic lines of what the therapist determines to be right or wrong. It is useful to remember the importance of neutrality as part of the psychoanalytic/dynamic stance. Therapists should strive to take a curious and empathic position by attempting to understand the subjective experience of their patient and their search for personal meaning, whatever their sexual orientation or gender identity.

In the recently published book, *Sexuality and Gender Now: Moving Beyond Heteronormativity* (Hertzmann and Newbigin, 2020), an anonymous transgender male patient has written a chapter entitled, "A person beyond gender: A first-hand account" in which he gives an account of his experience of transitioning as a trans man, having been assigned female at birth. The author writes honestly and movingly about his experience of feeling different, confused and distressed as a trans man in relation to societal prejudices and discomforts, and how he came to find some coherence in his identity with the help of psychodynamic psychotherapy. The book also includes psychoanalyst Suchet's (2020) account of her work with a patient transitioning from female to male, and her reflections of the process of change in her clinical understanding. These chapters offer useful examples of how psychodynamic psychotherapy helpfully provides an opportunity for exploration and understanding in this emerging area.

Some therapists, particularly those less experienced in working with sexual and gender diverse patients, express anxiety about making a mistake or saying something wrong. In terms of gender diversity and the use of pronouns, we are aware of clinicians' fear of making mistakes around terminology and pronouns. Mistakes and misattunements do happen. What is important is not to ignore those slip ups or brush aside their significance; rather it is important for the therapist to reflect on them and their possible meaning. Owning up to our mistakes can provide helpful avenues for further exploration, as the following clinical example illustrates.

> *Peter, 25 years old, identifies as a gay man. He came to see me because he was struggling to come to terms with his sexuality, having grown up in a conservative Catholic family. During the course of therapy, he began a relationship with Sam, who is gender non-binary, and thus uses the pronouns they/them. I noticed that in referencing his partner, Sam, I would at times revert to calling Sam he or him, and not use the appropriate pronouns. I was aware of the risk of repeating Peter's experience of not being understood through my mistake, and so decided to own it by saying, "I seem to be finding it difficult to find the right pronoun today, and I wonder what effect that is having on you?" Peter replied saying that he also struggled to use the right pronoun at times. It became possible for us to think about this as a shared experience, rather than the difference being located in me as the insensitive, biased therapist who was disappointing Peter. Not having to be the authority, and also being able to acknowledge a mistake without being overly apologetic or self-flagellating, reflected Peter's progress in therapy as he began to modify his own harsh superego, and step back from his sense of disappointing others.*

Racialised and classed identities

Racism is widespread, creating divisions along *us* and *them* lines, and leading to a hierarchy of superiority and inferiority. Although the term 'race' is used to refer to an objective 'reality', it too is a social construct, not a biological fact. Throughout history, people have been assigned to groups of races on the basis of arbitrary characteristics, such as skin tone, eye shape and hair colour or texture. It is more accurate to say that people's identities have been *racialised*, in that they are socially constructed and positioned as belonging to a particular category, then treated accordingly.

There has been much interest in understanding the sociology and psychology of racism and prejudice. From a psychoanalytic perspective, racism can be understood through the concept of projection. Frantz Fanon (1967) writing about the black psyche, argued that primitive anxieties about animalism and sexuality are disavowed by white men and women and projected onto black men and women who are then perceived as 'primitive', and 'animal-like', with a wild, unrestrained sexuality. These primitive and infantile anxieties are psychotic-like, irrational and resistant to reason (Davids, 2006; 2011). While we may typically think of racism in terms of individual attitudes, the Black Lives Matter movement of recent years has highlighted how racism is systemic and embedded in the structures of our society.

Davids (2011), a psychoanalyst of Asian descent who grew up in apartheid South Africa, argues that earlier psychoanalytic understandings of racism focused on pathological internal processes, and neglected to acknowledge an external, real and social account of racism. As he states in the first line of his book, *Internal Racism: A Psychoanalytic Approach to Race and Difference* (2011), "to be black in a white world is an agony" (p. 1). Davids (2011) posits that we are all racist rather than locating racism in particular parts of society; he argues that institutional and societal racism gives rise to an organised 'internal racist' in our minds. This is often a subtle form of racism that gives rise to micro-aggressions, as opposed to overt racism, with which we are familiar and which can be understood in terms of the primitive projections discussed above. He illustrates through clinical material how ordinarily rational and reasonable adults reveal their internal racist attitudes. Davids (2006) argues that following the projection of unwanted aspects of the self, an "organised internal template" (p. 72) is formed which then governs the dynamic relations between white people and people of colour, such that for whites, their interactions with people of colour must conform to that template, ensuring that 'non-white others' remain as the objects containing that which is unwanted and disavowed. When the 'non-white object' steps out of this organised template, racist anxieties will flare up when faced with the threatened return of that which is disowned and projected. Davids regards the internal racist part of the mind as a "normal developmental achievement, which, once attained, is sub-sequently available to the individual as a resource with which to manage over-whelming anxiety" (2006, p. 73). So, for example, a white individual may reveal their internal racism with an utterance that highlights difference, thus causing a momentary rupture in the relationship with the non-white person in the social exchange. It is often then left to the non-white individual to respond in a manner that conforms and accepts the utterance, rather than challenge it and be accused of not being able to take a joke, thereby ensuring that the problem remains with the non-white individual. Although Davids writes about white racism towards people of colour, he stresses that everyone has this internal racism, regardless of skin colour. In Box 13.1, we have provided a link to the Harvard University online research that powerfully illustrates this implicit and unconscious bias.

We all have our prejudices, including mental health professionals. As Davids (2011) states, "some of us know our racism while others project it […] if at first we cannot find it we probably have not looked hard enough" (p. 43). Our psychoanalytic, psychological and psychiatric theories are inevitably prejudiced to favour the perspective of 'white' European, mostly male practitioners. Early psychoanalytic writings made limited references to the 'primitive' and 'savage' peoples outside of Europe (e.g. Freud, 1914b; Jung, 1930). As mentioned earlier, we cannot think about racism without thinking about white privilege and what is constructed as the norm, and it is incumbent on white therapists to increase their awareness of these blind spots. Although much of contemporary psychoanalytic theory may not be overtly racist, it nevertheless has a prejudiced, European bias, with underlying racist assumptions. Alongside this, it is interesting to note that psychoanalysis itself has been the focus of racist critiques, having been labelled by some as a "Jewish science" (see Frosh, 2005).

Despite growing awareness, we can still observe the consequences and expression of biases and assumptions in contemporary mental health treatment. For example, in the UK, those of African Caribbean descent are more likely to receive a diagnosis of schizophrenia and be detained than their white English counterparts (McLean et al., 2003), because their behaviours are perceived as more problematic, disruptive and dangerous. Furthermore, McLean and colleagues (2003) found that African Caribbean and other minority ethnic groups in the UK are more likely to be prescribed psychiatric drugs, and much less likely to be offered psychotherapies. This may be a dated study, but as the increased awareness around the Black Lives Matter movement has shown, not much has changed. At the time of finalising this chapter, an article in *The Guardian* (Khan, 2020) highlighted this issue of unequal access to psychological therapies for black and ethnic minority patients as well as the biased assumptions therapists can hold about their patients that informed their decision about which issues were significant to explore. The article draws on research that suggests that while only 10% of black and ethnic minority patients felt that their therapists adequately considered their cultural background, 75% of practitioners surveyed considered their practices to be culturally inclusive. There is a clear discrepancy in perceptions here.

It is important to also note that in the UK, black and ethnic minorities are significantly under-represented in the psychological and psychotherapy professions. In clinical psychology trainings in the UK, for example, applicants from black and ethnic minorities are less likely to be selected for training than their white peers (Turpin and Coleman, 2010). Reasons for this include a number of systemic and prejudicial barriers to training (Bawa et al., 2019). In psychoanalytic and psychodynamic trainings in the UK, there is a similar significant under-representation of black and ethnic minority practitioners.

Class is another form of social structure and prejudice that often intersects with race. In many European societies, ethnic minorities are more likely to experience lower socio-economic standards. Psychoanalytic psychotherapy and psychoanalysis have often been criticised for being elitist by catering only to the more privileged classes. Expensive psychotherapy trainings may preclude those with less privileged backgrounds from training in the first place. This is unfortunately the case, particularly as NHS funding cuts have resulted in fewer psychotherapy departments with even less provision for publicly funded psychodynamic psychotherapy. Thus, potential patients wanting to have longer-term psychoanalytic psychotherapy may have little choice but to access private therapy that disadvantages those from less privileged class backgrounds. In the years after the First World War, Freud and his psychoanalytic colleagues advocated for free psychoanalytic clinics (Danto, 2005), recognising the need to make the 'talking cure' accessible to all who needed it. These days, there are a fair number of psychotherapists who reserve a percentage of their time to work at lower rates, or who offer their services at reduced fee psychotherapy clinics. In the UK, there is limited provision of intensive and once weekly individual and group psychotherapy available through the NHS without any charge. It is important for the therapist to reflect on the meaning that a reduced or absent fee may have on the analytic frame, and possible transference and countertransference feelings about fees, value and worth that will need to be explored in light of these unconscious biases.

Patients from less privileged classes may be excluded in other, less explicit ways. For example, in assessing suitable patients for psychotherapy, emphasis is placed on having 'psychological insight' and being 'psychologically minded', namely that patients have some capacity to reflect psychologically on how they may play a part in their current difficulties (Coltart, 1987). A rigid, uncompromising adherence to this view may exclude some disadvantaged, under-educated groups from being considered suitable for psychotherapy. In a similar vein, psychotherapy values the capacity to symbolise and make use of metaphor. This can lead to a bias in perceiving someone with low levels of education as overly concrete and unable to benefit from psychotherapy, when this may not be the case at all.

As with race, class is a social identity that may not be adequately thought about or explored in therapy, and where possible dynamics between therapist and patient may silence some aspects of the patient's experience. Joanna Ryan (2006) conducted an interview-based study of psychotherapists' reports of how class featured in their therapy work with specific patients. She then analysed the data in terms of four possible therapist-patient pairings: 1) working-class therapist and middle-class patient; 2) middle-class therapist and working-class patient; 3) both therapist and patient are working-class, and 4) both are middle-class. Interestingly, she found that class issues were reported in all pairings, except where the therapist and patient were both middle-class. Ryan (2006) interpreted this as reflecting "the taken-for-granted hegemonic nature of middle-class positionings and values within the profession and its discourses" (p. 52), namely that middle-class positions, which are regarded as the 'norm', are not thought about in terms of reflecting identity differences. In this way, *difference* tends to be located in working-class positions, in much the same way as *whiteness* (and its privileges) is often not considered to reflect any identity difference.

Ryan (2006) observed that therapists do report different transference and countertransference dynamics around class. In the first category (working-class therapist with middle-class patient), therapists in Ryan's study described what they regarded as the patient's "contempt, disparagement, and arrogance" (p. 52) in instances where their competence is questioned or their class is directly or indirectly criticised. For some of these working-class therapists, it hooked into their own feelings of inadequacy and shame. Other therapists reported grappling with feelings of envy about their patient's privilege and wealth. In the second category of middle-class therapists and working-class patients, therapists reported struggling at times with feelings of guilt, as well as fearing class-based anger or attack which inhibited them clinically.

Disability and ableism

There are many societal assumptions, myths and misconceptions about disability and people with disabilities (Watermeyer, 2012). These may involve problematic ideas about weakness, damage and dependency, anxieties about vulnerability and mortality, feelings of pity, fear, horror or revulsion, to name just a few. Those with disabilities may be perceived as 'lesser' men and women, since ideas about bodies and attractiveness may challenge some people's notions of masculinity and femininity. People with disabilities may also be assumed to be asexual or have diminished interest in, or capacity for, sexual or romantic intimacy (Rohleder et al., 2019). There is ample evidence to suggest that disability stigma and oppression are significant issues, particularly for people with visible or severe disabilities.

There are many models for understanding 'disability' (outlined in Shakespeare, 2017). A medical model understands disability in terms of physical or psychological impairment; that is people are 'disabled' because they have an impairment. A social model of disability, advocated by the disability rights movement, locates 'disability' in the experience of social and environmental exclusion; that is, a person with an impairment is 'disabled' because they are excluded from full participation in a society typically built for people without disabilities.

Some disability scholars have critiqued the relative exclusion of people with disabilities in the counselling and psychotherapy literature (e.g. Reeve, 2014). Criticisms have also been made that psychotherapy and counselling approaches to disability typically draw on a 'tragedy' or 'loss' model of disability, regarding grief and mourning as a necessary process in psychological adjustment. It is argued that such an approach makes assumptions about the focus of psychotherapy, which may not properly consider the actual experiences of people with disabilities, some of whom may "locate the source of emotional distress in the failure of the environment to take account of their needs", rather than in their bodies (Reeve, 2014, p. 256).

Drawing on psychoanalytic theory, Deborah Marks (1999) refers to disability as an 'embodied relationship' between the physical body, the social and cultural environment and the individual psyche. She notes that "denigration and exclusion [are] the two key forms of psychic oppression suffered by disabled people" (Marks, 1999, p. 25). Such oppressive and prejudiced views about disability may be internalised by people with disabilities, impacting on their self-esteem and self-identity. Sinason (1992), in writing about learning disabilities that she refers to by the outdated term 'handicap', describes the 'secondary handicap' that occurs where a person with disability defends against the emotional pain of being different by attempting to manage the anxiety their disability causes in others by, for example, being submissive, compliant or overly friendly.

Patients with a disability may come for therapy wanting to talk specifically about this stigma and its impact on their self-esteem. Psychotherapy can provide a space to work with issues of self-esteem and self-worth as a result of these social prejudices and internalised oppression (Reeve, 2014; Watermeyer, 2012). Other patients may not refer to their disability much at all, concerned about other aspects of their lives instead. Therapists should also be looking for possible defences of avoidance or denial of an exploration of pain related to the experience of disability. It may be difficult to know what significance the patient places on their experience of disability for their psychic health, with therapists and patient holding differing ideas about the weight to place on their disability.

Therapists who do not have a disability may not always be aware of the ableist views and practices that they implicitly hold. This may be outside the immediate control of the therapist, but nevertheless is not always consciously considered or thought about. For example, our physical surroundings are typically built without holding disability in mind, thereby excluding people with disabilities from accessing facilities. Therapy rooms may be inaccessible to wheelchair users or other patients with mobility difficulties, for example, or they may lack appropriate bathroom facilities. This may arise unexpectedly should the patient, or indeed, the therapist, suddenly acquire a mobility disability during the course of treatment.

Talking about a serious impairment, illness or other disabling experience may be difficult for the patient as well as the therapist, possibly feeling like something disturbing cannot be changed and therefore cannot be thought about. Some illnesses, such as cancer and HIV, can also carry connotations around causality and blame (Sontag, 1991). For the patient, there may be feelings of loss and grief not only in relation to health and mortality, but also with regard to 'social death' as a result of stigma or others' fears about their illness or disability. Disability may be seen as a 'tragedy' which it can represent for some; notwithstanding this, it is important for the therapist to bear in mind that this may not be the patient's understanding.

Working with differences

Thinking about sameness and differences

Whenever we meet someone for the first time, we make assumptions about their identity and background that leads to notions of sameness and difference. This takes place when therapists meet their patients for the first consultation and vice versa, and forms part of the transference and countertransference. We may make assumptions about a person's nationality or culture based on their name or accent. We observe the clothes and jewellery they wear, including whether there is the presence of a wedding band. We notice their way of talking including vocabulary and use of language. We discern their mannerisms and gestures. We inevitably collect these sources of information, and they become cues for us as we consider who this person is and where they come from. This involves assumptions about class, nationality, ethnicity and culture, age, gender and sexuality, political views and so forth. On this basis, we inevitably compare ourselves to them, noting those points of sameness and difference. A good psychodynamic and psychoanalytic training includes observation as a core skill, often with an infant observation at the heart of acquiring this competence. While these perceptions are potentially important sources of information, therapists need to be mindful of what assumptions they make on the basis of these and how to keep them in check.

In Chapter 4, we discussed the importance of maintaining a neutral stance as part of the analytic attitude, and this extends to issues of diversity and difference. When it comes to working with patients from diverging cultural and social contexts to our own, we need to remain equidistant from the values and mores of our own culture as well as those of our patients. Some differences cannot be neutralised or erased (such as the colour of our skin, age or gender). Cultural neutrality coexists with ethnic differences, without becoming biased or prejudiced.

When a patient comes from a cultural or social context that differs significantly to our own, we may feel anxious about not being able to understand or relate to them. For example, the therapist may come from a Western cultural context that gives prominence to ideas of independence and individualism of the self. Furthermore, psychoanalytic theories have evolved largely in a Western context where such values are emphasised. A patient may come from a cultural context with a far more relational view of the self that cannot be thought of as separate to the familial and group network, as is evident in many Eastern and African cultures. Hofstede (1984) refers to these as cultural dimensions of individualism versus collectivism. Thus, the unit of identity is not an individual internal identity, but rather a collective identity involving family and community. These notions of the self and what it means to be a person or individual should be considered when arriving at a formulation of the patient's difficulties. Therapists need to take care not to impose their own values and ideas about identity on to their patients.

Part of the process of reflectiveness fostered through personal therapy and close supervision ensures that therapists continue to pay attention to their potential blind spots. For example, the therapist may focus on a perceived difference and assume that it is mutually experienced (such as the therapist and patient having differing racialised identities) and may not consider other aspects of difference that are preoccupying the patient (such as religion). There may be an assumption of sameness when both therapist and patient have aligned identities (e.g. both identify as gay) that may block the opportunity to explore the patient's unique experience. Where there is assumed sameness, the therapist may be pulled into a collusive dyad where a blind eye is turned to overtly shared areas of experience. Similarly, there may be assumptions around areas of differences that lead the therapist to shut down exploration because they feel they cannot properly understand the internal world and experience of the patient. There is an element of truth to this; of course, we cannot truly understand what it is like to live with an identity that we don't hold. However, this does not preclude us from empathically understanding some of that person's lived experiences. Otherwise, this leads to the conclusion that we can only be helped by someone who has had the identical experience we have had. It is important to explore assumptions of sameness and difference in sessions as they arise. This is all grist for the analytic mill, so to speak.

Maintaining an analytic attitude involves adopting a curious, not-knowing stance, as we discussed previously in relation to the analytic setting as well as mentalising techniques. This allows us to learn from our patients and gain a better understand of their subjective experiences, including their cultural and social contexts. The patient is likely to be anxious about the therapist not understanding them or being able to relate to their experience. We would explore this throughout the course of therapy, including how it plays out in the transference and countertransference. Maintaining a 'not knowing' stance is particularly important when the therapist and patient come from apparently similar cultural and social contexts. The mind of an other is opaque and we would not want to fall into the *psychic equivalence* trap (see Chapter 7) of great certainty about our patients' experiences.

When considering perceived differences, therapists may feel inhibited in commenting or offering an interpretation for fear of enacting some difference or saying something perceived as inappropriate or offensive (Ryan, 2006). This inhibition and silence may lead to stuckness in therapy, where projections and emotions about difference and inequality become unable to be faced and worked through. This anxiety may arise partly because we tend to consider identity differences of race, age, gender, religion and so forth as 'extra' variables that need to be held in mind. However, these are not additions but rather essential components of all our subjective and interrelational experiences. We live these differences every day, so it should not be seen as surplus to the regular work of psychotherapy.

As Davids (2011) reminds us, we all hold prejudices and have inescapable blind spots. As therapists, we need to be as aware as possible of our own prejudices. In exploring the internal worlds of our patients who are likely to have different social and cultural backgrounds to our own, we typically focus in psychodynamic psychotherapy on their intrapsychic dynamics, internal conflicts and internalised object relations. However, our mental representations are formed within a wider social, political and historical context, and this history suffuses the transference dynamic between therapist and patient.

We often think of biases in terms of prejudiced, negative biases. But we may also have biases towards people that we consider to hold abhorrent views that lie in opposition to our own. For example, if you have political views that could be classified as left-wing, would you feel able to work with a patient who holds strong far-right, nationalist views? If you are anti-abortion, could you work with someone who is pro-choice? While we strive to be neutral and non-judgmental, it would be idealistic to claim we could work with absolutely any patient group. It is important to be informed by your own biases and views that may interfere with your ability to deliver therapy to particular patients, and to act accordingly. We would encourage you to explore these strong feelings through supervision and your own psychotherapy before acting overly hastily and risking enacting an aspect of your and/or the patient's dynamics.

Patient preferences

A patient may deliberately seek out a therapist with certain characteristics or identity, either seeking sameness or difference in the therapist. These may be conscious choices, but of course, are often unconscious. For some, this may involve fantasies and assumptions about expertise and status. For example, a patient may express reservations about seeing a 'black' therapist, perceiving them not to be 'as good' as a 'white' therapist (Tummala-Narra, 2007).

Patients from some cultures may have a deferential attitude towards the therapist as the all-knowing 'doctor', expecting the therapist to advise them about their problems. Part of entering into therapy may be bringing these different, culturally informed expectations out into the open so that they can be explored and understood. This forms part of the scaffolding of building a therapeutic alliance and acculturating our patients to this very unique type of relationship in psychodynamic psychotherapy.

Some patients accessing private psychotherapy may make the choice to see a therapist of a certain demographic. For example, a straight female patient may seek a male patient because they have the thought that there is something that can be worked through in their relationships with men. Or, a man may seek a male therapist because they hope it will help address their difficult relationship with their father. A gay or lesbian patient may actively seek a therapist who is out as gay or lesbian, with the assumption that this will ensure an affirmative therapy. Many times, patients do not make such conscious choices, but it is always interesting to explore what drew them to come and see a particular therapist. There is probably some unconscious dynamic informing their choice.

In some cases, there may be a need to match patients with certain therapists, for example, where language barriers are an issue, it may be important to refer the patient to a therapist who speaks the same language fluently. An assessor may also take into consideration not referring a patient who has experienced a recent sexual assault to a therapist of the same gender as the perpetrator, as this may trigger further trauma. In all cases, the meanings of patients' choices and preferences for particular therapists are not only fruitful areas of exploration, but should also be respected in terms of the patients' right to receive the care they need.

Addressing an actual experience

A patient may come to a session reporting an experience that occurred outside the therapy room, for example a racist, sexist, homophobic, transphobic or ableist experience. In psychodynamic psychotherapy, we are usually concerned with the internal world of the patient. Indeed, Davids (2011) describes such an attack as a psychic assault, evocatively conveying how a hate attack causes the person to be forcefully tossed "into an arid area of non-being from which he has, somehow, to gather together once more the now-fractured strands of his being" (p. 3). However, in such cases, it is important to acknowledge the emotional impact of their actual experience, before attempting to explore the meaning of that experience. The assault is a trauma, and someone cannot enter into a reflective mental space while they are traumatised. The painfulness of the experience needs to be empathically addressed, before attempting to explore further links with the patient's internal world, if indeed there are any to be made. A therapist who moves too quickly in trying to make links with an internalised sense of oppression, for example, may be quite rightly perceived as minimizing the reality and significance of the assault that has occurred. This may involve the therapist stepping slightly away from their usual neutral stance to acknowledge the traumatic reality of the incident. The therapist could say, for example, "What happened sounds awful and unacceptable, and I can hear how traumatic it was for you". It may be that the patient relays an incident but seems to downplay its importance. Rather than collude with the denial of its significance, the therapist may consider saying, "I have listened to what you have described and it sounds awful and unacceptable, and I wonder whether you are protecting yourself from really feeling the full impact of it?"

Therapists themselves may have had traumatic experiences that cannot be denied. We have made numerous references to the neutral stance of the psychodynamic psychotherapist. However, given that some differences cannot be neutralised, the psychotherapist cannot always maintain a neutral stance and keep 'politics' out of the therapy room in moments of trauma, as some black psychologists, psychotherapists and counsellors have reflected on following the murder of George Floyd and the Black Lives Matter protests (e.g. Turner, see Box 13.1).

Using personal therapy and supervision

Therapists may explore and understand their own internal prejudices and blind spots in their personal therapy. An essential part of being a competent and reflective psychodynamic therapist is to be cognisant of your prejudices, not to ignore them. As Davids (2011) states, if you feel you do not have any sort of prejudice or bias, then you probably have not looked hard enough!

Supervision is an important space to think about diversity and difference from the perspective of the transference and countertransference. However, some therapists, in particular trainees and newly qualified therapists may feel cautious about raising countertransference thoughts and feelings that they perceive as 'problematic', for fear of being perceived by the supervisor as not-good-enough, incapable or of being judged. This can occur in a parallel process, where issues around diversity in the consulting room find their way into the supervisory relationship. A female therapist may experience difficulty in describing her feelings of attraction towards a female patient with a supervisor, for example.

Diversity and difference exist in the supervisor-supervisee relationship too. As Richards (2020) points out, writing from the perspective of sexual orientation, issues of sameness and difference may not always be adequately raised or explored in supervision, and perceived issues of sameness and difference may inhibit what the supervisee and supervisor comment on. Supervisees may feel reluctant to reveal uncomfortable countertransferences they may be grappling with, for fear of offending the supervisor whom they perceive to have similar characteristics to their patient.

Working with diversity and difference can feel like tricky terrain. The therapist who rushes in to highlight and explore difference may be at risk of 'othering' the patient. 'Othering' refers to the process of attributing characteristics onto an individual in a manner that sets them apart as representing something opposite to them (Rohleder, 2014). By pointing out the differences, the therapist is pointing a finger at the patient. At the other extreme, ignoring difference leads to silencing the patient. Care needs to be taken to create a safe space where difference can be named and explored as it emerges in the transference and countertransference. This again indicates the value of supervision in helping the therapist through this.

Box 13.1 Useful resources

Readings

We recommend the following books that cover some of the topics covered in this chapter:

Davids, M. F. (2011). *Internal racism: A psychoanalytic approach to race and difference*. Basingstoke: Palgrave Macmillan.
Ryan, J. (2017). *Class and psychoanalysis: Landscapes of inequality*. Abingdon: Routledge.
Hertzmann, L. and Newbigin, J. (2020). *Sexuality and gender now: Moving beyond heteronormativity*. Abingdon: Routledge.

Online resources

The Memorandum of Understanding on Conversion Therapy in the UK, signed by various UK professional bodies, is available online at: www.bpc.org.uk/sites/psychoanalytic-council.org/files/MoU2_FINAL_0.pdf
We mentioned this newspaper article in the chapter which reports on black and ethnic minority patients' experiences of therapy in the UK: Khan, C. (2020, 10 February). 'I thought I was a lost cause': How therapy is failing people of colour. The Guardian. Available from: www.theguardian.com/lifeandstyle/2020/feb/10/therapy-failing-bme-patients-mental-health-counselling
Dr Dwight Turner, a psychotherapist and academic in the UK reflects on his experience of being a black male psychotherapist in this powerful blog: http://www.bmevoices.co.uk/black-steel-in-the-hour-of-chaos/.
The website Race Reflections, founded by Guilaine Kinouani, is an online community engaging with issues of inequality, oppression and injustice. It has a closed membership with subscription for the community discussion aspects; the website features a number of useful resources and links to other websites: www.racereflections.co.uk
Project Implicit (website: https://implicit.harvard.edu/implicit/aboutus.html), led by scientists from Harvard University, University of Virginia and University

of Washington, has a number of implicit association tests that you are able to take (you need to register on their website), with the goal of seeing the potential hidden biases that you may have. Different tests look at topics such as race, gender, and sexual orientation. Some readers may be uncomfortable at the thought of doing this, or the suggestion at being prejudiced. We do so in the recognition that we are all embedded in a social and cultural context in which some prejudice is inevitable.

14 Technology and social media

We live in a world that is speeding up, where messages are sent in the swipe of a finger and information discovered in seconds. Indeed, there has been a humorous digital revision of Maslow's (1943) hierarchy of needs that introduces 'WiFi' followed by 'Battery' at the base of the triangle, below physiological survival needs of food, air, shelter and so on (Figure 14.1).

All this poses challenges to psychodynamic psychotherapy with its limits on gratification and emphasis on deliberate, careful exploration. The instrument of communication in psychotherapy is most often the word, by which we mean analysing both the verbal and non-verbal language of the therapist-patient relationship (Etchegoyen 1991). Despite technological advances in communication, what goes on in the consulting room remains largely unchanged since Freud pioneered the approach over a century ago. Balick (2018) underlines that "the *optimal* condition for a traditional psychotherapeutic space is that it lacks modern

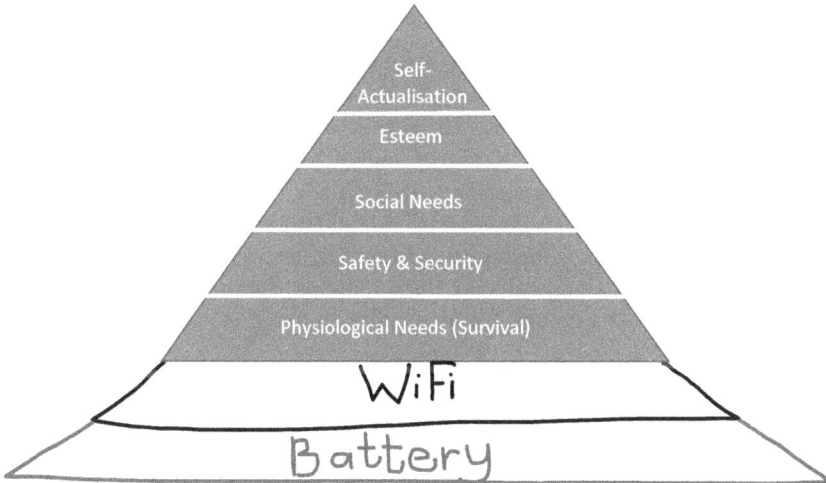

Figure 14.1 Updated Maslow's (1943) hierarchy of needs
Source: Adapted from *The Poke*: www.thepoke.co.uk/2016/02/15/maslows-hierarchy-needs-updated-2016/

technology completely, and is all the better for it" (p. 23). Notwithstanding this, we can't avoid the impact of technology in and outside the consulting room. Recent events with the Covid-19 pandemic have meant that we have been forced to engage with technology in order to continue working with patients through this time of social distancing and lockdown. These developments have made this chapter even more relevant to our profession. More than ever, we need to find ways to approach technology from a psychodynamic perspective, including our own use of technology to support the delivery of treatment as well as the ways our patients engage with technology and social media. Lemma (2017) writes that engagement with this area is essential: "communication technologies ought to be of great interest to contemporary psychoanalytic practitioners" (p. 8) and "[i]t is incumbent on us as therapists to be receptive to the possibility that technological developments can be used to support psychic development as much as they can be used to foreclose experience" (p. 8).

Technology and the internet have fed the illusion that we can know all and that nothing is off limits. Cohen (2013) writes about this disavowal of the realm of privacy in today's world of exhibitionism and voyeurism in his book, *The Private Life: Why We Remain in the Dark*. He reminds us of the inscrutability of the unconscious: "a region of yourself that even you can't enter freely, as private to yourself as to others, locked, alarmed, watched over by dangerous guard dogs of one kind or another" (2013, p. 80). He goes on to point to the paradox that Freud identified in his 1915 essay, 'The Unconscious', that our inner lives are more accessible to others than ourselves, and that we can't know our true selves until we acknowledge that this is largely outside our own awareness and if anything, belongs to someone else: "However hard you try to bring it to light, something always remains in the dark." (Cohen, 2013, p. 90). Psychoanalytic theories of the structural and topographical models of the mind, defence mechanisms and resistance, repetition compulsions and transference enactments provide a context for inevitable conflicts around privacy and insight that technology gives rise to. In thinking about the impact of technology on the psychotherapy setting, we want to acknowledge that this final chapter should be read in the context of the rest of the book and we don't want to pretend that we can ever provide conditions for perfect privacy or unassailable boundaries in psychotherapy; rather it is about our continued efforts to understand and interpret these events. Some psychoanalytic writers have begun to consider the impact of technology and the digital age on development, with the focus ranging from topics such as IVF, the Internet as a play space in child analysis (Chung and Colarusso, 2012), on-line pornography and sexual desire (Wood, 2011), social connectivity and gender identity.

In this chapter, we will think about the therapist's own online presence and how to apply the analytic frame to this area of modern life. We will also consider aspects of the frame in relation to our patients' use of technology to contact us between sessions by email, phone or text, and how to set up the parameters of our practice in relation to technology. Finally, we consider the ways of offering psychodynamic psychotherapy remotely through online platforms and telephone and what we need to bear in mind when working in these altered ways. We will make links to the relevant aspects of the set of competences developed by the British Association for Counselling and Psychotherapy (2020) for telephone and e-counselling.

The therapist's online presence

Zur et al. (2009) state that "the Internet blurs the line between what is personal and what is professional, as well as between self-disclosure and transparency. With the click of a mouse, most psychotherapists' personal lives can be easily viewed" (p. 24). Our traditional notions of anonymity are fast becoming archaic. We have to embrace how we manage this unavoidable self-disclosure rather than pretend it isn't happening. We have a growing online presence, the full extent of which we may not always be aware. It is becoming increasingly likely that this digital presence will pre-date aspiring therapists' decision to train in this field and most likely cannot be erased once it has entered cyberspace. While we should all take care to protect our online identities, as therapists it is incumbent on us to be even more vigilant about our online presence and privacy settings. We need to be mindful of the amount of information we put online in the service of protecting analytic neutrality and facilitating the development of the patient's transference without too much interference from external reality. Interestingly, this aspect of managing the therapist's boundaries is not one of the British Association for Counselling and Psychotherapy identified competences, yet we feel that this awareness is increasingly important in our digital age.

Consider your privacy settings on social media platforms, such as Facebook and Instagram as well as your professional presence on sites such as LinkedIn and Twitter. It can be easy to lose track of the digital footprint we leave behind; after all can you remember what you posted on social media ten years ago? Zur et al. (2009) warn therapists that "all their online postings, blogs or chats may be viewed by their clients and will stay online, in some form, forever" (p. 25). It is best to maintain a boundary between what is personal and private on the one hand, and what is professional and public on the other. When using Twitter, for example, therapists are better doing so in their professional capacity rather than posting their personal views and they should be mindful that their audience can include present, past and future patients.

It is accepted that many patients will google their therapists, particularly when deciding on which therapist to approach for help, in much the same way they conduct research for other purchases and important decisions. A key aspect of the analytic frame is therapeutic anonymity, namely the so-called blank slate clinician onto whom the patient can project their conflicts and fantasies. However, as we have shown, this is an impossible ideal because we can never truly be anonymous. We do, after all, convey all kinds of things in person through our dress, consulting room décor and accent while our social and professional lives probably include some public elements. We may serve on boards or committees in our community or be affiliated to a church, mosque or synagogue. We may have published papers in journals or spoken at conferences. Our previous professions may have had significant public profiles. Our online presence can reveal considerable information about us. For example, a LinkedIn profile often includes details of your qualifications including year and place, which in turn provides clues about your age and background. Your online connections probably reflect your particular interests. On Twitter, we may knowingly or unknowingly reveal our political views, the newspapers we read and our wider interests. You may make a conscious choice to be associated with particular causes or to demonstrate your support for psychological issues that you focus on in your practice.

If we are not careful about our privacy settings on platforms like Facebook, photos of ourselves could be available to be found by our patients. This includes being tagged in family and friends' photos, particularly when they may not have the same security settings as us. We may also not be aware of which social media networks we share with patients, as the following example illustrates.

> *Nassim came to a session and reported that they had seen my name pop up on Facebook as a suggested friend request, because, unbeknownst to both of us, we had a shared Facebook friend. My Facebook profile was set to private so they could not see my profile, and Nassim did not act on the suggestion to send a request to connect, but nevertheless an unexpected connection was brought to both of our awareness by the online platform we shared. We were able to discuss what that meant to them and the fantasies it raised about my private life as well as address their concerns about boundaries and confidentiality.*

In smaller psychoanalytic communities around the world, this level of overlap of psychotherapists and patients' lives is inevitable and, in some ways, they are all better placed to deal with this level of transparency from the outset as compared to larger cities where anonymity seems guaranteed. However, as the above example illustrates, there are times when we may not be aware of how our lives intersect with our patients.

We do not intend to suggest that therapists need to be paranoid, or that all patients stalk their therapists, but research suggests that many patients do, reasonably, at least look online to find out about their therapists and their expertise as part of the consumer culture we live in (Eichenberg and Sawyer, 2016, Zur et al., 2009), and in doing so, various online information about therapists is likely to crop up. Patients can search for information about their therapists in a variety of ways from visiting the therapist's professional websites, to carrying out an Internet search, searching for therapists through social networks, joining professional chatrooms, paying someone to conduct an online background check to the more extreme end of cyberstalking, illegal and invasive online searches (Zur et al., 2009). Patients have been known to even go so far as to assume false identities in order to gain access to greater levels of data.

The mirror experience of online googling is "patient-targeted googling", a term coined by Clinton et al., (2010) for the practice of psychotherapists looking up information about their patients online. We are ethically bound to respect our patients' right to privacy and as such need to keep any intrusions on privacy to a minimum. A therapist should be mindful as to why they feel a need to google a patient. Is this curiosity a function of the countertransference and a pull to be drawn into a prurient position of voyeurism, perhaps in response to the patient's own exhibitionism? Does the therapist have patient consent for this type of online activity? Is the therapist concerned about the legitimacy of what the patient is presenting to them and wants to fact-check this? Do they need to get contact information for the patient, perhaps in connection with an unpaid bill? Do they have concerns about danger to the patient and/or others? And if so, how factually truthful is the information that is found online? If something significant is found, what is to be done with that information? A study by Eichenberg and Hertzberg (2016) into patient-targeted googling in Germany found that over a third of surveyed therapists had looked for patient information online and that psychodynamic therapists are less likely to sanction online searching than other therapeutic modalities. We have to weigh up the potential damage that online patient searches will have to the therapeutic alliance as well as the way it will interfere with our own countertransference, thereby muddying the water for unconscious processes to be communicated and understood. However curious we may feel, the rules of abstinence that apply to the analytic frame should inhibit our curiosity from being enacted rather than considered.

We suggest that you regularly search for your name (in various combinations including with key words) to understand what can be found out about you online. You can use Google alerts (www.google.com/alerts>hl) to be notified when new Internet content about you becomes available. Therapists do need to reflect on what information is available about them online, including making choices about what to reveal on social media. This includes checking the online settings for any of your social media platforms to ensure you have the highest level of security. Even then, you will also need to explain this to friends and family who, with their less stringent privacy settings, may be a gateway to information about you. Some therapists opt to use nicknames, pseudonyms or a different surname to their professional identity to keep their online presence separate and confidential.

You should also consider your wider privacy and safety online. Is your home address hidden from searches? Have you taken your name off the public electoral roll? Have you included a mobile phone number on your website? If so, is this a dedicated work number or a line you use for both personal and professional use? Without realising it, you may find yourself answering a work call outside of hours when you are caught off-guard. It is worth letting unrecognised numbers go directly to voice mail rather than finding yourself explaining to a prospective patient that you are unable to speak to them on the weekend – after all, you did answer the phone! You can make it clear on your website that you are available during office hours, or you can specify a time period in the week when you can speak to prospective patients. It is important to be consistent with this when replying to any other patient communications outside session time, including text messages and emails. Unless you have the option of electing a time when your email will send, we suggest it is best to leave these in draft form for the morning, rather than be tempted to hit send late at night or over the weekend. Ideally, it is best to restrict communication to session time so that these communications take place within the analytic setting.

Some therapists have clear social media guidelines and policies, such as the International Society for Mental Health Online (2000) and Kolmes' (2013) on-line resource of Internet policies for her private practice. The therapist, in laying out the terms and conditions of the work, may state that they do make use of social media, but will not accept requests to connect via these platforms, thereby limiting the therapist-patient communication to formal channels (which may or may not include email or text). Thus, they would not accept requests to connect on LinkedIn or other platforms. We have included an example of a social media contract that some readers may find useful in Appendix 4 although we do acknowledge that the existence of a contract does not exclude this form of tech-nological acting out. Indeed, some psychotherapists are reluctant to introduce unnecessary prohibitions on the analytic frame that may invite acting out and interfere with patient liberty. Rather than providing overly explicit instructions or contracts, a psychodynamic approach would be to consider any patient's acting out in relation to technology (or otherwise) as material to be understood.

Certain social media platforms may be more difficult to ensure that therapists are not connected to their patients. For example, with Twitter you may not be able to control who follows you. Therapists can choose to set their Twitter to private mode, so that their tweets are not visible, and users have to request to follow them. There are available options to block specific users from following you, but the therapist does need to consider what message this sends a patient who may be following you. Blocking particular people also requires you to list their names. This is a more active step that needs careful thought and justifica-tion since it does reveal patient confidentiality by making this report. If you have a patient you feel is unable to adhere to the usual therapeutic boundaries, it may raise the question of their suitability overall for psychodynamic work. It does flag the matter of therapist safety, something that is paramount for therapy to continue effectively.

The British Psychological Society (2012) has published guidelines for therapists on professionalism and social media. The guidelines cover issues of professional-ism in relation to communicating with existing or previous patients on social media, much of which is covered in this chapter. Another key area of guidance addresses patient confidentiality. It goes without saying that therapists are expec-ted not to post details of patients they work with online, however, research has shown that therapists may describe casework in blogposts with sufficient detail to allow patients to be potentially identifiable, as found for example, by Lagu et al., (2008) in their analysis of medical blogposts written by nurses and physicians. The British Psychological Society guidelines go on to warn that even where thera-pists think their posts are private (such as in Facebook) a written comment nevertheless leaves a digital trace and may be viewed or forwarded to someone else. A further key area considered by the guidelines is the nature of personal material made available on social media, particularly whether it is appropriate professional conduct, for example, to have photos or video clips of therapists engaging in inappropriate or problematic behaviour. What is posted may not be grounds to question the therapist's professional conduct (e.g. being drunk at a private party), but it could create feelings of mistrust in the patient or even colleagues and employers. The therapist needs to be mindful about anything that may blur the boundary between their private and professional lives.

There are those Luddites and puritans who take the position that the only way to be safe online is to have no digital presence whatsoever. However, this is increasingly impossible and not always desirable. It is helpful to remember that in the past, people were resistant to the introduction of telephone answering machines, now obsolete! Many therapists were *digital immigrants* who moved into the world of technology, as opposed to *digital natives* who grew up in this milieu (Prensky, 2001) and so we have to reconstruct our online lives with care as we enter the field of psychotherapy. Analytic supervisors and seminar leaders are often less technologically aware than their supervisees and trainees, an inverse experience that many families now face with children being more tech-savvy than their parents. This is an area that is often ignored in psychotherapy trainings, leaving therapists to work this out themselves. Indeed, digital natives will need support in examining their online activity and rethinking what may have felt automatic through the lens of becoming a psychotherapist (Zur et al., 2009). Hopefully, this will start to change as recognition is given to this crucial aspect of the analytic frame in psychotherapy trainings going forward.

Privacy, confidentiality and data protection

We were all too familiar with the barrage of emails from companies requesting permission to use our personal data as part of their mailing lists when the EU's *General Data Protection Regulation* (GDPR) was legislated on 25 May 2018. This was one of the most wide-reaching changes to data privacy regulation that was intended for the digital era and has implications for therapists working in the field of mental health. According to GDPR regulations, all psychotherapists are probably *Data Controllers* by virtue of processing personal information for their patients, then using that information in particular ways (such as preparing invoices or writing patient notes), and carrying out this processing as part of a treatment contract, exercising professional judgement when processing that data, having a direct relationship with their patients who are the subjects of that data and having autonomy as to how they process that data. Being a *Data Controller* comes with stringent data protection obligations.

The Information Commissioners Office (ICO) is the UK's independent authority established to uphold information rights in the public interest, including transparency of public bodies and data privacy for individuals. Controllers shoulder the highest level of compliance responsibility, having to demonstrate concurrence with all the data protection principles as well as other GDPR requirements. You are also responsible for the compliance of your processor(s), namely anyone appointed to process data on your behalf, like an administrator, receptionist or accountant. Controllers in the UK must register with the ICO (www.ico.org.uk) and pay the data protection fee, unless they are exempt. If you are outside the UK, it is worth identifying whether you have to register with a similar type of agency. The ICO website contains useful information about how you need to keep patient information safe.

The GDPR legislation obligates us to:

a   Maintain an internal record of all processing activity;
b   Record the purpose of the processing;
c   Keep a description of the technological or organisational measures to ensure a level of security.

We are required to have clear consent from our patients to process their personal data for the specific purposes we have set out, for example, to contact them if you have to change their appointment time or to write to their GP to advise they have commenced treatment. Any concerns about the safety of your patient will override considerations of data security, however, it is still important to share only the absolute minimum amount of data necessary.

Patients have the right to be informed about the collection and use of their data. They should be notified of the purpose of the data collection, retention periods, the lawful basis for that processing and with whom the data will be shared. This can be done via a privacy notice, worded in clear and plain language (we have included an example in Appendix 5), which therapists can upload onto their practice websites. Patients can withdraw consent at any point. Again, the only exception to this consent is a safeguarding concern where the legal obligation to keep the patient or someone else safe overrides data protection. Patients can request to access their data, with therapists required to respond to those requests within 40 calendar days. This has a bearing on the type of clinical notes you keep. Increasingly, we need to think about writing notes that the patient could read. It is possible to redact certain information if you felt that reading this would be harmful to the patient. Consider also how you keep notes about your patients – are these typed or hand-written on a tablet or in a notebook? Paper notes need to be locked away securely while electronic notes can be password protected.

The patient also has a right to be forgotten. This means that all records should be destroyed once you have completed working with a patient or in the event that they drop out of treatment. If a patient does not want you to have any contact with their GP, for example, you will need to consider the risks attached to this and whether you feel able to continue seeing a patient in your private practice without that support. Box 14.1 has a list of useful prompts to apply these principles to your clinical practice.

Box 14.1 Some aspects of GDPR to consider for your practice:

- Do you keep all patient information under password or lock?
- Do you have a locked filing cabinet?
- Is your computer, laptop, iPad or mobile phone password protected?

- If you transfer files to anyone, do you encrypt and password protect them as well as sending the password by separate email?
- Do you have a privacy notice on your website or in your contract with patients? It is important to let your patients know how you will be using their personal data and the purpose of it.
- How long do you keep patient records for?
- Do you shred confidential information and dispose of it safely?

When working remotely with patients, we also have to consider the way confidentiality of the setting is now the shared responsibility for both patient and therapist to ensure. The ability to discuss issues relating to confidentiality and data protection is another British Association for Counselling and Psychotherapy (2020, p. 11) competence for remote working and includes the following aspects:

- Helping patients maintain and protect their confidentiality and data security when using their own equipment;
- Negotiating to ensure that any therapeutic records are kept confidential;
- Discussing how patient data will be protected, for example through encryption;
- Discussing limits of confidentiality, for example, making patients aware if you will be discussing anonymised clinical material with a supervisor;

To this we would add regularly updating virus protection and software, using an encrypted platform that offers a secure way of carrying out therapy, encouraging patients to use headphones to allow a greater degree of confidentiality during sessions, ensuring you have a reliable Internet service and a charger for your phone or laptop if needed. Just as with the revised hierarchy of needs, we cannot carry out this way of working unless we have WiFi and battery. The WiFi you have can be improved by signing up for a speedier broadband, by upgrading your router to a newer model and/or by using a WiFi extender where you are not plugging your computer directly into the router.

Patient's use of technology in the setting and the transference

Technological advances like texting and emails are an inevitable part of clinical practice today and present new challenges to the analytic frame, providing patients with direct access to psychotherapists in ways that were not previously possible and that produce considerable pressure on us to respond. We are interested in the way the patient uses technology and whether it is being used in a healthy way to promote object relatedness and separation, or whether technology is employed in fixed, pathogenic ways that constrict object-relating, defend against anxiety and provide concrete gratification. There isn't just one way of understanding the meaning of these technological manifestations of the transference, rather they need to be understood within the context of the therapy and the patient's development. One patient may be understood as pushing boundaries and being intrusive in sending the therapist an online friend request, while another may be considered to be expressing a wish for closer connections.

The British Association for Counselling and Psychotherapy (2020, p. 11) competences include the ability to establish "ground rules" and boundaries for telephone and e-counselling. These include:

- Therapist's availability and the limits around that (for example, not being available after hours or on weekends);
- Length of therapy sessions, perhaps having some flexibility if the patient finds it difficult to use the full fifty minutes;
- Where relevant, how many messages the patient can send the therapist and how quickly the therapist will respond to those messages;
- The importance of routinely acknowledging messages sent between therapist and patient;
- No online communication between therapist and patient outside the agreed therapeutic contact.

Some therapists have dedicated mobile phones for patients and only take text messages to avoid intrusions when working while others ask patients to leave voice messages if they cannot answer the call. If you do have a mobile phone for your work (rather than a landline or reception service), then you need to give some thought as to how you want your patients to use it. If you do accept text messages from patients, you also need to consider how you intend to respond to those messages. On the whole, it is advisable to keep extra-therapy communication to a minimum and it is best to avoid making any form of interpretation by text, email or letter when you don't know how it will be received. In keeping with this principle, it is acceptable to acknowledge that you have received the patient's message without elaborating further, for example by saying you will see them next week or wishing them well. A rule of thumb is that any message that can't be answered in a simple, straightforward way will need to be discussed during the session. If we do want to make contact with patients after a missed session, it is important to word what we say carefully in order to avoid sounding overly critical or complacent. Nina Coltart (1993, p. 60) gives this example of how she deals with patients who miss an assessment appointment by calling them:

NC: 'Is that Mr/Mrs X?'
P: 'Yes, speaking.'
NC: 'This is Dr Coltart here.'
P: 'Oh *hallo*! How are you?'
NC: 'I'm fine, thank you. How are you?'
P: 'Oh, keeping well – yes, thanks.'
NC: 'I was wondering where you were.'
P: 'Er – were you? Um – well – oh, heavens! What's the date? Oh my God, its not – the eighteenth. I'm meant to be seeing you …'

NC: 'Yes' (This response is cool, but at the same time rooted in interest, though not overdone).

While this is somewhat dated in that she writes about calling the patient on their home landline whereas nowadays we are more likely to phone on their mobile phone, it is worth noting the tightrope she describes walking between being firm yet interested in the meaning of this omission without becoming punitive.

In its most benign form, text messages serve to hold the therapist in mind at times of absence, facilitate reality-testing and assist with emerging independence. However, the use of technology can take on more fixed qualities that disavow the reality of separateness rather than allowing it to be borne. The way our patients interact with technology will inevitably be coloured by their own mental health difficulties, with the meaning differing moment to moment. We are encouraged to be curious about the particular meaning it has for our patients, both conscious and unconscious including how its use illuminates possible resistance to therapy. It is helpful to generalise existing psychoanalytic concepts into the new digital age. For example, 'pocket dial' and 'pocket text' (that is, unintentional calls or messages sent from mobile phones) can be thought of as technological parapraxes that may reveal unconscious material.

We can conceptualise the way our patients use the Internet, emails and texts as transitional phenomena to manage the frustration of absence and start accepting reality without the illusion of having magical control over the object (in this case the psychotherapist). However, for those patients with a persecutory internal world who have probably suffered environmental deprivation or abuse, the use of technology can take on a different function. Patients may defend against their claustrophobic-agoraphobic anxieties by creating an illusion of merger with the object while at other times, their use of technology functions to create distance and prevent the feared union. The following clinical example illustrates these issues:

> *My patient, Maya often sent texts to tell me she was running late. It left me wondering about her need to keep me in the picture and how she might experience me as critical of her lack of punctuality. I wondered if her texts about her lateness functioned to rid herself of guilt and fear at my anticipated reprisal as if she were trying to control me and deny her dependency. The physical act of texting itself may have soothed her in the face of out-of-control delays at the mercy of public transport and traffic.*
>
> *At times, Maya complained about how a friend tracked her movements through texts, yet his controlling behaviour felt like proof to her that he cared, in sharp contrast to her mother's self-absorbed behaviour. I took up the way Maya tried to control me through her texts while at the same time wanting to hold on to feeling she was cared for by me. She used texts to bridge her journey to therapy, conveying the illusion of closeness in my absence. During these transitions, Maya would reach out to fix me en route to her sessions.*
>
> *It seemed to me that her texts represented a concrete expression of her wish for a caring object who worries about her whereabouts. She sent her text to find me and stimulate me to think about her, something she couldn't trust would happen without her prompt. Her anxiety*

was then displaced on to me as her therapist, such that I became the object consumed with worry which she then has the power to relieve.

On another occasion, I received a fragmented text following a cycling accident that seemed to convey her disjointed state of mind. It communicated her distress that went beyond words, spelling and punctuation. When I explored it with her, Maya was unaware that she had messaged me. It was important to bring these extra-therapeutic communications back into the consulting room so they could be thought about, in the same way we would want to bring psychoanalytic thinking to bear on all acting out in the therapy setting.

As mentioned earlier, patients will be curious about their therapists. We are better equipped to explore our patients' curiosity when we encounter it in the consulting room. However, as we have seen, it can find expression through acting out between sessions, via Internet, email and text and these require interpretation. Being curious about what goes on in one's psychotherapist's life outside the constraints of the consulting room, can be construed as a variant of the primal scene and the wish to intrude beyond the proverbial bedroom door into areas outside the analytic relationship, including the psychotherapist's private life and professional world including published works. As Lemma (2017) puts it:

In this new technological context childish curiosity about what goes on in the parental/analyst's bedroom can quickly escalate into a perverse intrusion into it and, if unexamined, can undermine the analytic process, on occasions making it unviable. (pp. 120–121)

The intrusion of external reality can really interfere with the transference and this is part of the reason why we aim to hold a neutral analytic stance. While therapists are not always aware of these secret intrusions, slips occur occasionally in the technological field. Here are two clinical examples that illustrate this:

Brandon once sent me a Facebook friend request, apparently unaware that he had done so and when I brought it to his attention, it was far more shaming to him than a dream might be; it betrayed his curiosity together with his longing for more contact with me in the external world.

Wynne sent me a request to follow me on LinkedIn shortly after we concluded working together. I elected to write back to her, advising that while I received this request, it is not my policy to connect with patients in this way. I explained that this is as much to protect their confidentiality as my own need for appropriate boundaries. I said I would be happy to offer her a review appointment, in this way addressing her covert wish to remain in contact with me. We can understand her request as the patient's resistance to concluding the work together, wishing to remain in contact in some form or possibly, to subvert the patient-therapist relationship by converting me into a professional contact of hers.

Online communication: emails and texts

Letters (dubbed "snail-mail" by Bhuvaneswar and Gutheil, 2008, p. 243) are fast becoming obsolete now that many therapists communicate with their patients by email and possibly text. However, responding to electronic communication brings with it an urgency that is at odds with the reflective thoughtfulness of the psycho-dynamic stance. If we get caught up in the urgency of these requests and respond too quickly, we can circumvent exploring and understanding what is going on. Emails and texts can function at one-removed to deal with anxiety-provoking interactions and any implicit aggression, such as missed sessions, lateness, can-cellations and so on. Sending a text or email can represent a more detached way of interacting that is impersonal, two-dimensional and controlled. The advent of new technologies requires us to apply analytic understanding and even rethink therapeutic techniques, where appropriate.

Mobile phones offer a greater degree of immediacy and access, with phones mostly carried on, or close to, the body. We relate to our mobile phones like transitional objects using them both to connect to others as well as self-soothe; in many ways, our phones are our attachment devices. The speed of new forms of communication implies urgency and can compel us to respond with equal promptness. The Urban Dictionary includes evocative phrases like 'insta-regret', 'texter's remorse' and 'regrext' to convey the agonising feelings caused by impulsive or inadvertent communication. Writers suggest that the absence of the physical embodied setting both precludes the development and expression of erotic and aggressive responses to the psychotherapist (Sabbadini, 2013) as well as the converse: "indeed, the Internet disinhibits one's defence mechanisms and allows for greater disclosure than in ordinary discourse" (Uecker cited in Gabbard, 2001, p. 734). Suler (2005) termed this the *online disinhibition effect* that develops from the dissociative anonymity, physical invisibility and asynchronous com-munication offered by the Internet, without the checks provided by the real-life context. We will come back to this later in the chapter.

Patients can employ these new methods of communication defensively, for example to provoke concern or convey indirectly what is too difficult to say face-to-face. Bhuvaneswar and Gutheil (2008) are critical of emails for subverting boundaries, posing risk issues, and encouraging projections and role confusion. They point out that silence in a consulting room can feel empathic whereas non-response to emails is more likely to feel hurtful. By contrast, Gabbard (2001) warns of it being a "serious mistake" to view all written communication from our patients as resistance or acting out (pp. 729–730) and describes his personal struggle in allowing some email correspondence between face-to-face sessions with his patient: "Was I transgressing a boundary by incorporating e-mail commu-nication into analysis, or was I breaking new ground in the analytic frontier in a constructive and creative way?" (pp. 734–735). He concludes that "the use of email communication in the course of an analysis can have multiple meanings, just as can any other form of enactment" (p. 735).

In the strictest sense, any wish to make contact outside agreed session times breaches therapeutic boundaries and can be seen as acting out by the patient or therapist. However, Lingiardi (2008) suggests we cannot answer questions around whether or not to reply to patient's emails, for example, because "it's a question that cannot be manualized. The answer must be found within the context of the relationship and must be informed by the broader debate of enactment" (p. 121).

For some patients, the concrete response of a text or voice message can be proof of a caring therapist; the obverse also applies. This is teleological thinking in which action represents proof of concern. Bateman and Fonagy (2006) warn that we are deviating from the psychoanalytic template of therapeutic support when

> in accordance with the patient's wishes (giving them the illusion of control) that is experienced as meaningful; special acts such as checking in with patients between sessions, emailing offering weekend appointments, allowing between session contact, etc. are demanded as physical proofs of commitment. (p. 23)

When we are driven to respond by action and when the act of responding feels as important if not more important than the thought, we are operating in teleological mode. Greenacre (1950) warns of the disproportion between verbalisation and motor activity in acting out. We are ready to recognise this in our patients. However, the loss of mentalisation occurs in therapists too, notably when faced with a threat or when our emotions are overly aroused (Bateman and Fonagy, 2006, p. 24). When we are flooded with anxiety – our own or projected – it can result in a temporary failure in containment and we may find ourselves responding with less thoughtfulness than usual.

There are contradictory pulls for technology to foster too little as well as too much intimacy and we can see how this can map on to our patients' early experiences and quality of object- relating. In this way, being interested in our patient's use of digital technology provides a rich source of material for interpretation and the way they engage with the Internet gives insight into their preoccupations and unconscious conflicts.

Online banking

We have spoken about payment earlier in Chapter 4 in relation to the analytic setting, and in Chapter 12 we considered some of the difficulties that can occur around money. Here, we want to focus on technological aspects of payment and how remote payment can obscure this financial transaction from our view if we don't attend to it. The exchange of the bill at the end of the month, and payment at the subsequent session is symbolic of the formal, professional boundaries of the psychotherapy relationship. The transaction provides an important and necessary sense of reality into a relationship that is often laden with fantasies and unconscious projections. The exchange of money also may hold symbolic meaning for the patient, and provides a transference communication. Making an electronic bank payment allows for the exchange to be impersonal – just another payment to another payee. As we know, payment and delays in payment is an area that is often informed by transference. The patient may feel angry with us, short-changed or upset that they have to pay for therapy. We have heard of examples where a patient paid a cheque into the therapist's bank account, only then to cancel it, thereby creating the illusion that the therapist had been paid. Another patient left her last bill partly unpaid, creating a reason for the therapist to remain in touch with her. Electronic payment may have countertransference meaning too, as the therapist is then left checking their bank account to see whether a payment has been made or not.

This does not mean we should not use online banking. We live in a changing contemporary society, and we need to accommodate the times that we live in. What is important, however, is not to lose sight of the meaning of money and payment for a particular patient and it becomes easier to do so when this happens outside the therapy room. When working entirely remotely, this is even more the case, since the bill will be sent by email and not given to the patient in the session.

Distance psychotherapy

There is an emerging interest in psychoanalytic applications of technology, including distance analysis and remote supervision by online platforms like Zoom or Skype as well as by telephone (e.g. Carlino, 2011; Lemma and Caparrotta, 2013; Scharff 2013; Russell, 2015; Lemma, 2017). In order to introduce psychoanalysis into areas where there is a limited psychoanalytic community, like in China for example, candidates are offered remote analysis interspersed with occasional intensive periods of *in situ* psychoanalysis. In the NHS, technology-mediated therapy is being offered as an economical way of reaching a wider audience. Indeed, there have been attempts to set up a virtual online DIT group (Lemma and Fonagy, 2013). This inevitably raises concerns around confidentiality, protecting therapist anonymity and digital transference. More recently with the Covid-19 pandemic, remote ways of working have become a necessity in order to continue our clinical work and it has forced many clinicians who would not otherwise have chosen this way of working to engage with remote therapy. Carlino (2011) highlights many possible reasons for electing distance therapy, including extending patient choice, having rationally justified reasons for working remotely such as work transfers, needing a particular language skill for therapy, worrying about privacy in a small analytic community, and disabilities. Among the latter, he lists illness or travel restrictions for patient and/or therapist, physical disabilities, economic reasons, instability in one's living and work arrangements, time constraints, and as we can now add to this list, emergency lockdowns that prohibit any form of embodied contact.

Doing therapy online requires a variety of practical and technological considerations. As such, it can be considered "a fundamental modification of the process and setting" (Lemma, 2017, p. 87). This has implications for the nature of the work as well as the suitability of patients for this way of working. The frame of therapy is no longer the sole responsibility of the therapist but is shared by the patient too. While we are trained in the importance of holding an analytic frame, the patient does not have a nuanced appreciation of this, and we do need to discuss this with the patient in preparation for online therapy. For example, would we want to conduct therapy with the patient holding their iPad or mobile phone in their hand, giving us a close up, and wobbly, view? A colleague reported carrying out her first remote session with a patient who moved out of London and how unsettling it was that she could see his underwear drying on the washing line in the background. One of us had a Zoom call with a patient while she was away on holiday and the screen opened to her lying on her hotel bed, skimpily dressed with the iPad resting on her chest, thus creating a more informal and intimate scene than when she was seen in person. Remote access gives the therapist more information than we would obtain if we were seeing the patient in our own consulting room. Both therapists and patients who have moved to remote therapy during the Covid-19 pandemic have commented on feeling exposed during the work that provides a very personal window into their world. For this reason, it is important to always consider the best way forward for remote working. For some patients, the telephone will be preferable to an online platform and vice versa. It is also advisable to have an alternate way of working, should there be technological problems.

Normally, the therapist provides and manages the therapeutic setting, in the form of providing a confidential and dedicated space which includes the physical setting of a comfortable chair or analytic couch, box of tissues and so forth as well as the internal setting of the therapist's reverie, unconscious receptivity and containment. In the case of computer-mediated or telephone therapy, the patient now has to assume responsibility for protecting the therapeutic frame on their side of the connection, ensuring the necessary boundaries and confidentiality so that they can engage in their session. While the therapist can ensure a confidential setting for therapy, we cannot be sure that the space the patient is connecting from is confidential or even safe. The therapist may, quite reasonably, assume that the patient will be attentive to this, yet we have heard of a case where the patient revealed to the therapist that an unknown person had been sitting silently in their psychotherapy sessions for the past year. A patient one of us saw remotely found it very challenging when he had his remote session from his home study, reporting feeling more inhibited because of his anxiety that his children could overhear his conversation.

Earlier we discussed the disinhibiting effect of using social media. This pertains to distance psychotherapy too, where some patients may be quick to reveal or discuss something very personal, that they may not otherwise comfortably choose to do when in the physical presence of the therapist. The British Association for Counselling and Psychotherapy (2020, p. 1) competences include the ability to manage the impact of disinhibition when working remotely, as summarised below:

- An ability to draw on the knowledge that disinhibition can be encouraged by features of the online environment, such as having a sense of being anonymous and invisible, experiencing absence of external authority in the online environment and not experiencing others as real.

- An ability to draw on the knowledge that disinhibition can be a common feature of online interactions and where this happens, it can affect the therapeutic process, including: inappropriately disclosing sensitive information too rapidly, thereby leaving the patient feeling overwhelmed; overly rapid development of intimacy with the therapist followed by withdrawal or distancing; difficulty in pacing sessions including saying more than they would have in face-to-face sessions and subsequent regret at over-disclosure; as well as uninhibited expression of anger, hatred or criticism. To this, we would add sexual and erotic feelings that may find expression more easily in this remote way of working.
- An ability to help patients pace their communications so that they can process the material they are disclosing. This may include interjecting to slow the patient down and summarise what you have heard them say as well as asking patients to stop and reflect on what has developed in therapy.
- An ability to draw on knowledge that, without the face-to-face embodied therapy setting, both therapist and patient can easily develop inaccurate fantasies about the other and in the face of this, the therapist should be able to address and explore these unsubstantiated assumptions. While this is the bread and butter work of transference interpretations, there is an understanding that working remotely lends itself to greater inaccuracies and links with both Russell's (2015) and Lemma's (2017) observations about the noticeable absence of the therapist's bodily countertransference to ground this way of working.
- The ability to recognise that the therapist is also likely to experience disinhibition themselves during remote working which may lead them to making unhelpful interventions, for example by being too direct, forthright or insensitive, or even by making self-disclosures. After all, we should not consider ourselves unaffected by the change in the medium of working.

Russell (2015) describes various ways in which online therapy can lead to some casualisation of the therapist-patient relationship, for example, where changes in the environment may not be noticed, picked up or addressed. There may be an invitation for each to act more casually in their behaviour because it is easy to forget that our body language and facial expressions can still be seen when we are not physically present in the same room. The potential for distraction is also heightened when one is not physically in each other's presence. For example, a patient may glance at their incoming emails while in the session, or they may have the television on muted in the background. Most often, the patient may be calling from their home, giving the therapist some awareness of their private life that they would not otherwise be aware of. For example, there may be photographs of family or friends in the background, a family member may be enlisted to help them connect to the session or even brings the patient a cup of tea.

Filip had been in therapy with me for a little over a year before he moved to another country, for good reasons. We had various weeks to discuss the impact of this on the therapy and the options for us to consider: whether he would end therapy, whether he would start with a new therapist in the new country, or whether we would continue with therapy online. We agreed to continue online, because the move was a challenging one for Filip. With the many changes in his life that the move would bring, continuing with therapy would provide some helpful continuity. We also explored his wish to symbolically keep a piece of himself behind in the therapy space, keeping his connection to his most recent previous home. In order to prepare ourselves for the change, we agreed to have some sessions online before he moved, so we could connect again in person during the next session and think about how the online sessions felt. It was the first time I was going to be doing online therapy on a continuous basis, so this was something for me to get used to.

We spoke about what would be different. However, thinking about this and experiencing it are different. After his move, the difference in the therapeutic relationship in the move from face-to-face to online became more pronounced. Things were obviously different. Because of the different time zones, Filip was calling in from his home, late in the evening. His appearance and presentation were different. He was now calling having changed out of his work clothes, and was much more casual than he had been in sessions before. There were times when I decided to work from my office at home (ensuring that the space was kept confidential), and so we could both see into each other's private lives, to a certain extent. During one session, he got a glimpse of my pet who had snuck into my home office. After the initial few weeks, there was a growing sense of emotional distance in the therapeutic relationship. Most of the time the connection was fine, but there were moments when the connection froze or lagged and I had to ask Filip to repeat what he had said, and vice versa. We were in different social-cultural contexts, where there were different references to the outside world brought in that I would not be aware of. He now experienced me as somewhat remote. This had transference meaning in that he experienced his parents as remote and hard to reach, and in his personal relationships he found it difficult to open up and let people in, for fear of being humiliated. The remoteness of online therapy made it easier for him to retreat into privacy, and in turn he experienced me as less available to him. The sense of separation and loss was felt in the transference as well as in the reality of moving. After some months, we agreed to bring the therapy to an end, and we spent several sessions working towards this. While having some continuity and containment during a time of upheaval was helpful, the therapeutic frame was just not the same.

There are practical arrangements around scheduling sessions across different time zones, depending on the locations of both the therapist and patient. For example, the patient may be located at a time zone where it is late at night, and they are dressed casually, perhaps ready for bed, whereas it is the middle of the day for the therapist. While sometimes there can be a good connection, at other times there are time lags or freezes in the video or audio transmission that need to be worked with. How to start the session also needs to be agreed; it is not the same as the patient arriving at the consulting room and ringing the doorbell. Where possible, it is best to try and replicate the analytic setting where the therapist is waiting to receive the patient whose responsibility it is to arrive on time to the session. We suggest that the therapist is logged in and waiting on the agreed platform, so that the patient then dials in at the agreed time. With Zoom, the therapist can have a virtual waiting room where you can admit the patient as the session begins. Some contingency arrangements should be agreed if there are connection difficulties, and how that is to be communicated if across different countries.

Lemma's (2017) recommendations for how to structure sessions using new media like Skype, is particularly useful to therapists considering and employing this way of working. She extrapolates the principles of engagement and the analytic frame to this new modality in a thoughtful and containing way, providing clear clinical guidelines to create and safeguard the analytic setting as well as consider which patients are most suitable for working in this way and under which conditions one might consider using new media. We may want to think about where the patient sits – in more traditional analytic distance work, the patient is asked to position the camera so the therapist sees the patient as they would if they were using the couch (Weitz, 2018). Lemma cautions against using distance psychotherapy with particular patients including those who have never been seen in person by the therapist. Both Lemma (2017) and Russell (2015) emphasise the importance of the embodied experience in the consulting room, which is difficult to achieve through mediated psychotherapy. In an interview with the psychoanalyst Essig who has written extensively on the topic of screen relations, Russell (2015) reports his personal communication that

> The process of being with an other when you're in the same consulting room is a direct unmediated experience that evolution has primed us to be able to do, including affect attunement systems, mirror neurons, olfaction and bodily sensation. These whole series of things that are present in the consulting room are not present when we are trying to connect via technology. (p. 57)

Operating in the absence of these cues provides an explanation for the shared experience of the demanding and tiring nature of remote therapy. Essig describes screen relations as simulations of the experience of being embodied beings sharing the same space. When imagination or the suspension of disbelief comes together with an affective connection and the joint attention of patient and therapist, then there can be an "emotional illusion" of telepresence, something that requires a highly demanding emotional contribution of both therapist and patient (Russell, 2015, p. 57). We need to remain mindful of the real differences in these ways of working and to mark those differences for our patients rather than act as if we can continue uninterrupted. In response to the unprecedented move to remote working during the Covid-19 pandemic in the spring of 2020, we developed the following guidelines for patients about preparing to move to online sessions, which we include in Box 14.2.

Box 14.2 Guidelines for patients about remote working

Unlike when you come to see me in person, the responsibility for creating a safe and confidential space for psychotherapy is now shared with you when we move to working remotely. It requires being in a different mental space. Our habits are often hard to break if we are used to browsing online or watching tv in the background when speaking to family and friends. Here are some useful tips to make the most of this transition to remote therapy:

1   **Privacy** is crucial. Do your best to find a private space where you can feel free to speak, without worrying about anyone listening or walking in on your session. This includes telling others that you are unavailable during your session time.
2   **Turn off all devices** other than the one you are using for the video call. Turn off notifications. There is a Do Not Disturb option on most computers and smart phones that can be enabled to assist with this.
3   **Location matters**. When possible, try and meet from the same location each time.
4   Try to keep the setting as **professional** as possible. If you do need to use your bedroom, bring a chair to sit on rather than using your bed. Dress as you usually would for your session. Find somewhere to prop up your phone, iPad or computer, so that you don't have to hold on to it or rest it in your lap.
5   Arrange yourself as you would if you were meeting in person in the office. **Sit** in a comfortable chair, rather than reclining or lying down on furniture. If you have been using the analytic couch, you can place your device behind you, before lying down as you usually would; we also have the option of seeing each other at the start of the session and then disabling our cameras until the end of the 50 minutes.
6   Keep a box of **tissues** nearby. Pour a glass of **water** if you want, but don't eat or snack during your session.
7   Don't jump immediately from another activity into your session. Leave yourself a ten- to fifteen-minute **buffer** before your session to clear your head and mentally prepare, and a similar buffer afterwards to process and absorb. If possible, take a walk outside by yourself before or after sessions. If not, some gentle stretching indoors is useful. This before and after buffer time is in fact an important part of your session.

As we come to the end of this book, it is symbolic that we end on issues of technology and online psychotherapy. These are the new frontiers, and we cannot predict what the future holds for technology and the ensuing implications for psychotherapy. It is likely we will have much more sophisticated and faster means of communicating online, perhaps even with the use of holograms, that will change the feel of distance psychotherapy, bringing the hologram of the therapist or the patient into the room. Who knows! Psychoanalytic theory and psychodynamic psychotherapy have to move with the times. The profession began with

Freud, but it certainly has not remained there. While his influence and reach are significant, there have been numerous substantive developments in our thinking and practice, and there will continue to be.

Box 14.3 Useful resources

Readings

We recommend Alessandra Lemma's book which covers different aspects of technology and social media: Lemma, A. (2017). *The digital age on the couch: Psychoanalytic practice and new media*. London: Routledge.

Gillian Isaacs Russell's (2015) book provides an excellent exploration of distance psychotherapy: *Screen relations: The limits of computer-mediated psychoanalysis and psychotherapy*. London: Karnac Books.

Online resources

The BACP has a number of very useful resources for working online: www.bacp.co.uk/news/news-from-bacp/coronavirus/working-online-resources/

The UKCP has a helpful document addressing issues of privacy and confidentiality in a variety of contexts at www.psychotherapy.org.uk/wp-content/uploads/2018/08/UKCP-Security-and-Confidentiality-Guidelines-2018.pdf

Lecture by psychoanalyst Professor Josh Cohen on issues of privacy in the modern world, based on his book The private life, why we remain in the dark: https://youtu.be/LM7gBxtk6ml.

An expert in online and cross-cultural therapy, Anastasia Piatakhina Giré shares her tips with Victor Yalom around transitioning to online therapy now that more and more people are finding themselves sheltering in place during the Covid-19 pandemic of 2020: https://youtu.be/erDHige08sk.

Appendix 1

Specimen terms and conditions

Fees and payment

Bills are issued monthly in arrears at the end of the calendar month. Payment is due within seven days by electronic banking transfer to the account detailed on your bill. Cheques are also accepted. All available sessions must be paid for, including those that you do not attend, as this time is reserved for you on a regular basis. If you are unable to attend a session, I require at least 48 hours' notice. If there are frequent cancellations, I may need to bill you for these missed sessions too. If you are unable to attend, an alternative time in the same week may be offered, but this is not guaranteed. My fees are reviewed annually. However, this does not necessarily mean that your fee will change.

Breaks and holidays

Advance notice is given of my breaks and holidays. You are encouraged to take holidays to coincide with these dates, where possible. There are no sessions on bank holidays.

Privacy

I collect, store and process personal information about you to enable me to run my psychotherapy practice. Psychotherapists and psychologists are required to comply with the directives as set out by the General Data Protection Regulation (GDPR). I am a registered data controller with the Information Commissioner's Office (ICO). I collect personal data upon the legal basis of 'Legitimate Interests' and/or with your consent, according to the GDPR guidelines, as I need information about you in order to be able to work with you.

Under the GDPR, you have the right to:

- Ask for a copy of your personal data held by me, at no cost to you
- Ask me to correct any personal information that I hold about you, or inform me about any changes to your personal information

- Request that your personal data be transferred to another person (data portability)
- Ask to be informed of what data processing is taking place
- Right to be forgotten

Confidentiality

All aspects of your therapy remain fully confidential, and my practice is subject to the strict code of practice and ethical standards of my registering professional body. In line with best practice and requirements for continuing professional development, I regularly discuss my clinical work in supervision. However, all clinical material discussed is fully anonymised.

Communication with GP/other health professionals

All clients are asked to provide details of their GP and/or psychiatrist at the start of therapy. Once the work is underway, it is my practice to notify the GP that you have started working with me. If I am subsequently concerned about your safety or that of another person in connection with you, I may need to contact your GP and/or psychiatrist in order to help you receive the necessary support. I will endeavour to discuss this fully with you before I do so.

Professional communication

I keep professional communication limited to email, post and text messaging. I do make use of social networking platforms (such as LinkedIn), but I keep my practice communication separate from this. Thus, I do not as a rule accept requests to connect on social media platforms. This is also to ensure protection of your own anonymity.

Notice of ending

It is anticipated that the end of your therapy will be thought about and discussed between us during the course of the work, as this is an important part of the process. Should you decide to discontinue your therapy before a date for ending is agreed, two sessions' notice is required so that we may have a proper period of ending.

Undertaking therapy with me is deemed to be acceptance of the terms and conditions set out in the above paragraphs. These may be updated from time to time, and you will be notified accordingly.

Appendix 2
Specimen referral/pre-assessment questionnaire

We have designed this drawing on our experience of using different types of forms and questionnaires over the years in different services. We have found these to be useful preparatory questions to ask when someone is being referred or referring themselves for an assessment.

Psychotherapy referral questionnaire

When you come for your initial assessment consultation you will have an opportunity to discuss your difficulties in detail with me. Talking in person is the most important way of understanding them. However, it would help both of us to prepare, if you could provide some initial information prior to us meeting. If you could complete this confidential questionnaire with as much detail as you feel comfortable sharing now, and return it to me before you come, or bring it with you on the day if you feel uncomfortable sending it to me beforehand.

Personal details

Name:

Gender: Date of birth:

Sexual orientation:

Relationship status:

Children/dependents:

Occupation:

Address:

Telephone:

Email:

GP name and address:

Reasons for seeking therapy

1   How would you describe your current difficulties?

2   When do you feel these first started?

3   Are you having or have you recently had any thoughts of harming yourself or suicidal thoughts? Please describe.

4   Are you having or have you recently had any thoughts of harming someone else? Please describe.

5   Are you currently taking any medication (for mental or physical health problems)? Please provide name and dosage.

6   Can you say why you are seeking help now?

7   In what way do you expect therapy to help you?

A bit about you

1   How would you describe yourself as a person and how do you feel other people see you?

2   What are your most significant relationships?

_____
_____
_____

3   If you have a partner and/or family, do you have any difficulties or unhappiness in your relationship with your partner or family?

_____
_____
_____

4   What aspects of your life give you satisfaction, or help you to cope?

_____
_____
_____

Declaration

I understand that the above contact details and personal information will be stored securely and used only by you. The contact details provided are to enable you to contact me. I understand that my GP will only be contacted in cases of medical or safeguarding emergencies, and that this shall be discussed with me should such an occasion arise.

Signed:

Date:

Appendix 3

Specimen end of therapy report

Here is the format for a summary of the end of psychotherapy that you may find helpful. It has been adapted from a format that has been used in the NHS and adapted for general use.

Final summary of treatment

A: Details

Therapist's name:

Patient's name:

Supervisor's name (indicate any changes in supervision arrangements):

Date of initial meeting:

Psychotherapy Contract details (frequency, breaks, length of treatment):

Date of first session:

Date of last session:

Total number of sessions made available:

Number of sessions attended:

Number of sessions missed:

Nature of termination (e.g. planned, unplanned, ended early because of outside circumstances):

B: Summary of the work

1 **Summary of the assessment and referral process**: including the initial meeting and the reasons why the patient presented for help now.

2 **Psychodynamic formulation of the patient's history**: share your formulation of the development of the patient's difficulties, including consideration of the patient's likely defences and coping strategies.

3 **Themes of psychotherapy**: what issues were dealt with in treatment and what were the main themes and core conflicts that emerged and were explored.

4 **Changes in psychotherapy**: describe any changes that have occurred since the patient started therapy. These can include changes in symptoms, behaviour, intimate or personal relationships, changes in work and social life, changes in the patient's attitude to parents, siblings or other family members, changes in the therapeutic relationship.

5 **The experience of being with the patient**: This section should focus on your affective response to the patient and the transference-countertransference as it unfolded over the course of treatment.

C: Post-treatment considerations

1 **Areas of concern for the future**: Include here any areas of the patient's life where you feel there are still difficulties, indicating, if possible, the likely consequence if these remain the same.

2 **Future plans**: Describe what was said to the patient with regard to future treatment at the end of therapy. Include here your view about future treatment.

Appendix 4

Specimen social media contract

Social media

I do not accept contact/friend requests from current or former patients on any social networking site (Facebook, LinkedIn, etc). Adding patients as friends or contacts on these sites can compromise confidentiality and our respective privacy. It also blurs the boundaries of our therapeutic relationship. If you have questions about this, please bring them up when we meet and we can talk more about it.

I prefer using text messages or email only to arrange or modify appointments. Please do not email me content related to your therapy sessions, as neither of these methods is completely secure or confidential. If you choose to communicate with me by email, be aware that all emails are retained in the logs of your and my Internet service providers. While it is unlikely that someone will be looking at these logs, they are, in theory, available to be read by the system administrator(s) of the Internet service provider. You should also know that any emails I receive from you and any responses that I send to you become part of your legal record.

Emails, phone calls, and emergencies

For small administrative matters such as checking appointment times or changing them, you are welcome to email me [insert your email address]. I generally receive and return emails within 24 hours with the exception of weekends.

If you need to contact me between sessions about a clinical matter, please leave a message for me at [insert your phone number]. I usually check my messages each day unless I am on leave. Emergency phone consultations of five minutes or less are normally free. However, if we spend more than five minutes in a week on the phone, if you leave more than five minutes' worth of phone messages in a week, if I spend more than five minutes reading and responding to emails from you during a given week, or if I spend more than five minutes involved in case management or coordination of care, I will bill you on a prorated basis for that time.

If you feel the need for many phone calls and cannot wait for your next appointment, we may need to schedule more sessions to address your needs. If an emergency situation arises, please indicate it clearly in your message to me. If your situation is an acute emergency and you need to talk to someone right away, you should contact your GP during office hours or go to your nearest 24-hour Accident and Emergency department.

Confidentiality of e-mail and voice mail communication

E-mail and voice mail communication can be easily accessed by unauthorised people, compromising the privacy and confidentiality of such communication. Please notify me at the beginning of treatment if you would like to avoid or limit in any way the use of any or all of these communication devices. Please do not contact me via e-mail for emergencies.

Appendix 5

Specimen privacy notice for website

Privacy notice

I collect, store and process personal information about you to enable me to run my psychotherapy practice. Psychotherapists and psychologists are required to comply with the directives as set out by the General Data Protection Regulation (GDPR). I am a registered data controller with the Information Commissioner's Office (ICO). I collect personal data upon the legal basis of 'Legitimate Interests' and/or with your consent, according to the GDPR guidelines, as I need information about you in order to be able to work with you.

Use of my website

When you use my website, you do so at your own discretion. My website may collect information about the type of device you use to access the website, the Internet protocol (IP) address used to connect your computer to the Internet, and the date and time you access the website. This information is used to monitor the performance of the website. Like many websites, this website uses "Cookies" to enhance your experience and gather information about visitors and visits to the website. For detailed information on the use cookies and their purposes see [for example: https://www.counselling-directory.org.uk/cookie-policy.php]

By accessing and using the website, you consent to the processing of data about you in this manner and for the purposes set out in this Privacy Notice.

When you contact me by sending a message via my website, you are in control of how much and what type of information you choose to provide. Although I only require initial contact information from you, I accept that you may choose to provide me with further information.

Information collected

When arranging a consultation with me, the information you give me may include your name, address, e-mail address and phone number. Any contact details you provide me is saved electronically in a password protected document.

When making any cheque or electronic payments for my services, this may include your banking details.

Any notes that I take from our initial assessment meeting are anonymised and stored securely. I may make brief records of attendance and reference to content of sessions in order to track the progress of our work together or use it as the basis of reflection and guidance in professional supervision.

I will only share your personal data with a relevant authority or healthcare provider (e.g. your GP) where it is necessary for compliance with a legal obligation to which I am subject, or where it is necessary to protect the vital interests of you or another person (e.g. in a safeguarding concern).

Should anything happen to me that prevents me from attending a session and from communicating with you directly – such as illness or death – then I have appointed a Therapeutic Executor who would be able to access your contact details to inform you should this situation arise.

I will retain your personal information for as long as I provide services to you, and for a period of up to seven years thereafter. Once information is not needed, it shall be securely destroyed.

Your rights

Under the GDPR, you have the right to:

- Ask for a copy of your personal data held by me, at no cost to you
- Ask me to correct any personal information that I hold about you, or inform me about any changes to your personal information
- Request that your personal data be transferred to another person (data portability)
- Ask to be informed of what data processing is taking place
- Right to be forgotten

Changes

This Privacy Notice was last updated on [insert date]. If I change my Privacy Notice, I will post the changes on this page.

References

Abbass, A. A., Hancock, J. T., Henderson, J., & Kisely, S. (2006). Short-term psychodynamic psychotherapies for common mental disorders. *Cochrane Database of Systematic Reviews*, Issue 4, Article No. CD004687. doi:10.1002/14651858.CD004687.pub3

Ablon, J. S., & Jones, E. E. (1998). How expert clinicians' prototypes of an ideal treatment correlate with outcome in psychodynamic and cognitive-behavioral therapy. *Psychotherapy Research*, 8, 71–83.

Abrahams, D. (2017). Dynamic Interpersonal Therapy: Working with perceptions of the self and other. *BACP Healthcare Counselling and Psychotherapy Journal*, 7(3), 8–13.

Ainsworth, M. D. S., Blehar, M. C., Waters, E., & Wall, S. (1978) *Patterns of attachment: A psychological study of the strange situation.* Hillsdale: Lawrence Erlbaum Associates.

Akhtar, S. (2009a). *Comprehensive dictionary of psychoanalysis.* London: Karnac.

Akhtar, S. (2009b). *Turning points in dynamic psychotherapy: Initial assessment, boundaries, money, disruptions and suicidal crises.* London: Karnac.

Allen, J. G., Fonagy, P., & Bateman, A. W. (2008). *Mentalizing in clinical practice.* Washington DC: American Psychiatric Publishing.

Allison, E., & Fonagy, P. (2016). When is truth relevant? *The Psychoanalytic Quarterly*, 85(2), 275–303.

American Psychiatric Association (2013). *Diagnostic and statistical manual of mental disorders* (5th edition). American Psychiatric Association.

American Psychoanalytic Association (2019). American Psychoanalytic Association issues overdue apology to LGBTQ community. Available from: https://apsa.org/content/news-apsaa-issues-overdue-apology-lgbtq-community

Balick, A. (2018). How to think about psychotherapy in a digital context. In P. Weitz (ed.), *Psychotherapy 2.0: Where psychotherapy and technology meet* (pp. 23–40). Abingdon: Routledge.

Barber, J. P., Crits-Christoph, P., & Luborsky, L. (1996). Effects of therapist adherence and competence on patient outcome in brief dynamic therapy. *Journal of Consulting and Clinical Psychology*, 64(3), 619.

Barrett, M. M. (2003). Desire and the couch: Perspectives from both sides of the analytic encounter. *Psychoanalytic Psychology*, 20(1), 167–169.

Bartholomew, K., & Horowitz, L. M. (1991). Attachment styles among young adults: A test of a four-category model. *Journal of Personality and Social Psychology*, 61(2), 226–244.

Bateman, A., & Fonagy, P. (2006). *Mentalization-based treatment for borderline personality disorder: A practical guide.* Oxford: Oxford University Press.

Bateman, A., & Holmes, J. (1995). *Introduction to psychoanalysis: Contemporary theory and practice.* Hove: Routledge.

Bawa, H., Gooden, S., Maleque, F., Naseem, S., Naz, S., et al. (2019). The journey of BME aspiring psychologists into clinical psychology training: Barriers and ideas for inclusive change. *Clinical Psychology Forum*, 323(November), 3–7.

Beutel, M. E., Stern, E., & Silbersweig, D. A. (2003). The emerging dialogue between psychoanalysis and neuroscience: Neuroimaging perspectives. *Journal of the American Psychoanalytic Association*, 51(3), 773–801.

Beutel, M. E., Stark, R., Pan, H., Silbersweig, D., & Dietrich, S. (2010). Changes of brain activation pre-post short-term psychodynamic inpatient psychotherapy: An fMRI study of panic disorder patients. *Psychiatry Research: Neuroimaging*, 184(2), 96–104.

Bhuvaneswar, C. G., & Gutheil, T. G. (2008). Email and psychiatry: Some psychotherapeutic and psychoanalytic perspectives. *American Journal of Psychotherapy*, 62(3), 241–261.

Binder, J. L. (1999). Issues in teaching and learning time-limited psychodynamic psychotherapy. *Clinical Psychology Review*, 19(6), 705–719.

Binder, P. E., Holgersen, H., & Nielsen, G. H. S. (2010). What is a "good outcome" in psychotherapy? A qualitative exploration of former patients' point of view. *Psychotherapy Research*, 20(3), 285–294.

Bion, W. R. (1959). Attacks on linking. *International Journal of Psychoanalysis*, 40, 308–315.

Bion, W. R. (1962a). *Learning from experience*. London: Heinemann.

Bion, W. R. (1962b). The psycho-analytic study of thinking. *International Journal of Psychoanalysis*, 43, 306–310.

Bion, W. R. (1970). *Attention and interpretation: A scientific approach to insights in psychoanalysis and groups*. London: Tavistock.

Blagys, M. D., & Hilsenroth, M. J. (2000). Distinctive activities of short-term psychodynamic-interpersonal psychotherapy: A review of the comparative psychotherapy process literature. *Clinical Psychology: Science and Practice*, 7, 167–188.

Blatt, S. J. (1974). Levels of object representation in anaclitic and introjective depression. *The Psychoanalytic Study of the Child*, 29(1), 107–157.

Blatt, S. J., & Luyten, P. (2009). A structural–developmental psychodynamic approach to psychopathology: Two polarities of experience across the life span. *Development and Psychopathology*, 21(3), 793–814.

Blumenthal, S., Wood, H., & Williams, A. (2018). *Assessing risk: A relational approach*. Abingdon: Routledge.

Bogdan, R. J. (2005). Why self-ascriptions are difficult and develop late. In B. F. Malle & S. D. Hodges (eds.), *Other minds: How humans bridge the divide between self and others* (pp. 190–206). New York: Guilford Press.

Bollas, C. (2009). *The evocative object world*. Hove: Routledge.

Bowlby, J. (1969). *Attachment and loss, Volume 1: Attachment*. London: Hogarth Press.

Bowlby, J. (1973). *Attachment and loss, Volume 2: Separation*. London: Hogarth Press.

Bowlby, J. (1980). *Attachment and loss, Volume 3: Loss*. London: Hogarth Press.

Brenner, C. (1981). Defense and defense mechanisms. *The Psychoanalytic Quarterly*, 50(4), 557–569.

Breuer, J., & Freud, S. (1895). Studies on hysteria. In J. Strachey (ed.), *The standard edition of the complete psychological works of Sigmund Freud* (vol 2). London: Hogarth Press.

British Association for Counselling and Psychotherapy (2019). Good practice across the counselling professions 001: Gender, sexual, and relationship diversity (GSRD). Leicester: British Association for Counselling and Psychotherapy. Available from: www.bacp.co.uk/media/5877/bacp-gender-sexual-relationship-diversity-gpacp001-april19.pdf

British Association for Counselling and Psychotherapy (2020). Competences for telephone and e-counselling. Available from: www.bacp.co.uk/media/8113/bacp-competences-for-telephone-ecounselling-apr20.pdf

British Psychoanalytic Council (2011). Statement on homosexuality. Available from: www. bpc.org.uk/sites/psychoanalytic-council.org/files/6.2%20Position%20statement%20on% 20homosexuality.pdf

British Psychological Society (2012). *E-Professionalism: Guidance on the use of social media by clinical psychologists*. Leicester: British Psychological Society.

British Psychological Society (2019). *Guidelines for psychologists working with gender, sexuality and relationship diversity*. Leicester: British Psychological Society. Available from: www.bps.org.uk/ news-and-policy/guidelines-psychologists-working-gender-sexuality-and-relationship-diversity

Britton, R. (1989). The missing link: Parental sexuality in the Oedipus complex. In J. Steiner (ed.), *The Oedipus complex today: Clinical implications* (pp. 83–101). London, Karnac Books.

Britton, R. (2004). Subjectivity, objectivity, and triangular space. *Psychoanalytic Quarterly*, 73(1), 47–61.

Butler, J. (1990). *Gender trouble: Feminism and the subversion of identity*. New York: Routledge.

Campbell, D. (1995). The role of the father in a pre-suicide state. *The International Journal of Psychoanalysis*, 76, 315–323.

Carlino, R. (2011). *Distance psychoanalysis: The theory and practice of using communication technology in the clinic*. London: Karnac Books.

Casement, P. (1985). *On learning from the patient*. London: Routledge.

Castonguay, L. G., Goldfried, M. R., Wiser, S. L., Raue, P. J., & Hayes, A. M. (1996). Predicting the effect of cognitive therapy for depression: A study of unique and common factors. *Journal of Consulting and Clinical Psychology*, 64, 497–504.

Chung, C. J., & Colarusso, C. (2012). The use of the computer and the internet in child psychoanalysis. *The Psychoanalytic Study of the Child*, 66, 197–223.

Clinton, B. K., Silverman, B. C., & Brendel, D. H. (2010). Patient-targeted googling: the ethics of searching online for patient information. *Harvard Review of Psychiatry*, 18(2), 103–112.

Cohen, J. (2013). *The private life: Why we remain in the dark*. London: Granta.

Coltart, N. (1987). Diagnosis and assessment for suitability for psycho-analytical psychotherapy. *British Journal of Psychotherapy*, 4(2), 127–134.

Coltart, N. (1991). The silent patient. *Psychoanalytic Dialogues*, 1, 439–453.

Coltart, N. (1993). *How to survive as a psychotherapist*. London: Sheldon Press.

Coren, A. (2010). *Short-term psychotherapy: A psychodynamic approach* (2nd edition) Basingstoke: Palgrave Macmillan.

Coughlin, P. (2016). *Maximizing effectiveness in dynamic psychotherapy*. Abingdon: Routledge.

Dalal, F. (2018). *CBT: The cognitive behavioural tsunami: Managerialism, politics and the corruptions of science*. Abingdon: Routledge.

Damasio, A. R. (1999). *The feeling of what happens: Body and emotion in the making of consciousness*. New York: Houghton Mifflin Harcourt.

Danto, E. A. (2005). *Freud's free clinics: Psychoanalysis and social justice, 1918–1938*. New York: Columbia University Press.

Davanloo, H. (2000). *Intensive short-term dynamic psychotherapy*. Chichester: Wiley.

Davids, M. F. (2006). Internal racism, anxiety and the world outside: Islamophobia post-9/ 111. *Organizational and Social Dynamics*, 6(1), 63–85.

Davids, M. F. (2011). *Internal racism: A psychoanalytic approach to race and difference*. Basingstoke: Palgrave Macmillan.

Demos, V. C., & Prout, M. F. (1993). A comparison of seven approaches to brief psychotherapy. *International Journal of Short-term Psychotherapy*, 8, 3–22.

Domenici, T., & Lesser, R. C. (eds) (1995). *Disorienting sexuality: Psychoanalytic reappraisals of sexual identities*. New York: Routledge.

Douglas, A., Ablett-Tate, N., & Chadd, N. (2016). Dynamic interpersonal therapy in an NHS tertiary level specialist psychotherapy service. *Psychoanalytic Psychotherapy*, 30(3), 223–239.

Eichenberg, C., & Herzberg, P. Y. (2016). Do therapists google their patients? A survey among psychotherapists. *Journal of Medical Internet Research*, 18(1), e3.

Eichenberg, C., & Sawyer, A. (2016). Do patients look up their therapists online? An exploratory study among patients in psychotherapy. *JMIR Mental Health*, 3(2), e22.

Ellman, S. J. (2007). Analytic trust and transference: Love, healing ruptures, and facilitating repairs. *Psychoanalytic Inquiry*, 27, 246–263.

Erikson, E. H. (1963). *Childhood and society* (2nd edition). New York: Norton.

Etchegoyen, R. H. (1991). *The fundamentals of psychoanalytic technique*. London: Karnac Books.

Evans, M. O. (2005). Gift-giving in psychotherapy: layers of meaning and developmental process. *British Journal of Psychotherapy*, 21(3), 401–415.

Fairbairn, W. D. (1944). Endopsychic structure considered in terms of object-relationships. *International Journal of Psychoanalysis*, 25, 70–92.

Fairbairn, W. D. (1952). *Psychoanalytic studies of the personality*. London: Tavistock Publications Limited.

Fanon, F. (1967). *Black skin, white masks*. New York: Grove Press.

Fischer-Kern, M., Tmej, A., Kapusta, N. D., Naderer, A., Leithner-Dziubas, K., Löffler-Stastka, H., & Springer-Kremser, M. (2008). The capacity for mentalization in depressive patients: A pilot study. *Zeitschrift für Psychosomatische Medizin und Psychotherapie*, 54(4), 368–380.

Flanders, S. (1993). *The dream discourse today*. London: Routledge.

Fonagy, P. (2015). The effectiveness of psychodynamic psychotherapies: An update. *World Psychiatry*, 14(2), 137–150.

Fonagy, P., & Allison, E. (2014). The role of mentalizing and epistemic trust in the therapeutic relationship. *Psychotherapy*, 51(3), 372–380.

Fonagy, P., & Target, M. (1996). Playing with reality: I. Theory of mind and the normal development of psychic reality. *International Journal of Psychoanalysis*, 77, 217–233.

Fonagy, P., & Target, M. (2003). *Psychoanalytic theories: Perspectives from developmental psychopathology*. London: Whurr Publishers.

Fonagy, P., Bateman, A., & Bateman, A. (2011). The widening scope of mentalizing: A discussion. *Psychology and Psychotherapy: Theory, Research and Practice*, 84(1), 98–110.

Fonagy, P., Gergely, G., Jurist, E. J., & Target, M. (2002). *Affect regulation, mentalization and the development of the self*. New York: Other Press.

Fonagy, P., Lemma, A., Salkovskis, P., & Wolpert, L. (2012). Psychoanalysis: does it have a valuable place in modern mental health services? *British Medical Journal*, 344(7845), 18–19.

Fonagy, P., Rost, F. Carlyle, J., McPherson, S., Thomas, R., Pasco Fearon, R. M., Goldberg, D., & Taylor, D. (2015). Pragmatic randomized controlled trial of long-term psychoanalytic psychotherapy for treatment-resistant depression: The Tavistock Adult Depression Study (TADS). *World Psychiatry*, 14, 312–321.

Fonagy, P., Lemma, A., Target, M., O'Keeffe, S., Constantinou, M. P., Wurman, T. V., Luyten, P., Allison, E., Roth, A., Cape, J., & Pilling, S. (2019). Dynamic interpersonal therapy for moderate to severe depression: a pilot randomized controlled and feasibility trial. *Psychological Medicine*, 1–10.

Frank, E., Kupfer, D. J., Wagner, E. F., McEachran, A. B., & Comes, C. (1991). Efficacy of interpersonal psychotherapy as a maintenance treatment of recurrent depression: contributing factors. *Archives of General Psychiatry*, 48(12), 1053–1059.

Frank, M. C., Vul, E., & Johnson, S. P. (2009). Development of infants' attention to faces during the first year. *Cognition*, 110(2), 160–170.

Freeman, E. S. (1978). *Dream analysis: A practical handbook for psychoanalysts*. London: Hogarth Press.

Freud, A. (1954). *The ego and the mechanisms of defence*. London: Hogarth Press.

Freud, A. (1963). The concept of developmental lines. *The Psychoanalytic Study of the Child*, 18, 245–265.

Freud, A., (1965). *Normality and pathology in childhood*. Harmondsworth: Penguin Books.

Freud, S. (1896). Further remarks on the neuro-psychoses of defence. In J. Strachey (ed.), *The standard edition of the complete psychological Works of Sigmund Freud* (vol 3). London: Hogarth Press.

Freud, S. (1900). The interpretation of dreams. In J. Strachey (ed.), *The standard edition of the complete psychological works of Sigmund Freud* (vol 4/5). London: Hogarth Press.

Freud, S. (1901a). The psychopathology of everyday life: Forgetting, slips of the tongue, bungled actions, superstitions and errors. In J. Strachey (ed.), *The standard edition of the complete psychological works of Sigmund Freud* (vol 6). London: Hogarth Press.

Freud, S. (1901b). On dreams. In J. Strachey (ed.), *The standard edition of the complete psychological works of Sigmund Freud* (vol 5). London: Hogarth Press.

Freud, S. (1905a). Three essays on the theory of sexuality. In J. Strachey (ed.), *The standard edition of the complete psychological works of Sigmund Freud* (vol 7). London: Hogarth Press.

Freud, S. (1905b). Fragment of an analysis of a case of hysteria. In J. Strachey (ed.), *The standard edition of the complete psychological works of Sigmund Freud* (vol 7). London: Hogarth Press.

Freud, S. (1910). Five lectures on psycho-analysis. In J. Strachey (ed.), *The standard edition of the complete psychological works of Sigmund Freud* (vol 11). London: Hogarth Press.

Freud, S. (1911). Formulation of the two principles of mental functioning. In J. Strachey (ed.), *The standard edition of the complete psychological works of Sigmund Freud* (vol 12). London: Hogarth Press.

Freud, S. (1912). The dynamics of transference. In J. Strachey (ed.), *the standard edition of the complete psychological works of Sigmund Freud* (vol 12). London: Hogarth Press.

Freud, S. (1913). On beginning the treatment (further recommendations on the technique of psycho-analysis (I)). In J. Strachey (ed.), *The standard edition of the complete psychological works of Sigmund Freud* (vol 12). London: Hogarth Press.

Freud, S. (1914a). Remembering, repeating and working through. In J. Strachey (ed.), *The standard edition of the complete psychological works of Sigmund Freud* (vol 12). London: Hogarth Press.

Freud, S. (1914b). Totem and taboo. In J. Strachey (ed.), *The standard edition of the complete psychological works of Sigmund Freud* (vol 13). London: Hogarth Press.

Freud, S. (1915). The unconscious. In J. Strachey (ed.), *The standard edition of the complete psychological works of Sigmund Freud* (vol 14). London: Hogarth Press.

Freud, S. (1917a). Mourning and melancholia. In J. Strachey (ed.), *The standard edition of the complete psychological works of Sigmund Freud* (vol 14). London: Hogarth Press.

Freud, S. (1917b). On transformation of instinct as exemplified in anal erotism. In J. Strachey (ed.), *The standard edition of the complete psychological works of Sigmund Freud* (vol 17). London: Hogarth Press.

Freud, S. (1920). Beyond the pleasure principle. In J. Strachey (ed.), *The standard edition of the complete psychological works of Sigmund Freud* (vol 18). London: Hogarth Press.

Freud, S. (1923a). The ego and the id. In J. Strachey (ed.), *the standard edition of the complete psychological works of Sigmund Freud* (vol 19). London: Hogarth Press.

Freud, S. (1923b). Remarks of the theory and practice of dream interpretation. In J. Strachey (ed.), *The standard edition of the complete psychological works of Sigmund Freud* (vol 19). London: Hogarth Press.

Freud, S. (1926). Inhibitions, symptoms and anxiety. In J. Strachey (ed.), *The standard edition of the complete psychological works of Sigmund Freud* (vol 20). London: Hogarth Press.

Freud, S. (1931). Letter from Sigmund Freud to Sándor Ferenczi, December 13, 1931. In E. Falzeder & E. Brabant (2000) *The correspondence of Sigmund Freud and Sándor Ferenczi, Vol 3, 1920–1933* (pp. 421–424). Cambridge, MA/London: The Belknap Press of Harvard Univ. Press.

Freud, S. (1933). New introductory lectures on psycho-analysis. In J. Strachey (ed.), *The standard edition of the complete psychological works of Sigmund Freud* (vol 22). London: Hogarth Press.

Freud, S. (1935 | 1951). Letter to an American mother. *American Journal of Psychiatry*, 107, 786.

Freud, S. (1937). Analysis terminable and interminable. In J. Strachey (ed.), *The standard edition of the complete psychological works of Sigmund Freud* (vol 23). London: Hogarth Press.

Freud, S. (1938). Splitting of the ego in the process of defence. In J. Strachey (ed.), *The standard edition of the complete psychological works of Sigmund Freud* (vol 23). London: Hogarth Press.

Frosh, S. (2005). *Hate and the 'Jewish science': Anti-Semitism, Nazism and psychoanalysis*. London: Palgrave MacMillan.

Gabbard, G. O. (2000). A neurobiologically informed perspective on psychotherapy. *The British Journal of Psychiatry*, 177(2), 117–122.

Gabbard, G. O. (2001). Cyberpassion: E-rotic transference on the Internet. *Psychoanalytic Quarterly*, 70, 719–737.

Gabbard, G. O., Lazar, S. G., Hornberger, J., & Spiegelo, D. (1997). The economic impact of psychotherapy: A review. *American Journal of Psychiatry*, 154, 147–155.

Garelick, A. (1994). Psychotherapy assessment: Theory and practice. *Psychoanalytic Psychotherapy*, 8(2), 101–116.

Garelick, A. (2011). Finding a space to think and a way to talk. *Psychoanalytic Psychotherapy*, 25(1), 3–12.

George, C., Kaplan, N., & Main, M. (1996). *Adult Attachment Interview protocol* (3rd edition). Unpublished manuscript, Department of Psychology, University of California at Berkeley.

Gergely, G., & Unoka, Z. (2008). Attachment and mentalization in humans: The development of the affective self. In E. L. Jurist, A. Slade, & S. Bergner (eds), *Mind to mind: Infant research, neuroscience, and psychoanalysis* (pp. 50–87). New York: Other Press.

Gergely, G., & Watson, J. (1996). The social biofeedback model of parental affect-mirroring. *International Journal of Psychoanalysis*, 77, 1181–1212.

Glasser, M. (1986). Identification and its vicissitudes as observed in the perversions. *International Journal of Psychoanalysis*, 67, 9–16.

Glover, E. (1927). Lectures on technique in psycho-analysis. *International Journal of Psychoanalysis*, 8, 486–520.

Goss, P. (2015). *Jung: A complete introduction*. London: John Murray Learning.

Green, A. (1986). *On private madness*. London: Karnac.

Greenacre, P. (1950). General problems of acting out. *The Psychoanalytic Quarterly*, 19, 455–467.

Greenberg, J. R., & Mitchell, S. A. (1983). *Object relations in psychoanalytic theory*. Cambridge, MA: Harvard University Press.

Greenson, R. R. (1974). The decline and fall of the 50-minute hour. *Journal of the American Psychoanalytic Association*, 22, 785–791.

Greenson, R. R. (1978). *Explorations in psychoanalysis*. New York: International Universities Press.

Grosz, S. (2013). *The examined life: How we lose and find ourselves*. London: Random House.

Gustafson, J. P. (1997). *The complex secret of brief psychotherapy: A panorama of approaches*. Northvale, New Jersey: Jason Aronson Inc.

Gutheil, T. G., & Gabbard, G. O. (1993). The concept of boundaries in clinical practice: Theoretical and risk-management dimensions. *The American Journal of Psychiatry*, 150(2), 188–196.

Haby, M. M., Donnelly, M., Corry, J., & Vos, T. (2006). Cognitive behavioural therapy for depression, panic disorder and generalized anxiety disorder: A meta-regression of factors that may predict outcome. *Australian and New Zealand Journal of Psychiatry*, 40, 9–19.

Hartmann, H. (1939). *Ego psychology and the problem of adaptation*. New York: International Universities Press.

Hartocollis, P. (1983). *Time and timelessness: A psychoanalytic inquiry into the varieties of temporal experience*. Madison, CT: International Universities Press.

Heimann, P. (1950) On counter-transference. *International Journal of Psychoanalysis*, 31, 81–84.

Heimann, P. (1956). Dynamics of transference interpretations. *International Journal of Psychoanalysis*, 37, 303–310.

Henry, W. P., Strupp, H. H., Butler, S. F., Schacht, T. E., & Binder, J. L. (1993). Effects of training in time-limited dynamic psychotherapy: Changes in therapist behavior. *Journal of Consulting and Clinical Psychology*, 61(3), 434.

Hertzmann, L., & Newbigin, J. (eds) (2020). *Sexuality and gender now: Moving beyond hetero-normativity*. Abingdon: Routledge.

Hinshelwood, R. D. (1989). *A dictionary of Kleinian thought*. London: Free Association Books.

Hinshelwood, R. D. (1991). Psychodynamic formulation in assessment for psychotherapy. *British Journal of Psychotherapy*, 8(2),166–174.

Hinshelwood, R. D. (1995). Psychodynamic formulation in assessment for psychoanalytic psychotherapy. In C. Mace (ed.), *The art and science of assessment in psychotherapy* (pp. 155–166). London: Routledge.

Hofstede, G. (1984). *Culture's consequences: International differences in work-related values*. Newbury Park: Sage Publications.

Holmes, J. (1995). How I assess for psychoanalytic psychotherapy. In C. Mace (ed.), *The art and science of assessment in psychotherapy* (pp. 26–39). London: Routledge.

Holmes, J. (1997). 'Too early, too late': Endings in psychotherapy – an attachment perspective. *British Journal of Psychotherapy*, 14(2), 159–171.

Holmes, J. (2012). Seeing, sitting and lying down: Reflections on the role of visual communication in analytic therapy. *Psychoanalytic Psychotherapy*, 26(1), 2–12.

Horowitz, L. M., Rosenberg, S. E., & Bartholomew, K. (1993). Inter-personal problems, attachment styles, and outcome in brief dynamic psychotherapy. *Journal of Consulting and Clinical Psychology*, 61, 549–560.

Horowitz. L. M., Rosenberg, S. E., Baer, B. A., Ureno, G., & Villasenor, V. S. (1988). Inventory of interpersonal problems: Psychometric properties and clinical applications. *Journal of Consulting and Clinical Psychology*, 56, 885–892.

Horvath, A. O., & Luborsky, L. (1993). The role of the therapeutic alliance in psychotherapy. *Journal of Consulting and Clinical Psychology*, 61(4), 561–573.

Howard, K. I., Kopta, S. M., Krause, M. S., & Orlinsky, D. E. (1986) The dose-effect relationship in psychotherapy. *American Psychologist* 41(2), 159–164.

International Society for Mental Health Online (2000) Suggested principles for the online provision of mental health services. Available from: https://ismho.org/suggestions.asp

Isay, R. A. (1986). The development of sexual identity in homosexual men. *Psychoanalytic Study of the Child*, 41, 467–489.

Isay, R. A. (2010). *Being homosexual: Gay men and their development*. New York: Vintage Books.

Jackson, C., & Rizq, R. (eds) (2019). *The industrialisation of care: Counselling, psychotherapy and the impact of IAPT*. Monmouth: PCCS Books.

Jones, E. E. (2000). *Therapeutic action: A guide to psychoanalytic therapy*. Northvale, NJ: Jason Aronson.

Joseph, B. (1985). Transference: The total situation. *International Journal of Psychoanalysis*, 66, 447–454.

Jung, C. G. (1930). Your Negroid and Indian behaviour. *Forum*, 83(4), 193–199.

Kahr, B. (2019). *How to flourish as a psychotherapist*. Bicester: Phoenix Publishing House.

Kakar, S. (1985). Psychoanalysis and non-western cultures. *International Review of Psychoanalysis*, 12, 441–448.

Karlsson, H. (2011). How psychotherapy changes the brain. *Psychiatric Times*, 28(8), 1–5.

Kegerreis, S. (2013). 'When I can come on time, I'll be ready to finish': Meanings of lateness in psychoanalytic psychotherapy. *British Journal of Psychotherapy*, 29(4), 449–465.

Kernberg, O. F. (1976). *Object relations theory and clinical psychoanalysis*. New York: Aronson.

Kernberg, O. F. (1982). Self, ego, affects, and drives. *Journal of the American Psychoanalytic Association*, 30(4), 893–917.

Kernberg, O. F. (1987). An ego psychology-object relations theory approach to the transference. *Psychoanalytic Quarterly*, 56, 197–221.

Kernberg, O. F. (2016). The four basic components of psychoanalytic technique and derived psychoanalytic psychotherapies. *World Psychiatry*, 15(3), 287–288.

Khan, C. (2020, 10 February). 'I thought I was a lost cause': How therapy is failing people of colour. *The Guardian*. Available from: www.theguardian.com/lifeandstyle/2020/feb/10/therapy-failing-bme-patients-mental-health-counselling

Khan, M. (1963). Silence as communication. *Bulletin of the Menninger Clinic*, 27, 300–313.

Kim, S., Fonagy, P., Allen, J., Martinez, S., Iyengar, U., & Strathearn, L. (2014). Mothers who are securely attached in pregnancy show more attuned infant mirroring 7 months postpartum. *Infant Behavior and Development*, 37(4), 491–504.

Klein, M. (1932). *The psycho-analysis of children*. London: Hogarth Press.

Klein, M. (1935). A contribution to the psychogenesis of manic-depressive states. *International Journal of Psychoanalysis*, 16, 145–174.

Klein, M. (1937|1975). *Love, guilt and reparation and other works*. London: Hogarth Press.

Klein, M. (1946). Notes on some schizoid mechanisms. *International Journal of Psychoanalysis*, 27, 99–110.

Klein, M. (1957). *Envy and gratitude, the writings of Melanie Klein*. London: Hogarth Press.

Klein, M. (1959). Our adult world and its roots in infancy. *Human Relations*, 12(4), 291–303.

Kohut, H. (1971). *The analysis of the self*. New York: International Universities Press.

Kohut, H. (1977). *The restoration of the self*. New York: International Universities Press.

Kohut, H. (1984). *How does analysis cure?* Chicago: University of Chicago Press.

Kolmes, K. (2013). Articles for clinicians using social media. Available from: http://drkkolmes.com/for-clinicians/articles/

Kritzberg, N. I. (1980). On patients' gift-giving. *Contemporary Psychoanalysis*, 16(1), 98–118.

Kübler-Ross, E. (2009). *On death and dying: What the dying have to teach doctors, nurses, clergy and their own families*. Abingdon: Routledge.

Lagu T., Kaufman E. J., Asch, D. A., & Armstrong, K. (2008). Content of weblogs written by health professionals. *Journal of General Internal Medicine*, 51(10), 1642–1646.

Laplanche, J. (1999). *Essays of otherness*. Abingdon: Routledge.

Laplanche, J., & Pontalis, J. B. (1973). *The language of psycho-analysis* (Trans. Donald Nicholson-Smith). London: Hogarth Press.

LeDoux, J. (1998). *The emotional brain: The mysterious underpinnings of emotional life*. New York: Simon and Schuster.

Leichsenring, F., & Klein, S. (2014). Evidence for psychodynamic psychotherapy in specific mental disorders: a systematic review. *Psychoanalytic Psychotherapy*, 28(1), 4–32.

Lemma, A. (2000). *Humour on the couch: Exploring humour in psychotherapy and everyday life.* London: Whurr Publishers.

Lemma, A. (2003). *Introduction to the practice of psychoanalytic psychotherapy.* Chichester: John Wiley & Sons.

Lemma, A. (2013). The body one has and the body one is: Understanding the transsexual's need to be seen. *The International Journal of Psychoanalysis*, 94(2), 277–292.

Lemma, A. (2015). *Minding the body: The body in psychoanalysis and beyond.* Abingdon: Routledge.

Lemma, A. (2016). *Introduction to the practice of psychoanalytic psychotherapy* (2nd edition). Chichester: John Wiley & Sons.

Lemma, A. (2017). *The digital age on the couch: Psychoanalytic practice and new media.* London: Routledge.

Lemma, A., & Caparrotta, L. (eds) (2013). *Psychoanalysis in the technoculture era.* Hove: Routledge.

Lemma, A., & Fonagy, P. (2013). Feasibility study of a psychodynamic online group intervention for depression, *Psychoanalytic Psychology*, 30(3), 367–380.

Lemma, A., & Lynch, P. E. (eds) (2015). *Sexualities: Contemporary psychoanalytic perspectives.* Hove: Routledge.

Lemma, A., Roth, A., & Pilling, S. (2008). *The competences required to deliver effective psycho-analytic/psychodynamic therapy.* London: Research Department of Clinical, Educational and Health Psychology, University College London.

Lemma, A., Target, M., & Fonagy, P. (2011). *Brief dynamic interpersonal therapy: A clinician's guide.* Oxford: Oxford University Press.

Leonidaki, V., Lemma, A., & Hobbis, I. (2016). Clients' experiences of dynamic interpersonal therapy (DIT): Opportunities and challenges for brief, manualised psychodynamic therapy in the NHS. *Psychoanalytic Psychotherapy*, 30(1), 42–61.

Leonidaki, V., Lemma, A., & Hobbis, I. (2018). The active ingredients of dynamic inter-personal therapy (DIT): An exploration of clients' experiences. *Psychoanalytic Psychotherapy*, 32(2), 140–156.

Levenson, H. (2010). *Brief dynamic therapy.* Washington: American Psychological Association.

Levy, S. T. (1987). Therapeutic strategy and psychoanalytic technique. *Journal of the American Psychoanalytic Association*, 35(2), 447–466.

Lewes, K. (2009). *Psychoanalysis and male homosexuality* (20th anniversary edition). Plymouth: Jason Aronson.

Lingiardi, V. (2008). Playing with unreality: Transference and computer. *International Journal of Psychoanalysis*, 89, 111–126.

Lipsey, M. W., & Wilson, D. B. (1993). The efficacy of psychological, educational, and behavioral treatment: Confirmation from meta-analysis. *American Psychologist*, 48, 1181–1209.

Luepnitz, D. A. (2002). *Schopenhauer's porcupines: Intimacy and its dilemmas. Five stories of psychotherapy.* New York: Basic Books.

Lynch, P. E. (2015). Intimacy and shame in gay male sexuality. In A. Lemma & P. E. Lynch (eds), *Sexualities: Contemporary psychoanalytic perspectives* (pp. 138–155). Hove: Routledge.

Malan, D. H. (1975). *A study of brief psychotherapy.* New York: Plenum/Rosetta Edition.

Malan, D. H (2001). *Individual psychotherapy and the science of psychodynamics* (2nd edition). London: Arnold Publishers.

Marks, D. (1999). *Disability: Controversial debates and psychosocial issues.* London: Routledge.

Maslow, A. H. (1943). A theory of human motivation. *Psychological Review*, 50(4), 370–396.

McLean, C., Campbell, C., & Cornish, F. (2003). African-Caribbean interactions with mental health services in the UK: Experiences and expectations of exclusion as (re)productive of health inequalities. *Social Science and Medicine*, 56, 657–669.

McWilliams, N. (1999). *Psychoanalytic case formulation*. New York: Guilford Press.

McWilliams, N. (2011). *Psychoanalytic diagnosis: Understanding personality structure in the clinical process* (2nd edition). New York: Guilford Press.

Meltzer, D. (1983). *Dream life: A re-examination of the psychoanalytic theory and technique*. London: Karnac.

Menninger, K. (1958). *Theory of psychoanalytic technique*. London: Imago.

Messer, S. B., & Warren, C. S. (1998). *Models of brief psychodynamic therapy: A comparative approach*. New York: Guilford Press.

Michels, R. (1977). Treatment of the difficult patient in psychotherapy. *Canadian Psychiatric Association Journal*, 22(3), 117–121.

Mikulincer, M., Shaver, P. R., Cassidy, J., & Berant, E. (2009). Attachment-related defensive processes. In J. H. Obegi & E. Berant (eds), *Attachment theory and research in clinical work with adults* (pp. 293–327). New York: Guilford Press.

Milton, J. (1997). Why assess? Psychoanalytical assessment in the NHS. *Psychoanalytic Psychotherapy*, 11(1), 47–58.

Mitchell, J. (1974). *Feminism and psychoanalysis*. London: Allen Lane.

Mitchell, S. A., & Black, M. J. (1995). *Freud and beyond: A history of modern psychoanalytic thought*. New York: Basic Books.

Mitchell, S. A. (1988). *Relational concepts in psychoanalysis: An integration*. Cambridge, MA: Harvard University Press.

Mitchell, S. A. (1997). *Influence and autonomy in psychoanalysis*. Hillsdale, NJ: The Analytic Press.

Molnos, A. (1995). *A question of time: Essentials of brief dynamic psychotherapy*. London: Karnac.

Moncrieff, J., Wessely, S., & Hardy, R. (2004). Active placebos versus antidepressants for depression. *Cochrane Database of Systematic Reviews*, Issue 1, Article No. CD003012. doi:10.1002/14651858

Neuberger, J., & Tallis, R. (1999). Do we need a new word for patients? *British Medical Journal*, 318(7200), 1756–1758.

Nilsson, T., Svensson, M., Sandell, R., & Clinton, D. (2007). Patients' experiences of change in cognitive-behavioral therapy and psychodynamic therapy: A qualitative comparative study. *Psychotherapy Research*, 17(5), 553–566.

Norcross, J. C. (2005). The psychotherapist's own psychotherapy: Educating and developing psychologists. *American Psychologist*, 60(8), 840.

Ogden, T. H. (1992). Comments on transference and countertransference in the initial analytic meeting. *Psychoanalytic Inquiry*, 12, 225–247.

Ogden, T. H. (1994). The analytic third: Working with intersubjective clinical facts. *International Journal of Psychoanalysis*, 75, 3–19.

Panksepp, J. (1998). *Affective neuroscience: The foundations of human and animal emotions*. New York: Oxford University Press.

Pedder, J. R. (1988). Termination reconsidered. *International Journal of Psychoanalysis*, 69, 495–505.

Perry, P., & Graat, J. (2010). *Couch fiction: A graphic tale of psychotherapy*. Basingstoke: Macmillan International Higher Education.

Powell, A. D. (2001). The medication life. *The Journal of Psychotherapy Practice and Research*, 10(4), 217–222.

Prensky, M. (2001). Digital natives, Digital immigrants. *On the Horizon*, 9(5), 1–6.

Quinodoz, D. (2002). *Words that touch*. London: Karnac.

Quinodoz, J. M. (2002). *Dreams that turn over a page: Paradoxical dreams in psychoanalysis*. Hove: Routledge.

Racker, H. (1953). Contributions to the problem of countertransference. *International Journal of Psychoanalysis*, 34, 313–324.

Racker, H. (1957). The meanings and uses of countertransference. *Psychoanalytic Quarterly*, 26, 303–357.

Reeve, D. (2014) Counselling and disabled people: Help or hindrance? In J. Swain, S. French, C. Barnes & C. Thomas (eds), *Disabling barriers – Enabling environments* (3rd edition) (pp. 255–261). London: Sage.

Richards, D. (2020). Working with sameness and difference: Reflections on supervision with diverse sexualities. In L. Hertzmann & J. Newbigin (eds), *Sexuality and gender now: Looking beyond heteronormativity* (pp. 57–78). Abingdon: Routledge.

Robinson, L. A., Berman, J. S., & Neimeyer, R. A. (1990). Psychotherapy for the treatment of depression: A comprehensive review of controlled outcome research. *Psychological Bulletin*, 108, 30–49.

Rohleder, P. (2014). Othering. In T. Teo (ed.), *Encyclopedia of critical psychology*. New York: Springer.

Rohleder, P. (2020). Homophobia, heteronormativity and shame. In L. Hertzmann & J. Newbigin (eds), *Sexuality and gender now: Looking beyond heteronormativity* (pp. 40–56). Abingdon: Routledge.

Rohleder, P., Watermeyer, B., Braathen, S. H., Hunt, X., & Swartz, L. (2019). Impairment, socialization and embodiment: The sexual oppression of people with physical disabilities. *Psychoanalysis, Culture & Society*, 24(3), 260–281.

Rose, S. H. (2007). *Oedipal rejection: Echoes in the relationships of gay men*. Amherst, NY: Cambria Press.

Roth, A., & Fonagy, P. (2006) *What works for whom?: A Critical review of psychotherapy research* (2nd Edition). New York: Guilford Press.

Rothstein, A. (1998). *Psychoanalytic technique and the creation of analytic patients*. London: Karnac Books.

Russell, G. I. (2015). *Screen relations: The limits of computer-mediated psychoanalysis and psychotherapy*. London: Karnac Books.

Ryan, J. (2006). 'Class is in you': An exploration of some social class issues in psychotherapeutic work. *British Journal of Psychotherapy*, 23(1), 49–62.

Ryan, J. (2017). *Class and psychoanalysis: Landscapes of inequality*. Abingdon: Routledge.

Rycroft, C. (1995). *A critical dictionary of psychoanalysis* (2nd edition). London: Penguin Books.

Ryle, A (1990) *Cognitive analytic therapy: Active participation in change*. Chichester: John Wiley & Sons.

Sabbadini, A. (2013). New technologies and the psychoanalytic setting. In A. Lemma & L. Caparrotta (eds), *Psychoanalysis in the technoculture era* (pp. 23–32). Hove: Routledge.

Safran, J., Muran, J., & Shaker, A. (2014). Research on therapeutic impasses and ruptures in the therapeutic alliance. *Contemporary Psychoanalysis*, 50(1–2),211–232.

Safran, J. D., & Muran, J. C. (2006). Has the concept of the therapeutic alliance outlived its usefulness? *Psychotherapy: Theory, Research, Practice, Training*, 43(3), 286–291.

Sandler, J. (1976). Countertransference and role-responsiveness. *International Review of Psychoanalysis*, 3, 43–47.

Sandler, J., & Freud, A. (1981). Discussions in the Hampstead Index on 'The ego and the mechanisms of defence': II. The application of analytic technique to the study of psychic institutions. *Bulletin of the Anna Freud Centre*, 4(1), 5–30.

Sapolsky, R. M. (2004). *Why zebras don't get ulcers.* New York: Henry Holt and Company.

Schachter, J. (1997). Transference N countertransference dynamics in the assessment process. *Psychoanalytic Psychotherapy*, 11(1), 59–71.

Schafer, R. (1983). *The analytic attitude.* London: Karnac Books.

Schafer, R. (2002). On male nonnormative sexuality and perversion in psychoanalytic discourse. *Annual of Psychoanalysis*, 30, 23–35.

Scharff, J. S. (ed.). (2013). *Psychoanalysis online: Mental health, teletherapy, and training.* London: Karnac Books.

Schlesinger, H. J. (2014). *Endings and beginnings: On terminating psychotherapy and psychoanalysis.* New York: Routledge.

Schön, D. A. (1983). *The reflective practitioner: How professionals think in action.* New York: Basic Books.

Schön, D. A. (1987). *Educating the reflective practitioner.* San Francisco: Jossey-Bass Publishers.

Schore, A. N. (1994). *Affect regulation and the origin of the self: The neurobiology of emotional development.* Hillsdale: Psychology Press.

Searle, L., Lyon, L., Young, L., Wiseman, M., & Foster-Davis, B. (2011). The young people's consultation service: An evaluation of a consultation model of very brief psychotherapy. *British Journal of Psychotherapy*, 27(1), 56–78.

Segal, H. (1957). Notes on symbol formation. *International Journal of Psychoanalysis*, 38, 391–397.

Segal, H. (1990). *The work of Hanna Segal: A Kleinian approach to clinical practice.* New Jersey: Jason Aronson Inc.

Segal, J. (1992). *Melanie Klein.* London: Sage Publications.

Shakespeare, T. (2017). *Disability: The basics.* Abingdon: Routledge.

Shaver, P. R., & Mikulincer, M. (2007). Adult attachment strategies and the regulation of emotion. In J. J. Gross (ed.), *Handbook of emotion regulation* (pp. 446–465). New York: Guilford Press.

Shedler, J. (2010). The efficacy of psychodynamic psychotherapy. *American Psychologist*, 65(2), 98–109.

Shedler, J. (2018). Where is the evidence for "evidence-based" therapy? *Psychiatric Clinics*, 41(2), 319–329.

Sinason, V. (1992). *Mental handicap and the human condition: New approaches from the Tavistock.* London: Free Association Books.

Smith, M. L., Glass, G. V., & Miller, T. I. (1980). *The benefits of psychotherapy.* Baltimore, MD: Johns Hopkins University Press.

Sodré, I. (2005). The wound, the bow and the shadow of the object: Notes on Freud's 'Mourning and melancholia'. In R. J. Perelberg (ed.), *Freud: A modern reader* (pp. 124–141). London: Whurr Publishers.

Solms, M. (2018). The neurobiological underpinnings of psychoanalytic theory and therapy. *Frontiers in Behavioral Neuroscience*, 12, 294.

Solms, M., & Turnbull, O. H. (2002). *The brain and the inner world: An introduction to the neuroscience of subjective experience.* London: Karnac Books.

Solms, M., & Turnbull, O. H. (2011). What is neuropsychoanalysis? *Neuropsychoanalysis*, 13(2), 133–145.

Sontag, S. (1991). *Illness as metaphor and AIDS and its metaphors.* London: Penguin Books.

Spurling, L. (2003). On the therapeutic value of not offering psychotherapy: An account of an extended assessment. *Psychoanalytic Psychotherapy*, 17(1), 1–17.

Steele, H., Steele, M., & Fonagy, P. (1996). Associations among attachment classifications of mothers, fathers, and their infants. *Child Development*, 67(2), 541–555.

Steiner, J. (1993). *Psychic retreats: Pathological organizations in psychotic, neurotic and borderline patients.* London: Routledge.

Stekel, W. (1921). *The beloved ego: Foundations of the new study of the psyche.* New York: Moffat Yard.

Sterba, R. F. (1982). *Reminiscences of a Viennese psychoanalyst.* Detroit, MI: Wayne State University Press.

Strachey, J. (1934). The nature of the therapeutic action of psycho-analysis. *International Journal of Psychoanalysis,* 15, 127–159.

Suchet, M. (2020). Crossing over. In L. Hertzmann & J. Newbigin (eds), *Sexuality and gender now: Looking beyond heteronormativity* (pp. 213–239). Abingdon: Routledge.

Suler, J. (2005). The online disinhibition effect. *International Journal of Applied Psychoanalytic Studies,* 2, 184–188.

Sullivan, H. S. (1953). *The interpersonal theory of psychiatry.* New York: Norton.

Swartz, L., & Rohleder, P. (2017). Cultural psychology. In C. Willig & W. Stainton-Rogers (eds), *Handbook of qualitative research methods in psychology* (2nd edition). London: Sage Publications.

Target, M., & Fonagy, P. (1996). Playing with reality: II. The development of psychic reality from a theoretical perspective. *International Journal of Psychoanalysis,* 77, 459–479.

Thomä, H., & Kächele, H. (1987). *Psychoanalytic practice: 1 – Principles.* Berlin: Springer-Verlag.

Tronick, E., Als, H., & Adamson, L. (1979). Structure of early face-to-face communicative interactions. In M. Bullowa (ed.), *Before speech: The beginning of interpersonal communication* (pp. 349–370). Cambridge: Cambridge University Press.

Tuckett, D. (2011). Inside and outside the window: Some fundamental elements in the theory of psychoanalytic technique. *The International Journal of Psychoanalysis,* 92(6), 1367–1390.

Tummala-Narra, P. (2007). Skin color and the therapeutic relationship. *Psychoanalytic Psychology,* 24(2), 255–271.

Turner, E. H., Matthews, A. M., Linardatos, E., Tell, R. A., & Rosenthal, R. (2008). Selective publication of antidepressant trials and its influence on apparent efficacy. *New England Journal of Medicine,* 358, 252–260.

Turpin, G., & Coleman, G. (2010). Clinical psychology and diversity: Progress and continuing challenges. *Psychology Learning & Teaching,* 9(2), 17–27.

Van Ijzendoorn, M. H., Schuengel, C., & Bakermans-Kranenburg, M. (1999). Disorganized attachment in early childhood: A meta-analysis of precursors, concomitants, and sequelae. *Development and Psychopathology,* 11, 225–249.

Van Waning, A. (1991). 'To be the best or not to be, that is the question …' on enactment, play and acting out. *International Journal of Psychoanalysis,* 72, 539–550.

Ventura, T. (2019). *Therapist competence in dynamic interpersonal therapy and its association with treatment outcome.* Unpublished Doctoral thesis (PhD), University College London.

Watermeyer, B. (2012). *Towards a contextual psychology of disablism.* London: Routledge.

Weitz, P. (2018). Psychotherapy 2.0: For better or for worse? In P. Weitz (ed.), *Psychotherapy 2.0: Where psychotherapy and technology meet* (pp. 3–22). Abingdon: Routledge.

Will, H. (2018). The concept of the 50-minute hour: Time forming a frame for the unconscious. *International Forum of Psychoanalysis,* 27(1), 14–23.

Wille, R. (2012). The analyst's trust in psychoanalysis and the communication of that trust in initial interviews. *Psychoanalytic Quarterly,* 81(4), 875–904.

Winnicott, D. W. (1949). Hate in the counter-transference. *International Journal of Psychoanalysis,* 30, 69–74.

Winnicott, D. W. (1953). Transitional objects and transitional phenomena – A study of the first not-me possession. *International Journal of Psychoanalysis,* 34, 89–97.

Winnicott, D. W. (1955). Metapsychological and clinical aspects of regression within the psycho-analytical set-up. *International Journal of Psychoanalysis,* 36, 16–26.

Winnicott, D. W. (1960). The theory of the parent-infant relationship. *International Journal of Psychoanalysis*, 41; 585–595.

Winnicott, D. W. (1965). *The maturational processes and the facilitating environment*. London: Hogarth Press.

Winnicott, D. W. (1967). Mirror-role of mother and family in child development. In P. Lomas (ed.), *The predicament of the family: A psycho-analytic symposium* (pp. 26–33). London: Hogarth Press.

Winnicott, D. W. (1969). The use of an object. *International Journal of Psychoanalysis*, 50, 711–716.

Winnicott, D. W. (1971). *Therapeutic consultations in child psychiatry*. London: The Hogarth Press.

Winter, S. (1999). *Freud and the institution of psychoanalytic knowledge*. Stanford: Stanford University Press.

Wolberg, L. R. (1980). *Handbook of short-term psychotherapy*. New York: Thieme-Stratton.

Wolberg, L. R. (1995). *The technique of psychotherapy Part 1* (4th edition). Northvale: Jason Aronson Inc.

Wood, H. (2011). The internet and its role in the escalation of sexually compulsive behaviour. *Psychoanalytic Psychotherapy*, 25, 127–142.

World Health Organisation (1992). *International statistical classification of diseases and related health problems*, 10th revision (ICD-10). Geneva: WHO.

Wren, B. (2020). Notes on a crisis of meaning in the care of gender-diverse children. In L. Hertzmann & J. Newbigin (eds), *Sexuality and gender now: Looking beyond heteronormativity*. (pp. 189–212). Abingdon: Routledge.

Yeomans, F. E., Clarkin, J. F., & Kernberg, O. F. (2015). *Transference-focused psychotherapy for borderline personality disorder: A clinical guide*. Arlington: American Psychiatric Publishing.

Young, J. E. (1990). *Cognitive therapy for personality disorders: A schema-focused approach*. Sarasota, FL: Professional Resource Exchange.

Zeligs, M. A. (1957). Acting in: A contribution to the meaning of some postural attitudes observed during analysis. *Journal of the American Psychoanalytic Association*, 5(4), 685–706.

Zeligs, M. A. (1960). The role of silence in transference, counter-transference, and the psycho-analytic process. *International Journal of Psychoanalysis*, 41, 407–412.

Zetzel, E. R. (1956). Current concepts of transference. *International Journal of Psychoanalysis*, 37, 369–376.

Zur, O., Williams, M. H., Lehavot, K., & Knapp, S. (2009). Psychotherapist self-disclosure and transparency in the internet age. *Professional Psychology, Research and Practice*, 40(1), 23–30.

Index

For Product Safety Concerns and Information please contact our EU
representative GPSR@taylorandfrancis.com
Taylor & Francis Verlag GmbH, Kaufingerstraße 24, 80331 München, Germany

www.ingramcontent.com/pod-product-compliance
Lightning Source LLC
Chambersburg PA
CBHW050333270326
41926CB00016B/3442